W9-BVJ-665

Pharmacy Labs

FOR TECHNICIANS

Jason Philip Sparks
Lisa McCartney

Third Edition

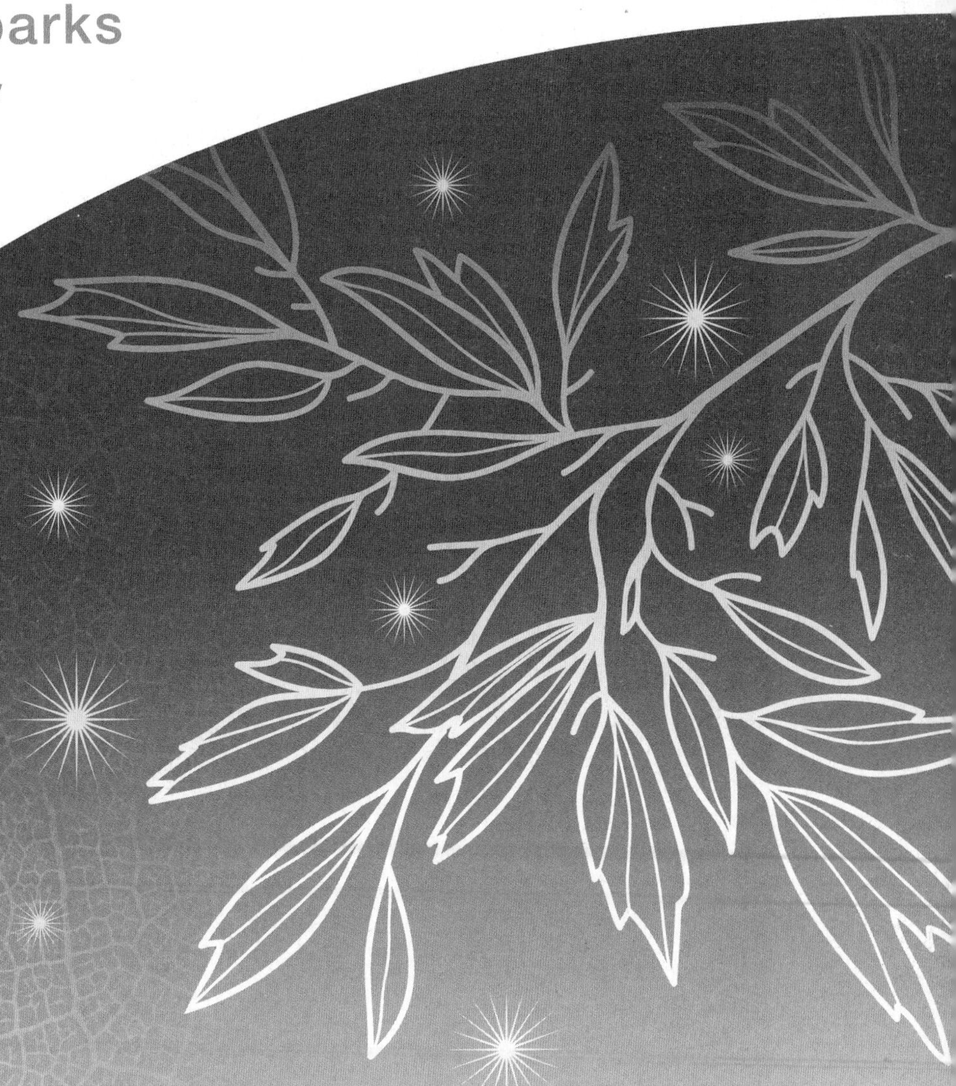

PARADIGM
EDUCATION SOLUTIONS

St. Paul

Senior Vice President Linda Hein
Managing Editor Brenda M. Palo
Developmental Editor Stephanie Schempp
Director of Production Timothy W. Larson
Production Editor Carrie Rogers
Copyeditor Peter Berry
Proofreader Suzanne Clinton
Cover and Text Designer Dasha Wagner
Layout Designer Dasha Wagner
Illustrators S4Carlisle Publishing Services
Indexer Terry Casey
Vice President Sales and Marketing Scott Burns
Director of Marketing Lara Weber McLellan
Digital Projects Manager Tom Modl
Digital Production Manager Aaron Esnough
Web Developer Blue Earth Interactive

Care has been taken to verify the accuracy of information presented in this book. However, the authors, editors, and publisher cannot accept responsibility for Web, e-mail, newsgroup, or chat room subject matter or content, or for consequences from application of the information in this book, and make no warranty, expressed or implied, with respect to its content.

Trademarks: Some of the product names and company names included in this book have been used for identification purposes only and may be trademarks or registered trade names of their respective manufacturers and sellers. The authors, editors, and publisher disclaim any affiliation, association, or connection with, or sponsorship or endorsement by, such owners.

Photo Credits: Following the index.

We have made every effort to trace the ownership of all copyrighted material and to secure permission from copyright holders. In the event of any question arising as to the use of any material, we will be pleased to make the necessary corrections in future printings. Thanks are due to the authors, publishers, and agents listed in the Photo Credits for permission to use the materials therein indicated.

978-0-76386-790-4 (Text)
978-0-76386-791-1 (eBook)

© 2017 by Paradigm Publishing, Inc., a division of EMC Publishing, LLC
875 Montreal Way
St. Paul, MN 55102
E-mail: educate@emcp.com
Web site: www.emcp.com

All rights reserved. No part of this publication may be adapted, reproduced, stored in a retrieval system, or transmitted in any form or by any means, electronic, mechanical, photocopying, recording, or otherwise, without prior written permission from the publisher.

Printed in the United States of America

18 17 16 1 2 3 4 5 6 7 8 9 10

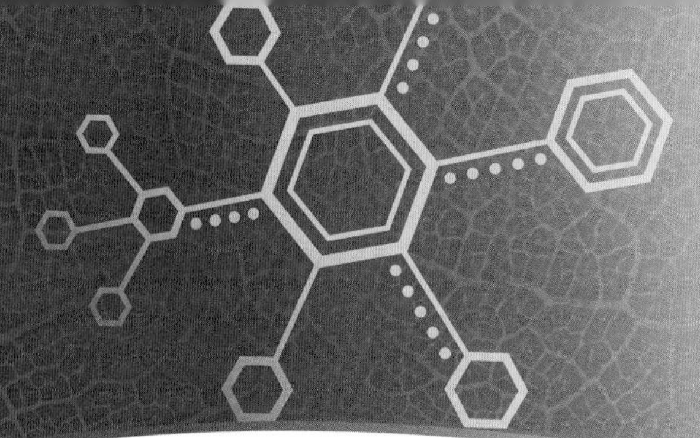

BRIEF CONTENTS

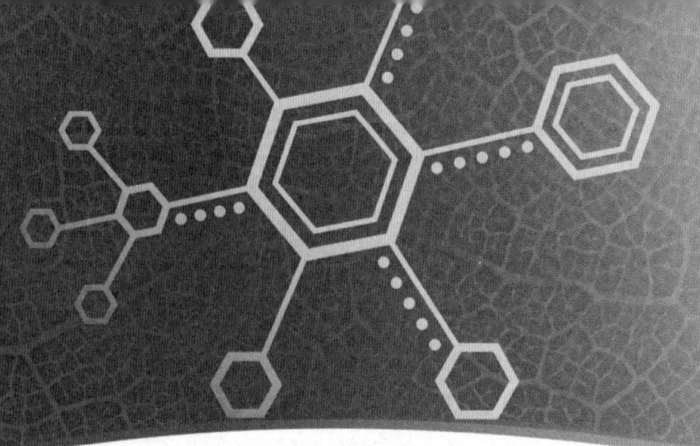

TABLE OF CONTENTS

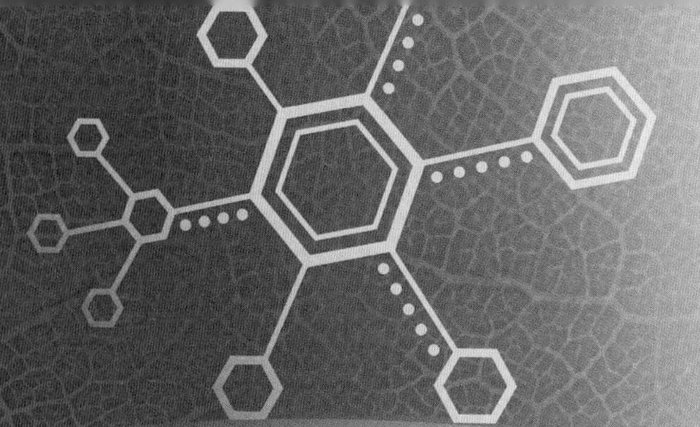

PREFACE

Pharmacy Labs for Technicians: What Makes This New Edition Exciting?

Pharmacy Labs for Technicians, Third Edition is a comprehensive lab manual designed to help students achieve success. This laboratory manual provides students the opportunity to practice key skills in the areas of using drug references, managing patient records and prescriptions, compounding medications, working with crash carts and cart-fill requests, and preparing oral syringes and aseptic parenteral dosage forms. *Pharmacy Labs for Technicians, Third Edition*, is designed to work in concert with Paradigm's *Pharmacy Practice for Technicians, Sixth Edition* or to stand alone as a labs course for pharmacy technician programs. The *Third Edition* features include:

- Alignment with new ASHP™ curriculum standards, covering accreditation topics in a logical order with easy-to-understand language.
- The web-based *Course Navigator* learning platform to assemble all student and instructor resources in one easy-access location.
- All new, web-based guided NRx tutorials and live assessments (based on QS/1's nationally recognized pharmacy management software).
- Brand new labs covering cutting-edge pharmacy topics such as medication therapy management and crucial pharmacy skills such as customer service and inventory management.
- All new margin features to help engage students and assist their learning.
- Numerous detailed labs that teach students pharmacy skills using hands-on practice.

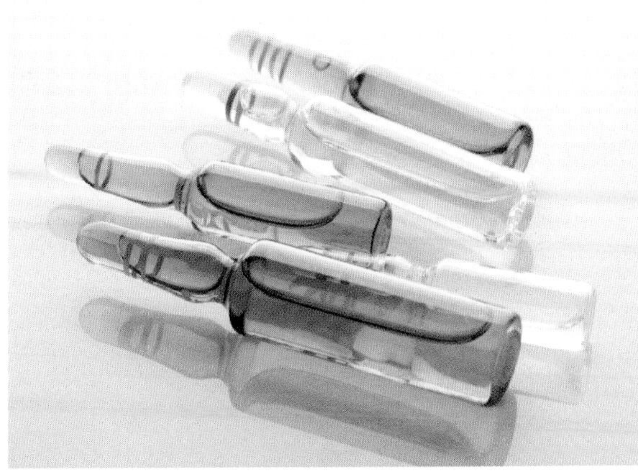

Study Assets: A Visual Walk-Through

Print and eBook

1 Learning Objectives

establish clear goals to focus each lab.

2 Supplies

are listed to help students prepare prior to completing each lab.

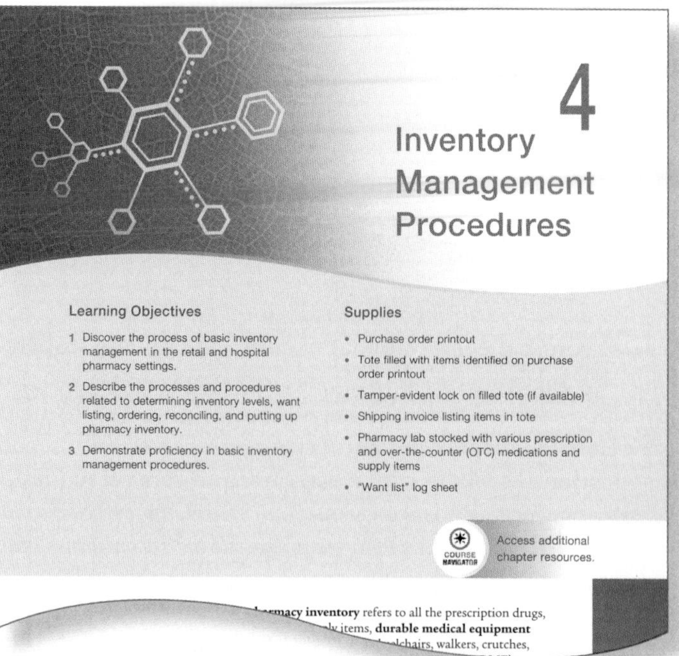
4

Inventory Management Procedures

Learning Objectives

1 Discover the process of basic inventory management in the retail and hospital pharmacy settings.
2 Describe the processes and procedures related to determining inventory levels, want listing, ordering, reconciling, and putting up pharmacy inventory.
3 Demonstrate proficiency in basic inventory management procedures.

Supplies

- Purchase order printout
- Tote filled with items identified on purchase order printout
- Tamper-evident lock on filled tote (if available)
- Shipping invoice listing items in tote
- Pharmacy lab stocked with various prescription and over-the-counter (OTC) medications and supply items
- "Want list" log sheet

Access additional chapter resources.

3 Online Resource Icons

callout digital resources.

Video

Web

3-D

4 Attractive Margin Features

spotlight important information.

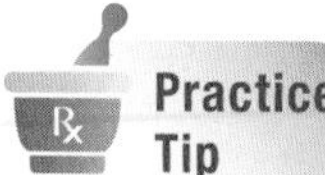

Provides reminders about key elements of pharmacy practice.

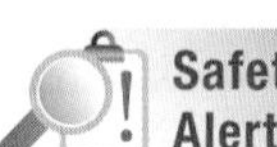

Serves as warnings to avoid problems in the field.

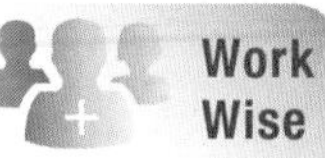

Gives advice on professionalism and soft skills.

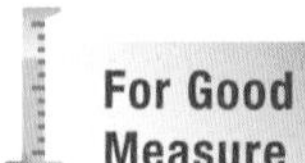

Assists in accuracy with measuring.

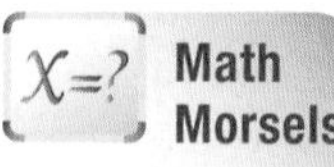

Supply calculating hints.

5 Steps

give clear instructions on how to perform lab tasks.

Procedure

1. Gather the filled and locked (if applicable) tote, purchase order receipt, and shipping invoice from your instructor.
2. Place the tote onto a tabletop or other suitable work surface.
3. If applicable, break open the tamper-evident lock, and remove it from the tote. Dispose of the lock in a waste receptacle.
4. Open the tote. Pick up the first item in the tote. Locate that item on the shipping invoice.

...and form listed on the exterior

6 Numerous Figures, Diagrams, Tables and Photographs

enhance visual learning, illustrate lab steps, and provide study tools.

FIGURE 8.1 Patient Profile and Insurance Card

PATIENT PROFILE

Patient Name
Donaldson | Vance |
Last | First | Middle Initial

12 Maple Leaf Trail
Street or PO Box

Round Rock | TX | 78664
City | State | ZIP

Date of Birth: 05/15/1987 (MM / DD / YYYY)
Gender: ☑ Male ☐ Female
Social Security No.: 000-00-0000
E-mail: vdonaldson@email.com

Home Phone: (512) 555-1212
Work Phone: (512) 555-1313
Other Phone: ( )

...cation dispensed in a child-resistant container.
...dication dispensed in a child-resistant container.

Cardholder Name: same
☑ Cardholder ☐ Child ☐ Disabled Dependent
☐ Spouse ☐ Dependent Parent ☐ Full-Time Student

...macy with your card.)

TABLE 3.1 Drug Schedules under the Controlled Substances Act of 1970

Schedule	Manufacturer's Label	Abuse Potential	Accepted Medical Use	Examples
Schedule I	C-I	Highest potential for abuse and addiction	For research only; must have license to obtain; no accepted medical use in the United States	Heroin, lysergic acid diethylamide (LSD)
Schedule II	C-II	High potential for abuse, which can lead to severe psychological or physical dependence	Dispensing is severely restricted; cannot be prescribed by telephone except in an emergency; no refills on prescriptions	Morphine, oxycodone, meperidine, hydromorphone, fentanyl, methylphenidate, dextroamphetamine, hydrocodone with acetaminophen
				Codeine with aspirin...

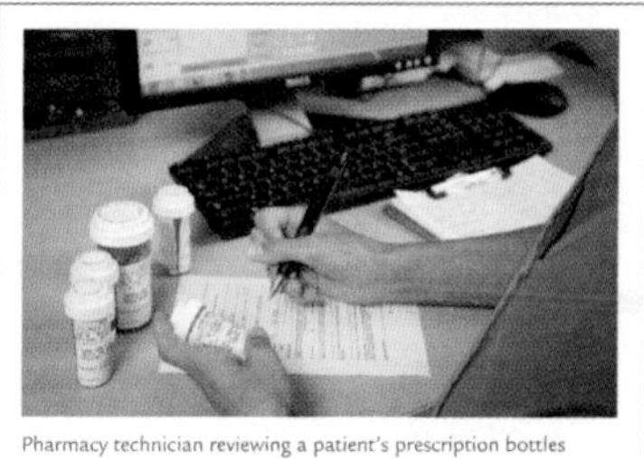

Pharmacy technician reviewing a patient's prescription bottles

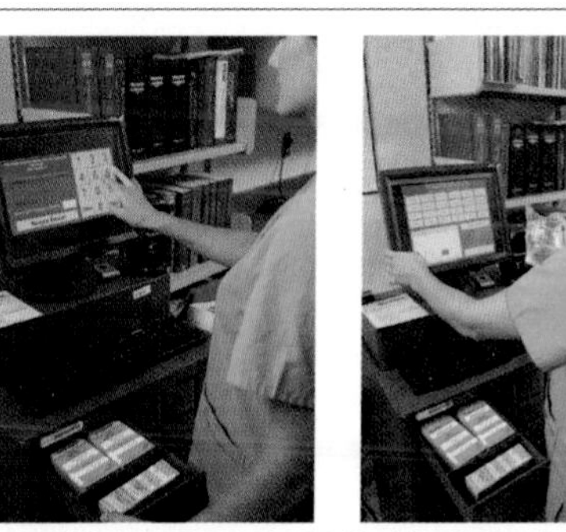

Pharmacy technician logging medications into the ADSDS (left) and placing drugs into specific drawers (right)

7 Take Note

features offer additional suggestions and warn of potential pitfalls in the field of pharmacy practice.

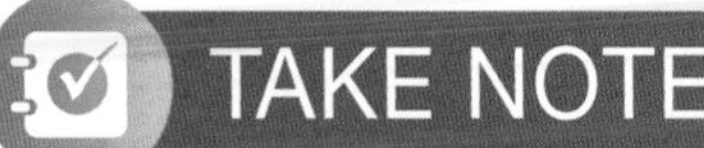

Schedule I drugs are not legally dispensed in the United States due to their high potential for abuse and addiction. Schedule II drugs are the most highly regulated, and sudden increases in usage in a particular pharmacy (or in prescriptions by a particular doctor) may cause the DEA to investigate. Schedule II drugs have no refills. Schedule III, IV, and V drugs have less potential for abuse and addiction than Schedule II drugs and have no limits on refills. See Table 3.1

8 Index

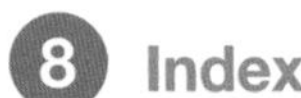

provides a quick location guide for terms and topics.

Course Navigator

Student Resources

- **NRx** interactive tutorials and assessments to accompany Labs 8-14.
- **Digital Flash Cards** make it easy to study key terms, common brand and generic drugs, and all core content.
- **Study Games** make it fun to practice key chapter concepts.
- **End-of-Chapter Review Exercises** align with Bloom's Taxonomy of learning and include fact-based quizzes, critical thinking questions, higher-level applications, problem solving, and research activities:

    Check Your Understanding Check Your Understanding–multiple choice (computer graded)

    Thinking Like a Pharmacy Tech critical-thinking and application assignments (with instructor rubrics)

    Your Career as a Pharmacy Technician short answer questions that address professionalism and soft skills (with instructor rubrics)

- **Supplemental Resources** include links to Top 200 Drug lists, Most Common Hospital Drugs, and other useful study resources from the most recommended pharmaceutical and medical websites.
- **Canadian Pharmacy Technician Supplement** addresses topics specific to Canadian pharmacy by Melissa Bleier, BscPharm, RPh. (For more information, see page xv.)

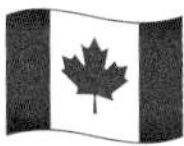

- **Practice Tests** provide computer-graded feedback, answers, and answer rationale.
- **Comprehensive Chapter Exams and Course Final Exam** test understanding of chapter topics and the complete course.

Instructor Resources

- **Alignment to ASHP Curriculum Goals and ASHP Accreditation Advice**
- **Course and Chapter Planning Tools** includes syllabus examples and chapter lessons and activities.
- **PowerPoint Slides** highlight key points of chapter content.
- **Computer-Graded Review Quizzes, Practice Tests, and Exams** have been developed by experts for preassembled and assemble-your-own quizzes and tests.
- **Simple, Adaptable Instructor Rubrics for Higher Level Learning Exercises** include presentations, discussions, short answer questions, and short essays.

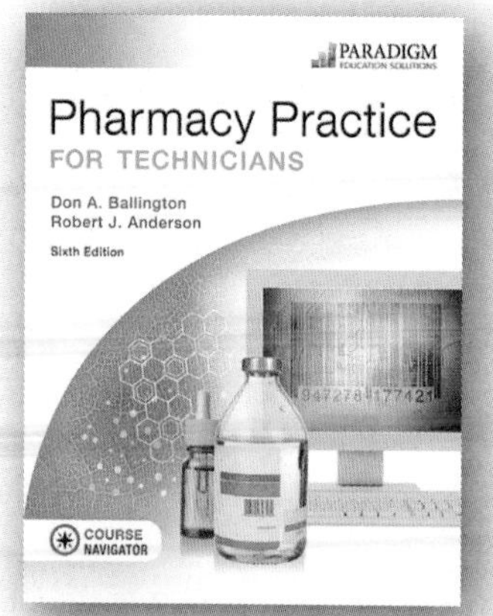

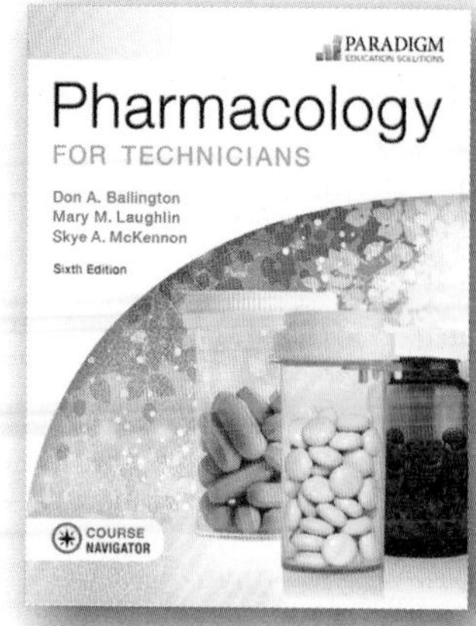

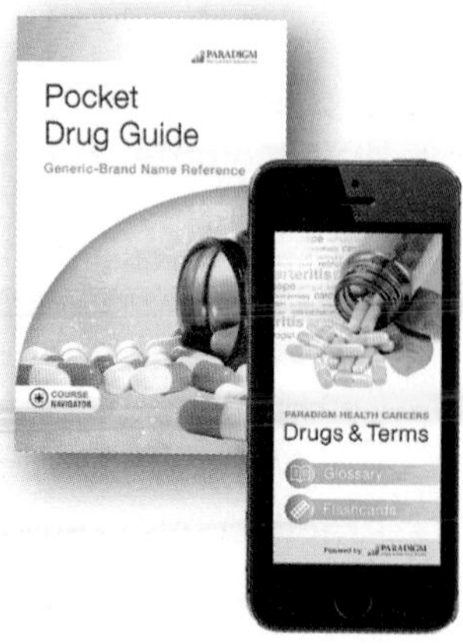

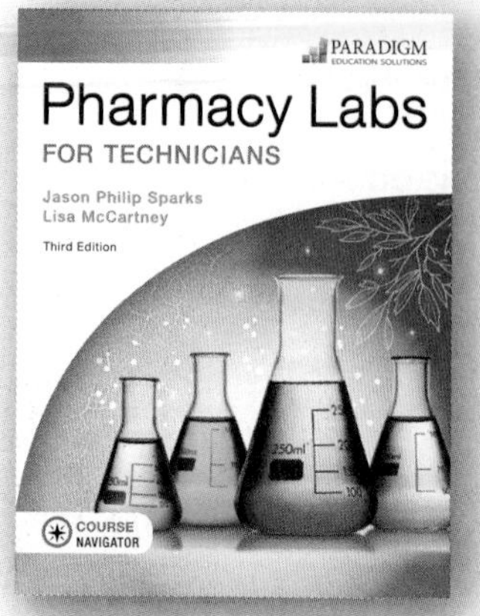

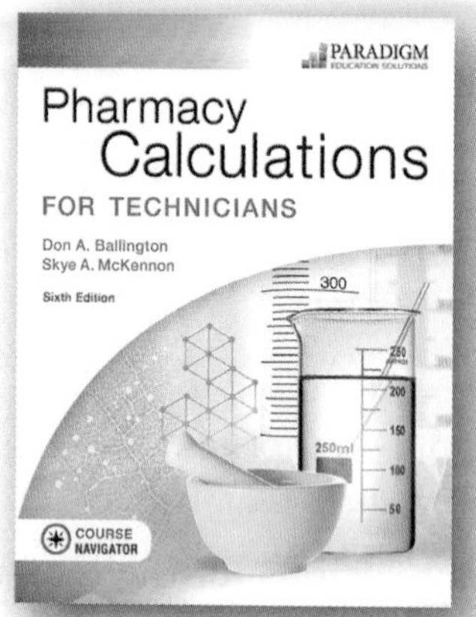

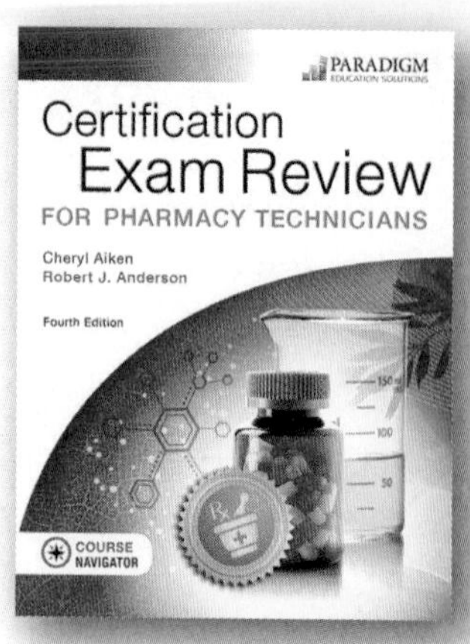

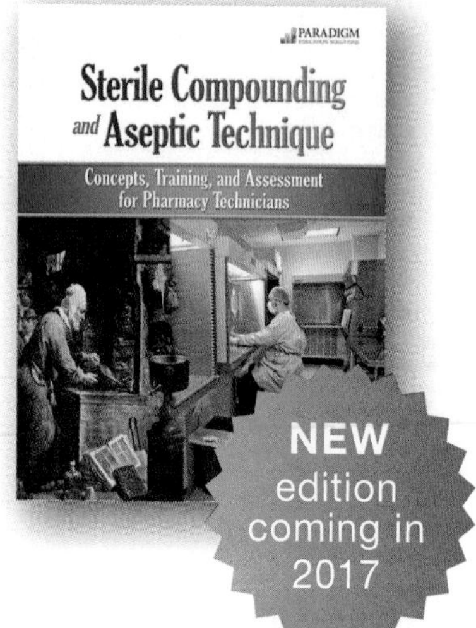

Paradigm's Comprehensive Pharmacy Technician Series

In addition to *Pharmacy Labs for Technicians, Third Edition,* Paradigm Publishing, Inc. offers other titles designed specifically for the pharmacy technician curriculum:

- *Pharmacy Practice for Technicians, Sixth Edition*
- *Pocket Drug Guide: Generic Brand Name Reference* and *SmartPhone App**
- *Pharmacology for Technicians, Sixth Edition*
- *Pharmacy Calculations for Technicians, Sixth Edition*
- *Certification Exam Review for Pharmacy Technicians, Fourth Edition*
- *Sterile Compounding and Aseptic Technique, Second Edition*

* For more information on Paradigm's new SmartPhone App on drugs and terms, see page xvi.

Related Health Career Titles

Additional titles in Paradigm's Health Career line of courses are particularly useful for pharmacy technicians:

- *Medical Terminology: Connecting through Language*
- *Pharmacology Essentials for Allied Health*
- *What Language Does Your Patient Hurt In?: A Practical Guide to Culturally Competent Care, Third Edition*
- *Exploring Electronic Health Records*
- *Deciphering Procedural Coding*
- *Introduction to Health Information Management*

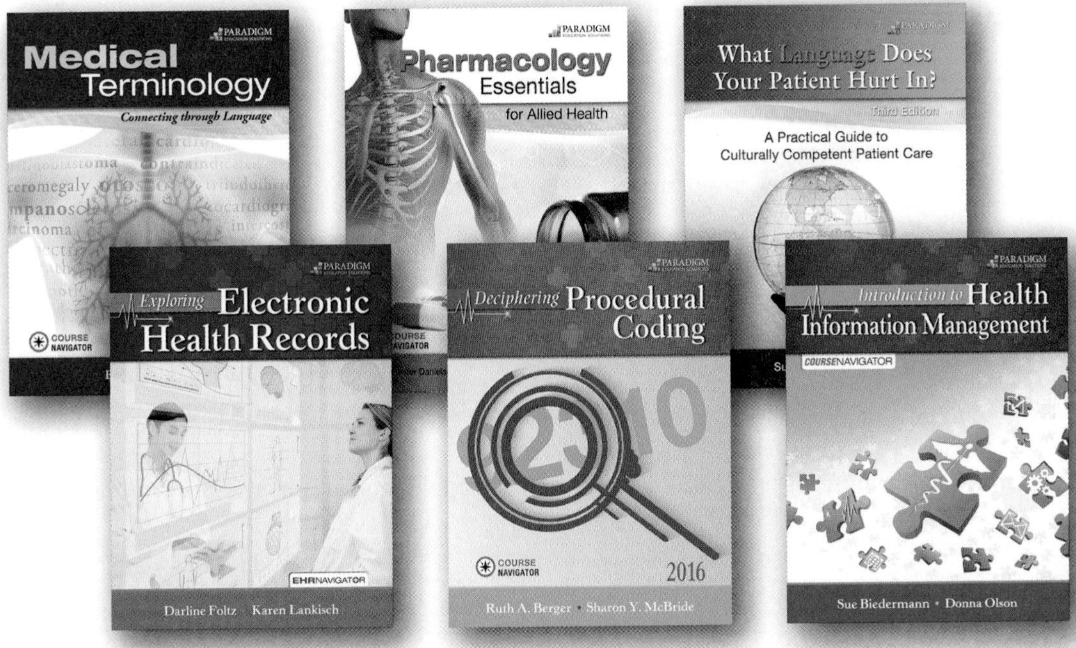

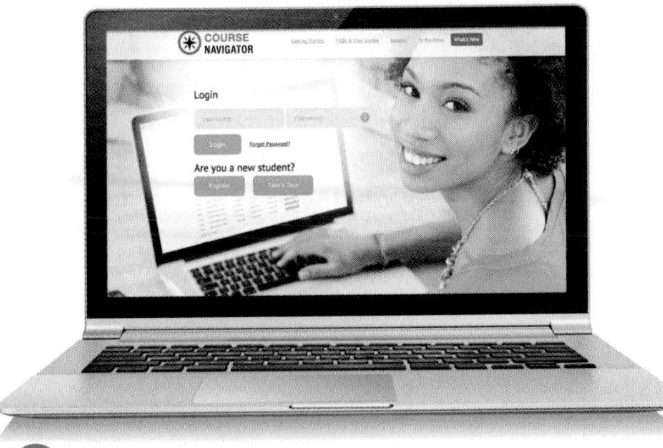

Course Navigator resources accompany all new editions.

About the Authors

Jason P. Sparks

Jason P. Sparks, MEd, CPhT, PhTR, is a data dork, educator, and problem solver with more than 17 years in education and pharmacy practice as a pharmacy technician. Sparks has taught courses in pharmacy practice, pharmacy law, mathematics, medical ethics, business, and academic success across the United States: Adjunct faculty at Cedar Valley College, Professorial Lecturer at the George Washington University, Division Chair/Coordinator at Arkansas State University–Mid-South (formerly Mid-South Community College), and Associate Professor at Austin Community College.

Sparks is published in the area of pharmacy practice and technology, including works for Paradigm Education Solutions, the American Society of Health-System Pharmacists (Getting Started... series), CriticalPoint, and the Journal of Developmental Education. Additionally, he has delivered a variety of presentations on pedagogy, student engagement, curriculum theory, instructional design, and digital learning to a variety of audiences across the US.

In 2007, the Texas Pharmacy Association named Jason Pharmacy Technician of the Year. He has served as President and Webmaster for the Pharmacy Technician Educators Council, a member of the Board and Chair of the Academy of Pharmacy Technicians for the Texas Pharmacy Association, and a Director of the Capital-Area Pharmacy Association in Austin, Texas.

Jason holds a Masters of Education in Management of Technical Education and Bachelor of Arts in English from Texas State University–San Marcos, and an AAS in Pharmacy Technology from Weatherford College. He became a PTCB-certified pharmacy technician in 2001 and registered with the Texas State Board of Pharmacy in 2004.

In his spare time, Jason loves to travel, read, and solve problems in assessment, assurance of learning, and programmatic and institutional improvement. Jason currently resides in Sugarhouse, Salt Lake City, Utah.

Lisa McCartney

Lisa McCartney, MEd, CPhT, PhTR, is the department chair for the ASHP/ACPE accredited pharmacy technician program at Austin Community College. She also serves as the CPE administrator for the department's ACPE accredited providership, which offers a variety of continuing pharmacy education activities for pharmacists and technicians. She became a PTCB-certified pharmacy technician in 1995 and has been registered with the State of Texas since 2005. She received her AAS degree in Pharmacy Technology from Weatherford College in 2008. In 2011, she received her BAAS Degree with an emphasis in Occupational Education, and in 2014, received her Master's degree in Education, both from Texas State University.

Lisa has been a pharmacy technician for more than 35 years, and has been educating pharmacy technicians since 1999. Lisa has a wide range of pharmacy experience, including employment in the community, hospital, home-healthcare, and oncology pharmacy settings. She is a regular presenter at pharmacy organization conferences around the United States, on topics such as: Emerging Roles in Pharmacy Practice, Specialty

Certifications for Pharmacy Technicians, and USP<797> Compliance. Lisa is a passionate advocate for the adoption of a single national standard requiring completion of an ASHP/ACPE accredited training program, PTCB certification, and State Board of Pharmacy registration for pharmacy technicians.

Lisa has served in a variety of leadership roles for the Texas Society of Health-System Pharmacists, and the Pharmacy Technician Educator's Council. Lisa is a 2011 International NISOD Award winner for Teaching and Leadership Excellence. Lisa received the 2012 Roy Kemp Award from the Pharmacy Technician Educator's Council, and the 2014 Mike Knapp Award from the Texas Society of Health-System Pharmacists. She is a subject matter expert in the area of sterile compounding and aseptic technique. In 2014, Lisa participated on the USP<797> Expert Panel which provided input on the latest USP chapter revision. In addition, she participated on two Texas State Board of Pharmacy committees regarding Pharmacy Technician Education and Sterile Compounding and Aseptic Technique. She has recently been selected to participate on the PTCB Task Force on Sterile Compounding.

Lisa is the author of Paradigm Education Solutions's, Sterile Compounding and Aseptic Technique: Concepts, Training, and Assessment for Pharmacy Personnel. The second edition is slated for release in 2017.

Acknowledgements

The quality of this body of work is a testament to the many contributors and reviewers who participated in the creation of Pharmacology for Technicians, Sixth Edition. We offer a heartfelt thank-you for your commitment to producing high-quality instructional materials for pharmacy technician students.

Reviewers, Textbook Content

Anne P LaVance, BS, CPhT
Delgado Community College

Brooke Stokely, BS, CPhT
Southeastern Institute

Contributing Writers, Digital Content

Gwyn Collier, CPhT, MCPhT, MBA
National American University

Brooke Stokely, BS, CPhT
Southeastern Institute

Paradigm's Health Career Drugs and Terms App

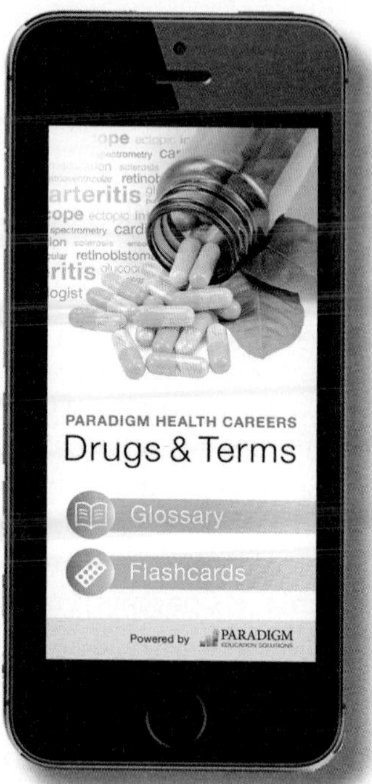

It identifies more than 3,000 drugs and terms. Students are able to:

- Search the terms database by drug class or body system.
- Use flashcards included in the app to review Schedule II drug classes and common medical terminology.
- Create their own flashcards to practice identifying drugs and terms.

This app also offers audio functionality to help students master pronunciation.

Canadian Pharmacy Technician Supplement

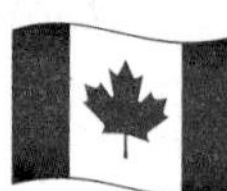

This supplement assists Canadian students in understanding the differences between US and Canadian pharmacy practice. The supplement has four parts that can be read alongside specific chapters in this textbook:

- Part 1: Scope of Pharmacy Technicians in Canada (Chapter 1: The Profession of Pharmacy)
- Part 2: Drug Regulation in Canada (Chapter 2: Pharmacy Law, Regulations, and Standards)
- Part 3: Controlled Substances (Chapter 2: Pharmacy Law, Chapter 7: Community Pharmacy Dispensing, and Chapter 14: Medication Safety)
- Part 4: Top 100 Drugs Dispensed in Canadian Pharmacies (Chapter 4: Introducing Pharmacology)

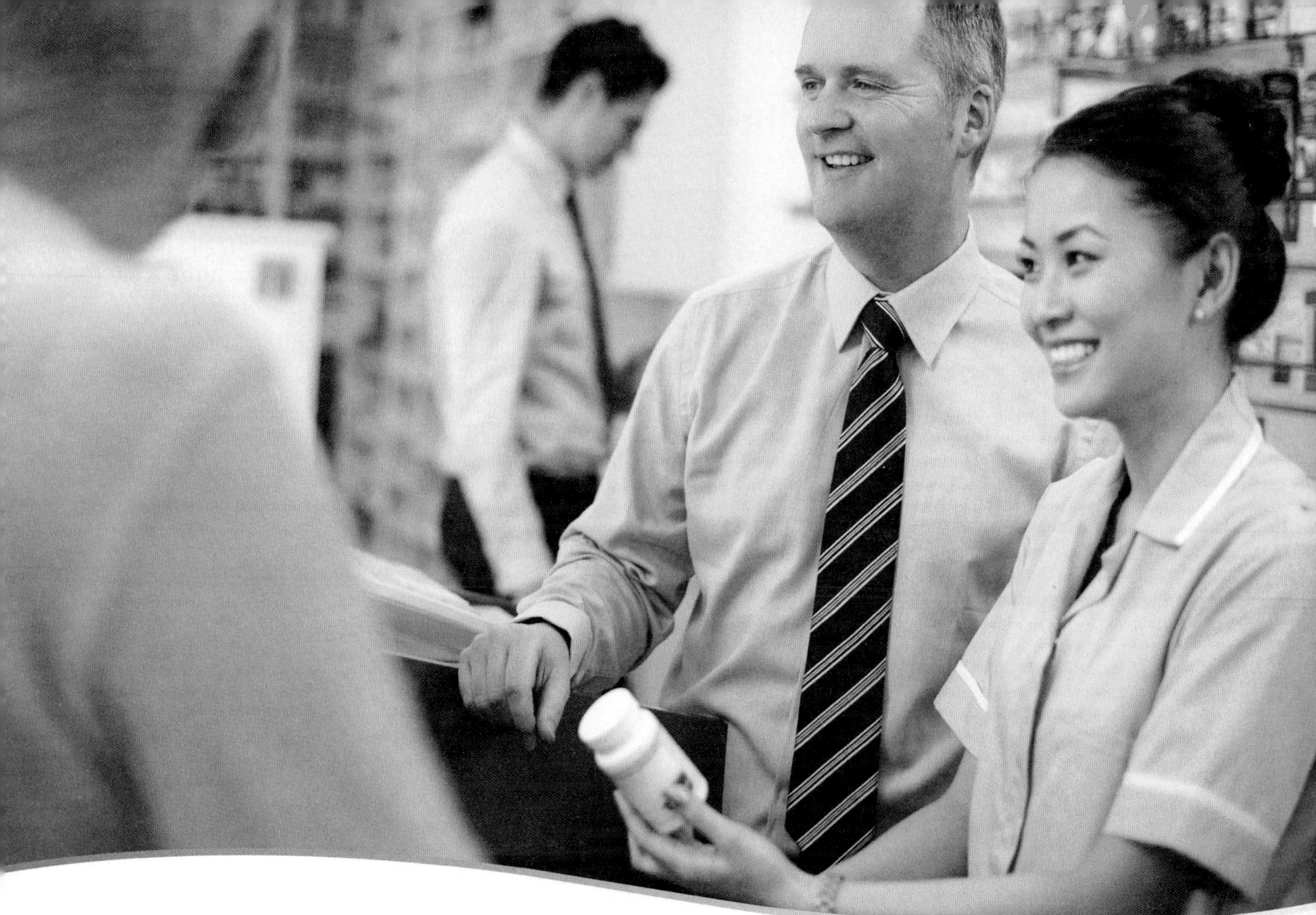

UNIT 1 Essential Pharmacy Skills

A day in the life of a pharmacy technician...

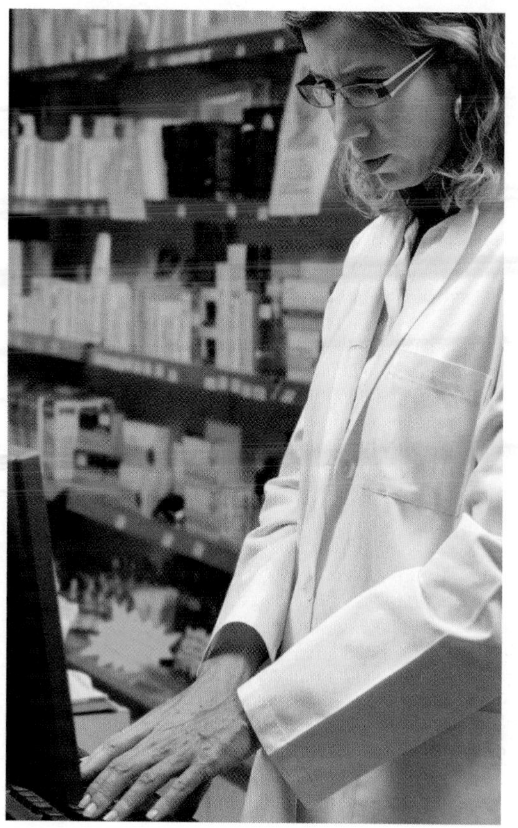

You arrive to the pharmacy and the pharmacist has a task for you: you are given a list of drugs and are asked to research the AWP for specific NDCs, identify any new labeling requirements, provide updates to any newly available dosage forms, identify a capsule found on the floor, determine if a particular NDC of Warfarin Sodium is at least an AB-rated therapeutic equivalent to Coumadin, and finally get the address for the nearest DEA office.

So, what do you do? Which references would you use? Is there a single comprehensive reference where all of this information is found? (hint: it's not a search engine on the Internet!)

A good pharmacy technician is a resourceful pharmacy technician: he or she knows how to get things done and where to locate valuable information at a moment's notice. Understanding how references work and organize information is a key skill for a pharmacy technician.

References come in a variety of types: printed books, online references, applications for personal computers, and apps for smart phones and tablets. Some of these are free while others require a subscription or annual purchase. A pharmacy technician should be familiar with using each reference type. You may find yourself in a pharmacy where only certain sources of information are available; for example, you may work in a pharmacy where only print references are available.

This unit guides you through how to determine if a resource is reliable, how to find accurate reference materials, and how to use some of the most commonly available references used in pharmacy practice. Many references were first published in print and are also now found only online for an annual subscription fee. However, many pharmacies continue to use the last printed version of these references. No matter which type of reference source you use in completing Lab 1, the importance of knowing how to use pharmacy references is vital. You never know where and when you will be asked to research information in your daily work as a pharmacy technician.

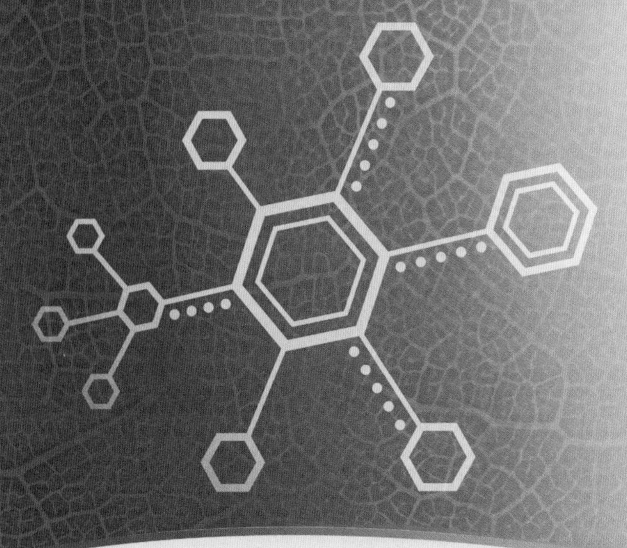

1 Using Reference Materials in Pharmacy Practice

Learning Objectives

1 Identify how pharmacy references contribute to pharmacy practice and patient safety.

2 Differentiate between reliable and unreliable sources of information.

3 Describe the differences among various pharmacy references and sources of information.

4 Collect information from various pharmacy references and sources of information.

Supplies

- Access to current editions of one or more of the following references: *Micromedex, United States Pharmacopeia Drug Information Volumes I and/or II*, the FDA's *Orange Book*, the FDA's *Redbook*, *Facts & Comparisons*, Trissel's *Handbook on Injectable Drugs*, and pharmaceutical manufacturers' drug monographs
- Customer-facing sites such as drugs.com, or online retailer sites such as costco.com, cvs.com, riteaid.com, or walgreens.com

Access additional chapter resources.

Among the many responsibilities of a pharmacy technician is the task of researching and providing information to pharmacists and fellow pharmacy technicians. The research, collection, and analysis of information contribute to the safety of patients. With so many references available, knowing which to use and when and how to use them will increase your value as a pharmacy technician. This lab provides an overview of the variety of resources available to pharmacy staff and patients, including the reliability of information, the general types of information available, and appropriate use of these resources.

As the digitization of information rapidly progresses, many comprehensive resources originally found only in print have transitioned to digital form. In many cases, these resources are now found *only* in digital form. Comprehensive reference texts, by definition, contain large amounts of information. To keep these resources easy to use and readable, the data is efficiently organized, and cross-references are often included.

A **cross-reference** is usually a word or phrase placed at the end of an entry, directing you to another part of the resource for related information. For example, when researching fluoxetine in *Drug Facts and Comparisons*, you would find this cross-reference under the individual product listing: "For complete and comparative prescribing information, refer to the Selective Serotonin Reuptake Inhibitors group monograph." Follow such leads to make the most of the reference and to better assist the pharmacist in the research of information. Remember, however, that the group monograph contains information about all drugs in the group, and you must read carefully to make sure that you are providing the correct information about the specific drug you are working with. Knowing how to use reference texts is a valuable skill when you are researching drugs or reviewing prescription information.

TAKE NOTE

As a pharmacy technician, you must remember that you should never provide drug information or counseling to patients; all patient questions requiring professional judgement must be referred to a pharmacist.

Reliable Sources of Information

With the power of the digital world and the Internet, anyone can create a website, make a social media page, or publish a document. When researching information for the care of a patient, it is important to consider the source of information. There are a variety of both reliable and unreliable sources of information, and it is your job as the pharmacy technician to understand the difference. A **reliable source of information** is a proven and maintained resource continually updated by an authoritative organization on the subject matter. When reviewing a resource for reliability, it is important to ask the following questions:

- Who is the author of the resource?
- When was the resource last updated?
- Is the resource from a known author or subject expert?
- Is the information verifiable by a second source?
- Does the author provide valid and up-to-date contact information?
- Does the material seem well organized?

Reliable sources of information are consistently maintained and actively updated with the most recent and accurate information, which is

© Paradigm Publishing, Inc.

based on verifiable fact. The resources often kept in your local pharmacy are considered reliable; examples include *Micromedex*, maintained by Truven Health Analytics, or *Drug Facts & Comparisons,* maintained by Wolters Kluwer Health, or the *Orange Book* maintained by the Center for Drug Evaluation and Research, a part of the US Department of Health and Human Services, Food and Drug Administration. These resources may be updated monthly, weekly, or even daily with the most current information.

A resource considered unreliable may at first look like the resources just mentioned; however, these unreliable resources are not likely to be up-to-date, well organized, well maintained, or from a recognized authority. Even if the source is well designed and easy to read, it could be a false source. For example, the fictional Cletus McTavish Online Compendium of Pharmaceutical and Homeopathic Remedies, last updated February 2012, is not likely a reliable resource due to the facts that Cletus McTavish is not a known authority, the resource is disorganized and appears to not be well maintained, and the resource is not regularly updated. Many researchers would consider this resource to be a **zombie reference**, which is a still-available reference, originally produced by an unknown source, that has not been updated for a significant period of time. Additionally, the use of a copyright symbol (©) does not guarantee quality.

A best practice of research is, "When in doubt, verify, verify, verify!" This means that when you find an answer to a question, it is best to verify that information using a second—or third, or fourth—source to ensure accuracy.

Pharmacy References

Management and organization of information has changed dramatically over the last 50 years. From printed books to microfilm, floppy disks, CD-ROMs, flash drives, mobile devices, and cloud storage, information today is available almost instantly. We can use a printed reference or an app on our mobile device to research a question. The references described in this chapter reflect the evolution of information organization. These references have been updated from print-only sources to Internet-based, mobile, and electronic references. While a few of these references are still available in print, all have been translated to modern technologies in an effort to provide more accurate and immediate access to information that can, and will, save countless lives.

Drug Facts and Comparisons

Drug Facts and Comparisons is a reference of clinical information for both prescription and over-the-counter (OTC) products. It provides important clinical and practical information for pharmacists and pharmacy technicians, ultimately enabling pharmacists to thoroughly and effectively counsel patients about their medications.

© Paradigm Publishing, Inc.

Drug Facts and Comparisons is available in three separate editions: a hardbound book, a perpetually updated loose-leaf binder, and an online edition. The hardbound edition (indexed at the back) is updated and published annually. The binder (indexed at the front) is updated by hand each month when a package of new and replacement pages is mailed to the pharmacy. A pharmacy staff member—most likely a pharmacy technician—follows the directions provided to remove some pages and to replace or add others. The online edition is updated more frequently.

The printed and online versions of *Drug Facts and Comparisons* are organized in different ways. Both printed editions are organized by body system and then by drug classification. Each classification begins with a **group monograph**, which is a discussion of all the drugs in the group, and then presents the drugs, one by one, in individual product monographs. The online edition is organized as a classic web-based reference with menus and search boxes to quickly locate relevant information.

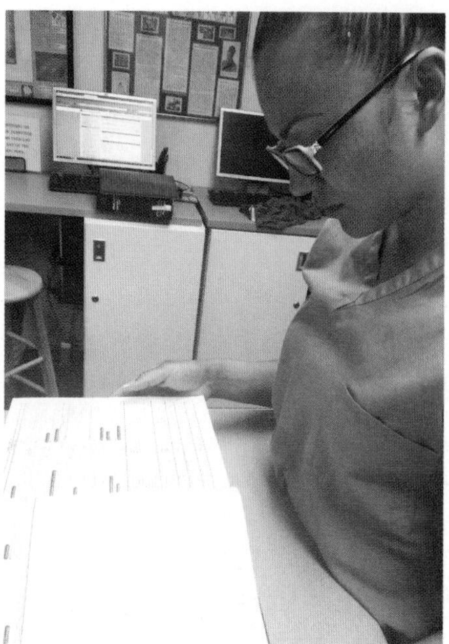

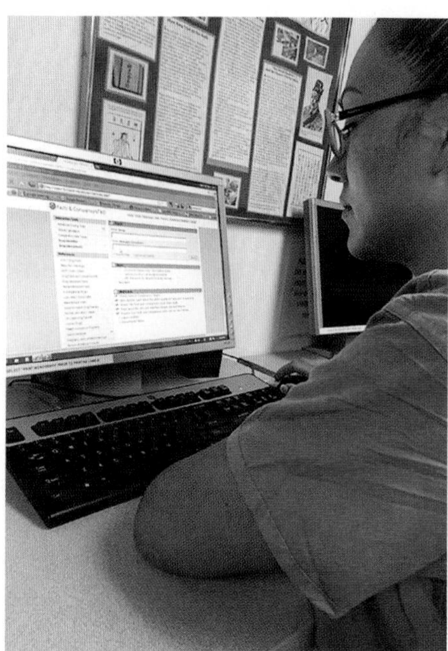

Drug Facts and Comparisons is available as both a print and web-based reference.

Micromedex Solutions

Multiple resources formerly in print, namely the *United States Pharmacopoeia* and the *Redbook 2000*, have been incorporated into a larger pharmacy resource known as *Micromedex*, a product published by Truven Health Analytics. A fully online and comprehensive resource, *Micromedex* provides data on pharmaceutical products, medication management, disease and condition management, pricing and product information, patient education, and information for medications often prescribed for pediatric and geriatric patients.

Micromedex provides a comprehensive collection of evidence-based pharmacy information, such as patient risk factors related to lab values,

© Paradigm Publishing, Inc.

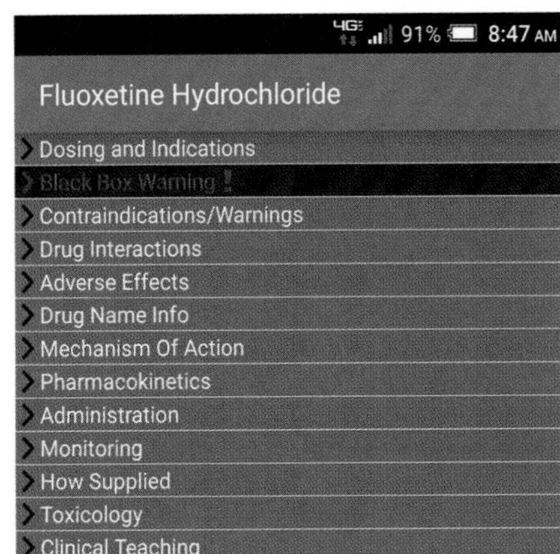

This is an example of Micromedex's mobile application.

medication therapy, and overall health issues. Further resources for the full continuum of healthcare practitioners are also available; such references provide common resources for all levels of healthcare practitioners, which then enables the discussion of patient matters at all levels, from pharmacy technician to pharmacist to physician. Beyond addressing issues related to patient intervention, *Micromedex* is also a resource for updates to average wholesale pricing (AWP) for legend and OTC drugs and for nondrug items (such as supplies and durable medical equipment).

The *Orange Book*

The *Orange Book* is published by the US Food and Drug Administration (FDA). It was originally printed with an orange cover, which explains its name. Now available as an online resource, the *Orange Book* provides information on the **therapeutic equivalency (TE)** of pharmaceutical products in the form of TE codes. TE occurs when drug products are pharmaceutically equivalent and are expected to have the same clinical effect with the same safety when administered to patients.

Pharmaceutical equivalence occurs when drug products contain the same active ingredient or ingredients, are of the same dosage form and route of administration, and are identical in strength or concentration.

TE codes are used to determine therapeutic equivalency of generic medications. In many instances, a rating of *A* must be earned for one product to be considered therapeutically equivalent to another. Drugs with a *B* rating have not yet undergone sufficient study to be granted an *A* rating by the FDA. It is important to note that generic equivalents have an *A* rating.

TAKE NOTE

Example TE Codes:

AA Active ingredients and dosage forms that are not regarded as presenting either actual or potential bioequivalence problems or drug quality or standards issues

AB Active ingredients and dosage forms that demonstrate adequate scientific evidence of bioequivalence through in vivo and/or in vitro studies

BD Products containing active ingredients with known bioequivalence problems and for which adequate studies have not been submitted

Searches for products may be conducted by active ingredient, proprietary name, patent number, applicant holder, or application number. This resource is updated as generic approvals occur.

Bioequivalence is a term used in the study of pharmacokinetics to describe the biological equivalence of two preparations of a pharmaceutical product. When two products are biologically equivalent, they are assumed to be the same. Bioequivalence is established through the in vivo study of the products. **In vivo** is a Latin term meaning "within the living;" in other words, a medication tested in vivo is tested on live subjects, such as plants, animals, or humans. In contrast, **in vitro** (Latin for "in the glass") studies are conducted on a partial or dead organism, such as tissue samples, cells, or molecules outside of their regular biological environment (in a test tube, petri dish, flask, etc.).

TAKE NOTE

Pharmaceutically equivalent drugs do not need to have the same outward characteristics as their equivalent products and may vary in qualities such as shape, score markings, release mechanism, packaging, color, flavoring, preservatives, expiration time frame, and certain labeling.

CALCIUM CHLORIDE
AHFS 40:12

; — Calcium chloride is available in 10-ml singl
efilled syringes containing 1 g of calcium chloride
ing 13.6 mEq (270 mg) of calcium and 13.6 mEq
er for injection. The pH may have been adjusted
: acid and/or calcium hydroxide. (1-4/02; 4; 29)

om 5.5 to 7.5. (1-4/02; 4)

ity — The 10% injection is labeled as having an c
ıOsm/ml. (1-4/02)
osmolality of a calcium chloride 10% solution wa
nometer to be 1765 mOsm/kg. (1233)

Compatibility

Solution	Mfr
ılsion 10%, intravenous	CU

Trissel's is a highly complex tool to help users make informed decisions.

Handbook on Injectable Drugs

The *Handbook on Injectable Drugs*, by Lawrence Trissel (commonly referred to as "Trissel's"), is a comprehensive guide on the compatibility, stability, pH, storage, and preparation of parenteral drugs. Parenteral medications bypass the GI tract during administration, often through injection or infusion. Each year, the reference is updated and **peer-reviewed** for accuracy and completeness. Peer-reviewed resources have been evaluated by experts in the relevant field. Within this resource, a researcher can find information on nearly 3,000 medications used in the preparation of parenteral fluids.

Trissel's is a printed and online reference intended for use as a guide for healthcare professionals engaged in the preparation and delivery of parenteral medications. Due to the nature of the subject, Trissel's is highly complex and should be used as a tool to help make informed decisions. Users of the text must carefully research their answers for accuracy to ensure patient safety.

© Paradigm Publishing, Inc.

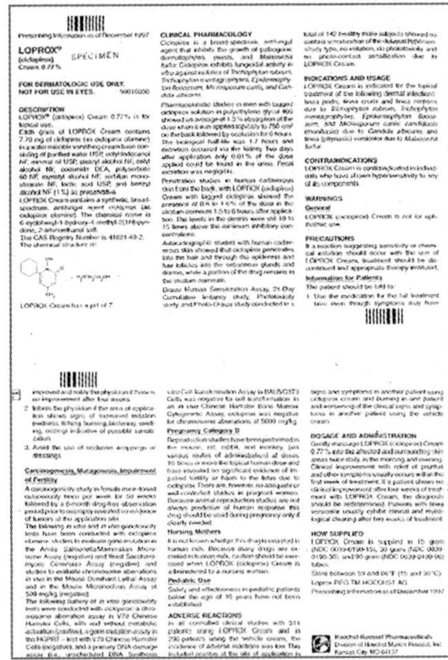

Monographs can be for prescribers or patients.

Pharmaceutical Monographs

A **monograph** is defined as a detailed, written study of a single specialized subject or as a written account of a single thing. In this context, the single thing or specialized subject is a pharmaceutical product. A monograph is a paper reference guide included with each stock bottle or box of product ordered by the pharmacy. The monograph contains many important facts about the associated product, including indication, usage, dosage forms, contraindications, warnings/precautions, adverse reactions, drug interactions, concerns for special populations (e.g., pregnancy risk, nursing mothers, and older adults), dependency/withdrawal effects, drug administration, information gathered during clinical trial, side effects, overdose effects, descriptions of the active ingredient, clinical pharmacology (pharmacokinetics and toxicology), counseling information, and other study information.

In many cases the medication also comes with a guide to provide to patients. The guide includes many similar facts but is written for the patients to easily understand. This patient guide, which is often required by law, helps address many serious questions and issues faced by patients who take these medications regularly. Although not intended as a replacement for counseling by a pharmacist, these guides provide a written reiteration of important information that is covered during patient education and counseling.

The information found in a monograph is also found in many of the previously named references. While in many instances, redundancy is considered a problem, the ongoing, redundant access (for both healthcare providers and patients) to information about a pharmaceutical product can save lives, both before and after a medication is dispensed.

Conclusion

Knowing how to use the reference materials covered in this lab is a valuable skill when you are researching drugs or reviewing prescription information. Consistent access to an abundance of information ensures the health and safety of all persons involved in the care of a patient. Although pharmacy technicians do not provide information directly to patients, you can help research and gather important information and affect the lives of those you care for on a daily basis.

Procedure

This lab will provide you with significant practice using a variety of pharmacy reference materials. You will become familiar with the information available in each reference (availability may vary in your program). When researching and locating information for the worksheet, be sure to note which references you used, including the date of access.

1. Identify which resources are made available to you through your program or institution.

2. Review the attached worksheet, and complete one worksheet each for four of the following (you may obtain additional copies of the worksheet from your instructor): atorvastatin, quetiapine, metformin, cephalexin, methylphenidate, atomoxetine, cefepime, clonazepam, phytonadione (for injection), furosemide, lactated Ringer's, clopidogrel, or duloxetine.

3. **Conclusion:** Tear out and turn in the completed worksheet pages to your instructor. Then go to the Course Navigator, answer all questions in the Lab Review section, and submit your answers to your instructor.

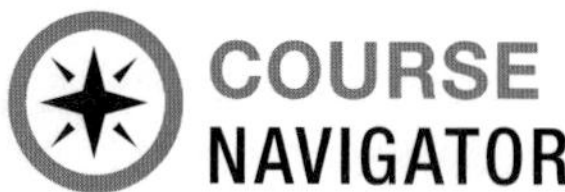

Access interactive chapter review exercises, practice activities, flash cards, and study games.

© Paradigm Publishing, Inc.

Name: ______________________ Date: ______________

Lab 1 Using Reference Materials in Pharmacy Practice

Reference used: ______________________

Generic name: ______________ Brand name: ______________

Pregnancy Category: ______________ Dosage forms: ______________

____

____

Drug class: ______________ Control schedule: ______________

Storage requirements: ______________________

Mechanism of action: ______________________

____

____

Adult dosage: ______________________

Pediatric dosage: ______________________

Geriatric dosage: ______________________

Adverse effects: ______________________

Special instructions for administration: ______________________

____

____

Drug interactions or precipitants: ______________________

____

____

Counseling information: ______________________

____

____

Patient information: ______________________

____

____

© Paradigm Publishing, Inc.

2

Customer Service and Processing Payments

Learning Objectives

1 Display positive communication skills while assisting a pharmacy customer.

2 Demonstrate proficiency in handling cash and operating a cash register.

3 Describe the procedures and rationale for employing appropriate skills related to pharmacy customer service.

Supplies

- Cash register stocked with register tape
- Simulated money with bills and coins, in multiple denominations
- Filled and labeled prescription(s), priced and ready for pickup
- One student who will act as a pharmacy customer in this role-play lab
- Customer service script to be used by the student who will play the customer in the role-play lab
- Prescription pickup signature log
- Controlled substance release log sheet
- Cash register instructions

Access additional chapter resources.

There are three basic types of communication: verbal, nonverbal, and written. In the pharmacy setting, **verbal communication** may take place face-to-face, by phone, or over the pharmacy intercom system. **Nonverbal communication** is composed of a variety of aspects that include eye contact, body language, and appearance. **Written communication** may take the form of a prescription or insurance information presented by a patient at the pharmacy counter or drive-through window or received from a prescriber via fax, e-mail, or scanner. All types of communication are equally important and must be effectively used and interpreted by the pharmacy technician.

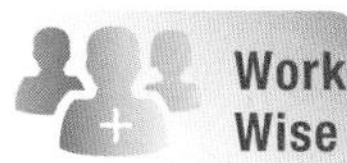

Work Wise

The process for verifying IDs varies between facilities; however, be sure to check that the ID photo matches the person presenting the ID. If you are doubtful, ask for their date of birth and address. If they cannot provide this information, it may be a fraudulent ID. If you have concerns about ID validity, consult the pharmacist on duty.

Whether communicating with a customer or with another healthcare practitioner, the pharmacy technician must always communicate clearly, display a positive attitude, and maintain a professional persona. This is especially true in situations that are challenging or stressful, as patients' lives may depend on the pharmacy technician's accurate and timely communication of information.

Clear communication is ensured by confirming understanding between the communicator and the person being communicated with. One way to verify understanding of communicated information is through repetition. For example, you might ask, "My understanding is that you are calling to request a refill on the furosemide 10 mg prescription for Gabriel Garcia, date of birth, 04/21/1963. Is that accurate?" Repeating information to confirm understanding is an important step toward avoiding a medication error. It should be noted that language barriers, cultural differences, disabilities, age, and literacy issues can create potential communication problems. It is the pharmacy technician's responsibility to ensure that information is communicated effectively.

Displaying a friendly and positive attitude is essential, no matter how busy or stressful the workday is. The technician is often the most visible member of the pharmacy team, and a positive, welcoming attitude, along with a genuine smile and eye contact, can communicate caring, empathy, and a desire to be of service. Making the customer feel cared for and understood is an important aspect of any successful business; it goes a long way toward ensuring repeat customers, which in turn helps the business to grow.

Another way of gaining customer trust and loyalty is to maintain professionalism in all aspects of communication. **Professionalism** refers to conducting oneself with responsibility, integrity, accountability, and excellence in the workplace. Professionalism is displayed by maintaining good personal hygiene, wearing a uniform or professional clothing that is neat and clean, and wearing an employee identification badge. Professionalism is also communicated by speaking in a volume and tone that is appropriate, is clearly understood, avoids slang or jargon, and respects patient confidentiality.

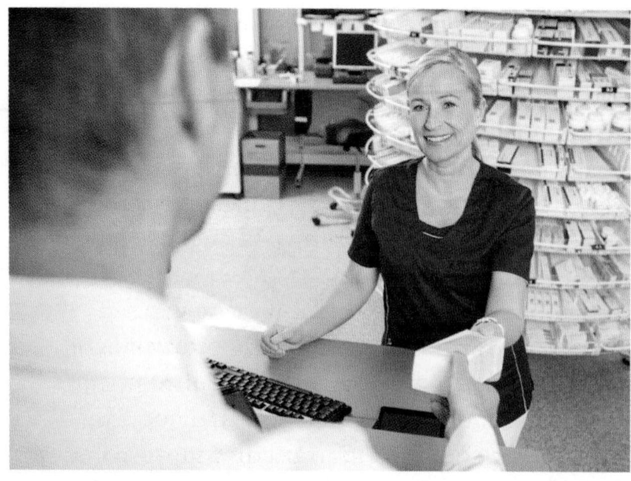

Being friendly, speaking clearly, smiling, and making eye contact are important aspects of professionalism and good customer service in a pharmacy.

Customer service is the assistance and other resources provided by a company to the people who buy or use its products or services. This assistance may take place before, during, and after the sale or use of the product or service. For example, a pharmacy technician must employ good customer service skills when receiving a phoned-in prescription from a doctor's office, when referring a patient's medication question to a pharmacist, and when ringing up a sale on the cash register.

© Paradigm Publishing, Inc.

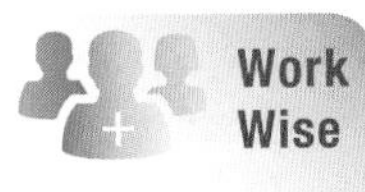

While employing excellent customer service skills, the pharmacy technician must also be able to multitask. Working the cash register in a pharmacy provides an excellent opportunity to employ effective customer service skills, as the pharmacy technician will be called upon to assist customers, answer phones, ring up customer orders, and process multiple transactions, all during the course of a single shift.

Pharmacy technicians must have excellent communication and customer service skills regardless of the pharmacy environment in which they work. In the hospital pharmacy environment, the pharmacy technician will most frequently interact with nurses, pharmacists, doctors, and other healthcare professionals. In addition to healthcare professionals, retail pharmacy technicians will interact extensively with patients, patients' family members, and others who might act as the designated agent for the patient when picking up prescriptions. A **designated agent** is a person who is the legal guardian of or is otherwise designated by the patient to make healthcare decisions on the patient's behalf should the patient be unable to make decisions for himself or herself. All of the people pharmacy technicians interact with are considered to be pharmacy customers and should be treated with the utmost respect and professionalism and in a manner that is welcoming and kind.

Retail pharmacy technicians have multiple opportunities every day to interact with a variety of customers. It is the pharmacy technician's responsibility to provide exceptional customer service when collecting accurate payment for prescriptions and goods and while ensuring that appropriate pharmacy laws and procedures are followed. This includes things like safeguarding cash and controlled substances, maintaining patient confidentiality, and performing verification procedures designed to confirm that the right medication is dispensed to the right patient. In addition, retail pharmacy technicians are often called upon to effectively deal with patients who are not feeling well, are experiencing difficulty paying for their prescriptions, or have language barriers or other issues that may present challenges. It is the pharmacy technician's responsibility to find ways to effectively serve all customers, no matter how challenging the situation may be.

Using a cash register is one of the primary tasks of pharmacy technicians in the retail or community pharmacy environment. Cash handling must be done accurately to ensure that correct money is taken in, correct change is counted out, and counterfeit bills are not accepted. Technicians may also be called upon to perform simple but important maintenance tasks such as changing out the register receipt tape, refilling the register's ink reserves, running transaction reports, voiding charges, processing returned merchandise, and counting the money in the register at the end of a shift (a process sometimes referred to as "counting," "balancing," or "reconciling" the cash drawer).

Like most other businesses, pharmacies often have a specific way in which they want pharmacy personnel to greet customers and answer the phone or drive-through intercom. This is referred to as a **script**. In practice, pharmacy personnel will utilize the same basic script every time they interact with customers. While the script is used primarily when greeting the customer, the pharmacy technician must also be prepared to handle inquiries from various healthcare professionals, respond to phone calls, assist customers at the drive-through window intercom, answer a multitude of customer questions, and determine which of those questions must be referred to a pharmacist for professional judgment. Pharmacy technicians must provide all of these crucial elements of customer service while also performing a variety of other job-related tasks.

Procedure

In this lab, you will have an opportunity to practice your customer service skills in the prescription pickup area. This lab provides you with an opportunity to hone your customer service skills while using the cash register and accurately handling cash transactions with customers who are picking up prescriptions. You will accomplish three primary tasks in this lab procedure: customer service, cash handling, and cash register operation.

Customer Service

The customer service portion of this lab will require you to respond to various customer service role-play interactions in an appropriate and professional manner, based on a variety of scenarios that are similar to what you will encounter in retail pharmacy practice. You will engage in appropriate eye contact, and while maintaining a smile and friendly vocal tone you will greet the customers, locate and verify their filled prescriptions, offer them pharmacist counseling, have them sign a signature log, ring up their prescriptions, answer any questions they may have, and thank them for their business.

Once a prescription has been filled, it is generally placed into a bag. The patient instruction leaflet is printed and either stapled to the bag or placed inside the bag with the prescription. Bags with completed prescriptions are usually filed alphabetically by the patient's last name in labeled bins or another storage area located near the pharmacy pickup window. Verification that you have selected the correct prescription is essential to patient safety; however, it is also important to maintain **Health Insurance Portability and Accountability Act of 1996 (HIPAA)** privacy regulations. The verification procedure should be conducted in as quiet and private a manner as possible, while still being able to communicate clearly and effectively.

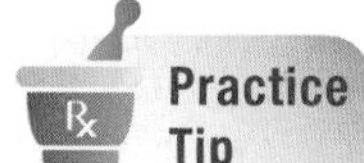

Log sheets are used in a variety of ways in the pharmacy department. They may be used to track verification procedures, to indicate a customer's refusal of counseling, or as a method to track inventory and determine what replacement stock to order.

Once you have verified that you have selected the correct prescription, you must determine whether or not the patient needs to be counseled. At a minimum, every new prescription should be a signal to you to offer pharmacist counseling to the patient. Many pharmacies have patients sign a pickup log to verify that the prescription has been received or to indicate that the patient has been offered (or has refused) counseling. In addition, most pharmacies require you to confirm identification and/or have the customer sign when picking up controlled substances, especially in the case of Schedule II medications. Refer to your pharmacy's policy and procedure manual for site specific requirements.

Operating a Cash Register

The second task in this lab will require you to use a cash register to ring up the patient's prescription(s). Cash register drawers have a removable plastic tray that is divided into multiple separate sections to accommodate different bill and change denominations. In general, cash drawers are set up with $1s in the upper right section, and pennies in the section directly below. Then,

 © Paradigm Publishing, Inc.

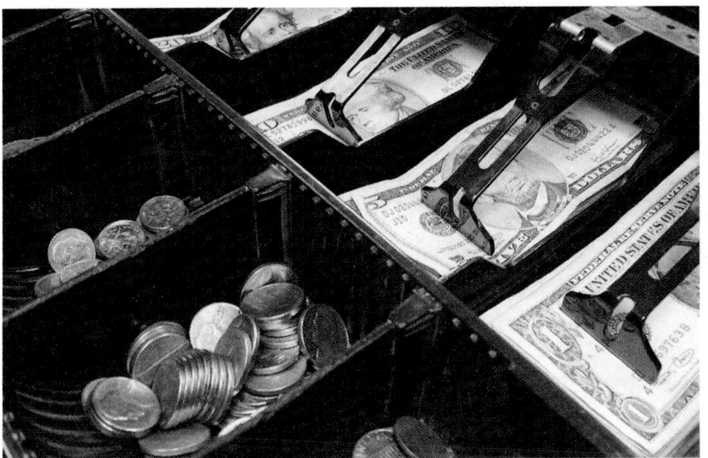

A typical cash drawer with a removable tray.

moving from right to left, the second section accommodates $5s with nickels in the section directly below, followed by $10s with dimes directly below, and finally $20s with quarters directly below. The final, left-most section is used for checks and/or coupons, and as a receptacle for rolled coins, with half-dollars kept directly below that. Bills larger than $20.00 are generally kept underneath the removable tray in the cash drawer. See Figure 2.1. It is important that all payments are kept securely in the cash drawer and that you place each bill and coin in it's proper place within the drawer. Bills should be placed face up, and pointing the same direction. Most cash registers are relatively simple to operate and have similar steps that include the following: typing in the patient's prescription cost, pressing the Subtotal key, typing in the amount of money given to you by the customer, pressing Cash or Amount Tendered, and then counting out the customer's change, if applicable.

Practice Tip

In most cases the cash drawer will be set up with the lowest denominations furthest to the right. This is because most people are right-handed, and the majority of change will be either $1 bills or pennies. However, this practice varies between facilities.

It should be noted that each cash register has specific, step-by-step procedures of operation. Some cash registers use bar code scanners or other technology and may be used as **point-of-sale (POS)** devices that accurately keep track of inventory being sold from the pharmacy. A POS device refers to a computerized network of cash registers or computers that accurately record each transaction made. Pharmacies use these networks to track and reorder medications and supplies, initiate automatic refills, monitor sales, determine inventory levels, and gather reporting information for tax purposes. You should familiarize yourself with the operating procedures of the cash register that you will be using for this lab procedure.

FIGURE 2.1 Cash Placed in Drawer Correctly

A typical cash drawer has the most accessed change—ones and pennies—on the right.

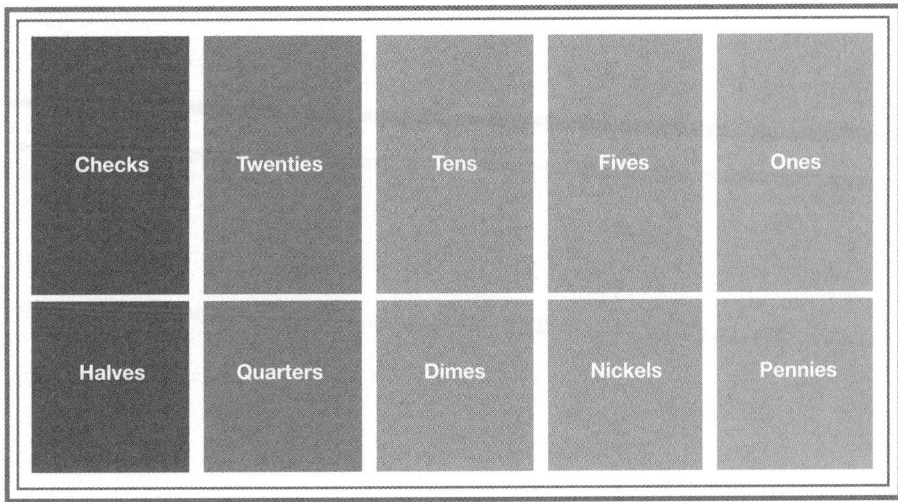

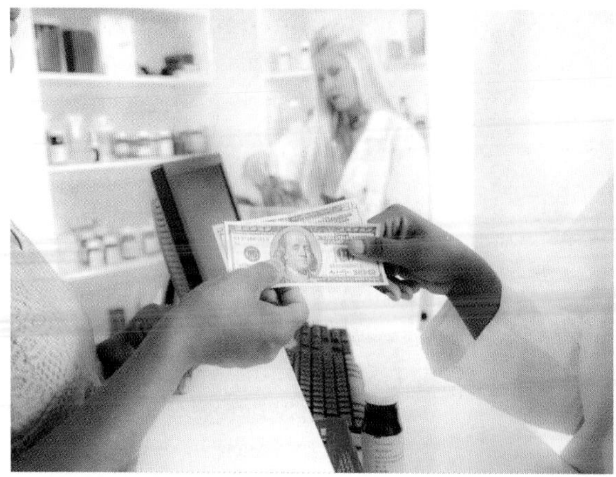

Processing cash payments is an important part of customer service in the pharmacy.

Processing Cash Payments

The third task that you will accomplish in this lab will be the accurate processing of customer cash payments. Collecting payment and returning change accurately are vital to a successful business. There is a specific method you can employ to assist you in this process. First, you will want to verify with the customer the payment amount he or she has handed you. For example, if a customer handed you a ten dollar bill, you would say, "Out of ten dollars," while keeping the bill in an area visible to the customer, preferably on the ledge of the cash register, just above the closed cash drawer. Once you have pressed the Cash or Amount Tendered key, the cash register will display the amount of change to be returned to the customer (if applicable), the cash drawer will automatically open, and a customer receipt will print. Retrieve the customer's payment from the ledge of the cash register, and place it into the appropriate slot in the register drawer. In the event that there is no change to return to the customer, you will close the cash drawer, tear the receipt off of the register, and give it to the customer.

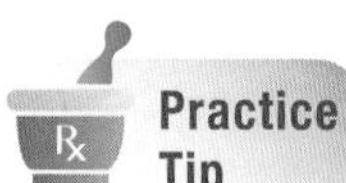

Practice Tip

Technicians must learn how to determine if counterfeit money has been presented for payment in the pharmacy. This might include examining the bill for evidence of security features such as watermarks, holographic images, or security threads that are contained in US treasury bills but not in counterfeit money.

While it may seem easiest to return the amount of change that is shown on the register by piling it into the customer's hand all at once, this is not the most accurate or efficient method of counting change. This method can be rendered completely ineffective should you make an error in entering in the amount tendered or should the customer decide to give you a different denomination after you have rung up the sale. Failing to accurately count returned change can lead to significant accounting errors that can negatively affect your job security and the pharmacy's bottom line.

Giving appropriate change is best accomplished using a method sometimes referred to as **counting up**. To use this method, start with the lowest applicable denomination and recite the amount out loud while systematically counting up (from the lowest applicable denomination to the highest) to the total that was given to you by the customer. For example, if the sale was for $13.56 and the customer gave you a $20 bill, you would then proceed through the process of counting up by doing the following:

- Place the $20 bill on the cash register ledge, and then say out loud, "That's $13.56 out of $20."
- Starting with the lowest applicable denomination (in this case, pennies), count out loud: "Four cents makes $13.60."
- Follow this by counting out the next applicable denomination (in this case, dimes), by saying, "plus forty cents makes $14."
- Follow this by counting out loud the next applicable denomination (in this case, singles), by saying, "plus one dollar makes $15."

 © Paradigm Publishing, Inc.

- Next, count out loud the next applicable denomination (in this case, fives), saying, "plus five dollars makes $20."
- Then, place the entire amount you counted into the customer's hand, tear off the receipt, and give it to the customer.
- Finally, place the $20 that the customer gave you for payment into the appropriate spot in the cash register drawer, and then close the drawer.

TAKE NOTE

Once you become proficient at the counting up method, you may choose to combine several steps (such as gathering all of the coins and returning it to the customer as one sum, versus counting pennies, then nickels, then dimes, etc.) This will make the process of counting up change much quicker.

For this lab, each of the customers you interact with will have a role-play script, which will guide them through a series of interactions typical of what you might encounter in a retail pharmacy. The procedure below will provide you with a basic script that is similar to a pharmacy script that you might use in practice. You will also be required to apply significant critical thinking skills in order to respond appropriately to a variety of customer questions and situations that may arise during the course of the role-play interaction.

Your instructor may choose to make this lab experience even more realistic by interrupting the role-play interaction with various situations that require your attention, such as simulated phone calls from customers or healthcare professionals. If the scenario requires you to interrupt your interaction with the customer that you are role-playing with, you should use appropriate customer service skills to momentarily excuse yourself from dealing with the customer while you address the person or situation that has been presented. Once you have finished addressing this situation, return to your face-to-face customer, apologize for the interruption, and complete your role-play transaction.

Practice Tip

Prescriptions may sometimes be picked up by a patient's family or other designated agent. You will need to consult your pharmacy's policy and procedure manual to determine its rules regarding who can pick up a prescription, especially with regard to picking up controlled substances, as these procedures may vary significantly among pharmacies.

1. Greet the customer by saying, "Welcome to ABC pharmacy. My name is ________ (your name). How may I assist you?" The customer will respond with his or her name and some information about the prescription that he or she is picking up.

2. Respond with "You are picking up a prescription for ________ (patient's name), for ________ (drug name and strength). Is that accurate?" The customer will respond with either "yes"–in which case you will move to Step 3–or "no." If the customer responds "no," verify the patient's name, drug name, and strength with the customer prior to moving to Step 3.

3 Go to the appropriate pickup bin, and find the filled prescription(s) for that patient. Ask the following questions to verify that you have retrieved the correct prescription:

3a "Would you please confirm the patient's last name?" The customer will provide the patient's last name as confirmation.

3b "Would you please confirm the patient's address?"The customer will provide the patient's address as confirmation.

TAKE NOTE

Each pharmacy has its own procedure for verifying prescription pickups. For example, some pharmacies will request the patient's date of birth instead of the address. In practice, you will need to refer to your pharmacy's policy and procedure manual for specific verification instructions. In addition, some patients have multiple prescriptions, including some that may be automatically refilled without the customers' awareness. Be sure to check the entire bin to ensure that you have retrieved all of the prescriptions for a patient. If there are additional prescriptions (other than what the customer has requested for pickup), ask the customer if he or she wishes to pick up all of the patient's filled prescriptions at the same time.

4 Once you have confirmed that you have retrieved the correct prescription(s), have the customer sign and date the prescription pickup log sheet.

5 Retrieve the prescription pickup log sheet from the patient, and record the prescription number and your initials next to the customer's signature.

6 Determine if the prescription is for a controlled substance. If so, ask the customer for identification. If the customer is not picking up a prescription for a controlled substance, go directly to Step 7. If applicable, the customer will produce identification. You should then write down today's date, the customer's name and date of birth, the patient's last name, the controlled substance's prescription number, and your initials on the controlled substance release log sheet.

7 Following the specific instructions for the cash register you are using, ring up the customer's prescription(s) and any other items he or she may be purchasing. Inform the customer that "The total due for your purchase is $______. How would you like to pay for that?"

© Paradigm Publishing, Inc.

TAKE NOTE

In practice, the pharmacy technician is the first line of security with regard to preventing controlled substance diversion. Controlled substance diversion is the theft of a controlled substance, or the transfer of a controlled substance from the individual for whom it was prescribed to another person for illegal use or sale. It is especially important that controlled substance prescriptions be kept behind the counter until the patient's information has been verified and payment has been rendered. This will help prevent someone from grabbing a controlled substance from the pharmacy counter and running off. In addition, there are a variety of procedures that pharmacies use to track controlled substances in an effort to prevent diversion. Be sure to refer to your pharmacy's policy and procedure manual to determine the procedures you are to follow.

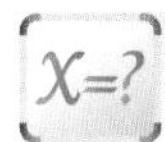

Math Morsels

Remember to count out loud so that the customer can hear and see the counting up process. This will help you to avoid accounting errors, which often occur with cash transactions that are not carefully counted.

8 Upon receiving the customer's cash payment, say, "That will be $_______ (amount due) out of $_______ (amount the customer gave you)."

9 Place the money that the customer gave you on the ledge of the cash register, just above the closed cash drawer.

10 Using the *counting up* method, in a clear voice begin counting back change out loud, starting with the lowest applicable denomination, until you have gathered the correct amount of change.

11 Tear the customer receipt off of the cash register.

12 Return the correct change and the receipt to the customer.

13 Place the customer's payment in the appropriate place in the cash register drawer, and close the drawer.

TAKE NOTE

In practice, you will become skilled in processing transactions that are paid by check or credit cards. In addition, you will sometimes process cash transactions in which the customer provides you with payment in the exact amount due. However, for the purposes of this lab, you will process only cash payments requiring you to return change to the customer, in order to allow you an opportunity to practice your cash-handling skills.

TAKE NOTE

In practice, you would then ask the customer to step to the counseling window so that the pharmacist can counsel him or her. However, for the purposes of this role-play interaction, the customer will not actually be counseled. It is considered best practice that any patients who are new to the pharmacy or have new prescriptions must always receive pharmacy counseling, and that even patients receiving long-time, often-refilled, maintenance medications must be asked if they have any questions for the pharmacist. This is the best way to ensure that patients receive important drug information, which can only be delivered by a registered pharmacist. The requirements for offering counseling vary among pharmacies, so be sure to review your employer's policy and procedure manual for specific instructions.

14 Inform the patient that the pharmacist needs to speak with him or her about the medication(s).

15 Once the counseling interaction is complete, ask the customer, "Is there anything else I can do for you today?" *The patient will respond to this question based on the instructions in the role-play script.*

16 Once you have determined that the customer is completely satisfied and has had his or her questions answered, close your interaction by saying, "Thank you for visiting us today; we appreciate your business. Have a great ___________ (morning, afternoon, or evening). Goodbye."

17 Repeat Steps 1–16 for all of the role-play scenarios given to you by your instructor. Your instructor will fill out the scoring rubric for this lab, available in the instructor resources on the Course Navigator.

18 **Conclusion:** After completing the role-play scenarios, go to the Course Navigator, answer all the questions in the Lab Review section, and submit your answers to your instructor.

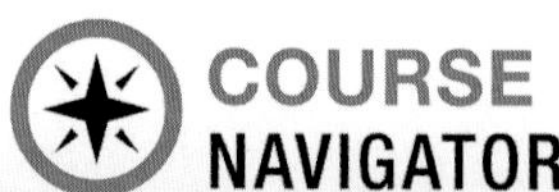

Access interactive chapter review exercises, practice activities, flash cards, and study games.

 © Paradigm Publishing, Inc.

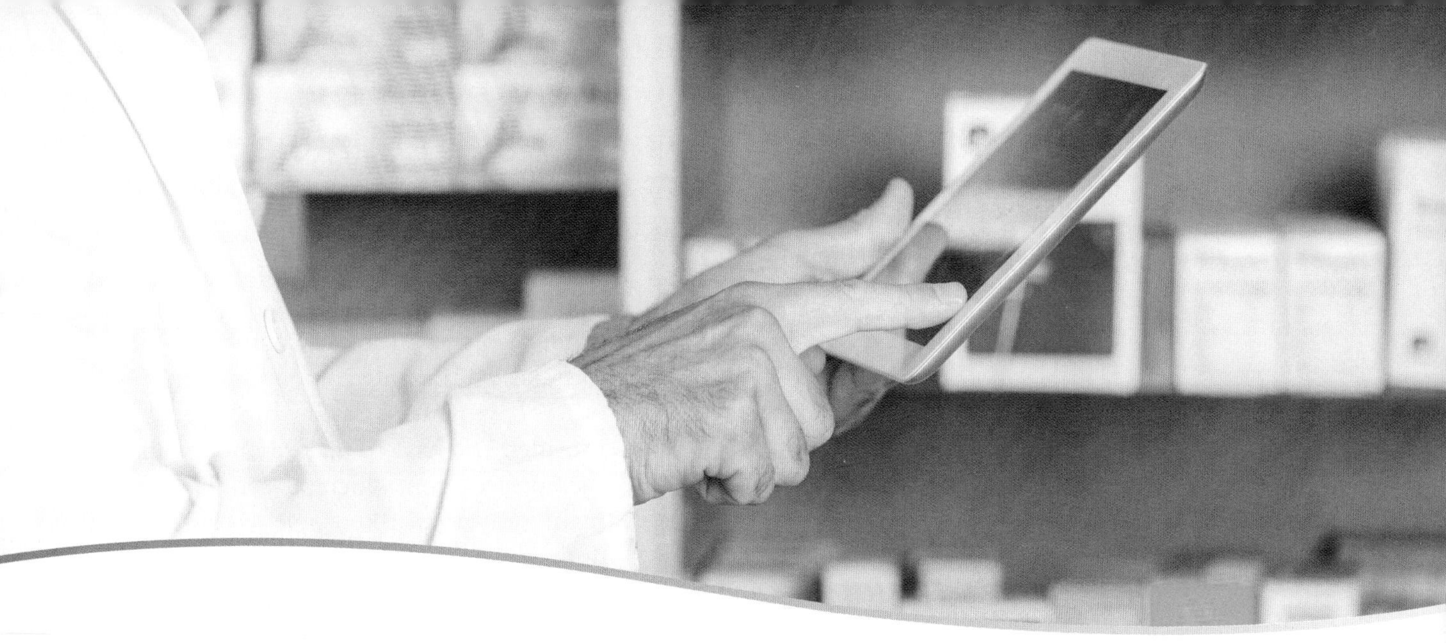

UNIT 2 Community Pharmacy Practice

A Day in the Life of a Pharmacy Technician...

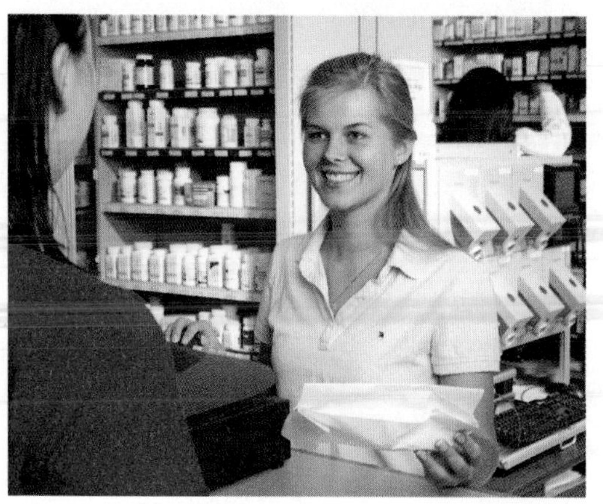

It's the first of the month. It seems like every single person in town wants to fill a prescription—some have refills, some don't, some are expired, some are too early, some have mistakes on the prescription form, and others have issues with the third-party provider. You have to make a phone call on each prescription, which takes time. Overnight, more than 100 people requested a refill online or via the telephone system. You've only been open for 15 minutes, the wait to fill a prescription is already over an hour, and the phone just keeps ringing.

What are you going to do?

The important thing to remember is that you should not panic. This is a common day for many pharmacy technicians working in community or retail pharmacies across the country. The knowledge to effectively process prescriptions, handle any sort of issue (called *exceptions*), and work as a member of the healthcare team to provide accurate and efficient pharmacy services is all acquired with practice and experience. As a new pharmacy technician, you will gain the skills to multitask and resolve complex issues encountered in the pharmacy on a daily basis.

From reviewing a patient profile for completeness and accuracy to working with the pharmacy team to accurately process each prescription, you play a vital role in the foundation of pharmacy operations. The pharmacy technician is an essential member of the pharmacy team, and it is important to remember that while you do a lot of work and take a lot from customers, you are working to help everyone feel better and to improve their health.

Pharmacy technicians must also be adaptable. Many aspects of the job are constantly changing: new laws are enacted, new brand name drugs come to the market, generics become available for popular drugs, and technology changes, such as doctors writing more e-prescriptions instead of patients bringing in handwritten forms. Pharmacy technicians should always be ready to learn new skills.

Task management (effective management of the assigned task) and working to meet the needs of each patient are the keys to success as a pharmacy technician. This unit will help you acquire the foundational knowledge of patient data management, prescription processing and management, and how to resolve some of the more common situations encountered in the daily work of a pharmacy technician.

While it may seem like a lot at first, practice and repetition will help you build the skills you need to ensure smooth operations and provide the best service possible to each patient at the pharmacy.

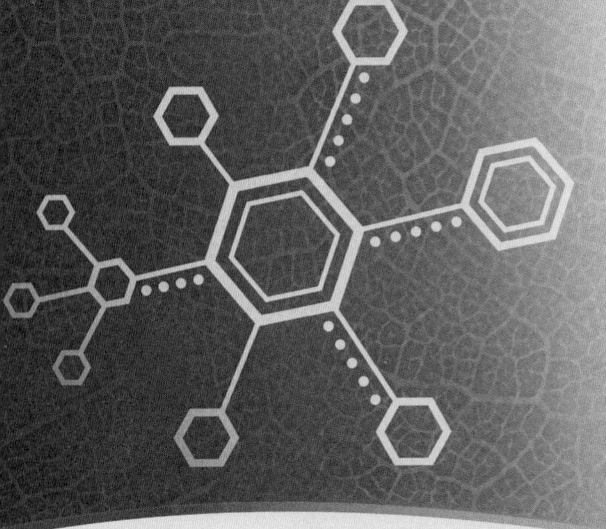

3

Validating DEA Numbers

Learning Objectives

1 Describe the purpose of a DEA number.

2 Describe the components and features of a DEA number.

3 Determine the validity of a prescriber's DEA number.

Supplies

- Calculator

Access additional chapter resources.

A **Drug Enforcement Administration (DEA) number** is a unique identifier assigned to prescribers, pharmacies, hospitals, and other entities (such as drug wholesalers and manufacturers) by the US Drug Enforcement Administration, a branch of the US Department of Justice. This number allows for tracking the authorized prescribing, preparation, storage, and dispensing of controlled substances.

In accordance with the law of the state in which the practitioner resides, having a DEA number grants him or her the ability to legally work with controlled substances pursuant to his or her area of responsibility. In other words, a DEA number means that a prescriber with a DEA number may write prescriptions, a wholesaler may store and sell controlled substances, a pharmacy may store and distribute controlled substances pursuant to prescription orders, and a hospital may do likewise in response to medication orders.

The DEA number consists of two letters and seven numbers. The first letter indicates the level of practice and responsibility. For example, physicians, dentists, podiatrists, veterinarians, pharmacies, and hospitals will have DEA numbers that begin with *A*, *B*, or *F*. Midlevel practitioners such as nurse practitioners, physician assistants, or optometrists will be assigned DEA numbers starting with *M*. As noted earlier, other DEA number prefixes exist for manufacturers (*E*), importers (*J*), and exporters (*K*). As a pharmacy technician, you will primarily work with prescribers, so this lab focuses only on those entities with prescriptive and housing authority (DEA numbers starting with *A*, *B*, *F*, and *M*).

The second letter of a DEA number represents one of two things: If assigned to a business, the second letter will be the first letter of the name of the business or of the company that owns the business. If the number is assigned to an individual, the second letter will be the first letter of the last name of that individual.

The first six digits are used as part of a checksum equation to verify the validity of the DEA number itself. The seventh digit is used as the validation number for the checksum equation.

Procedure

Using the following process described, validate the DEA numbers on Worksheet 3.1. If the number is correct, mark it as valid. If the number is incorrect, mark it as invalid, and describe the corrections needed to make it a valid number.

To validate a DEA number, follow this checksum equation:

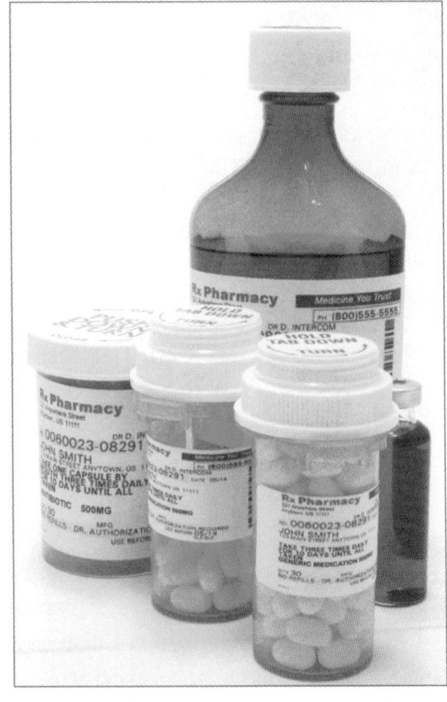

A DEA number allows a pharmacy to house and distribute controlled substances pursuant to prescription orders.

1. Add the first, third, and fifth digits.
2. Add the second, fourth, and sixth digits, and then multiply that sum by 2.
3. Add the results from Steps 1 and 2.
4. The last digit of the result of Step 3 should be the same as the seventh digit of the DEA number.
5. **Conclusion:** Complete Worksheet 3.1, validating all the DEA numbers on the worksheet. Tear out the worksheet and turn it in to your instructor. Then go to the Course Navigator, answer all questions in the Lab Review section, and submit your answers to your instructor.

© Paradigm Publishing, Inc.

Example 1: Pollard's Pharmacy has been assigned DEA number FP1234563

A pharmacy has the authority to order, store, and dispense controlled substances. It has been assigned a "primary level of practice" DEA number starting with the letter *F*. The name of the business starts with the letter *P*, so that is the second letter in the DEA number. Using the checksum equation above, the DEA number can be validated:

$$1 + 3 + 5 = 9$$

$$2 + 4 + 6 = 12 \times 2 = 24$$

$$9 + 24 = 33$$

The last digit of the DEA number (3) matches the last digit from the last step of the checksum equation (3). The DEA number is valid.

TAKE NOTE

In the case of an invalid DEA number, alert the pharmacist and seek guidance on how to proceed. There is a high level of liability in acting on a potentially forged prescription. Contacting local law enforcement should be handled by appropriate personnel, after consulting the pharmacist on duty and/or the pharmacy manager. Be sure to comply with company policies on the detection of forged prescriptions.

Example 2: Spencer Brown, PA, has been assigned DEA number MB1178690

Mr. Brown, a physician assistant, has been assigned a DEA number starting with the letter *M* because he is a midlevel practitioner. Depending on state law, a physician assistant may have limited authority to write prescriptions for controlled substances. The prescriber's last name starts with the letter *B*, which is the second letter in the DEA number. Using the checksum equation above, the DEA number can be validated:

$$1 + 7 + 6 = 14$$

$$1 + 8 + 9 = 18 \times 2 = 36$$

$$14 + 36 = 50$$

The last digit of the DEA number (0) matches the last digit from the last step of the checksum equation (0). The DEA number is valid.

Example 3: Lisa Tierny, DDS, has been assigned DEA number AT6379241

Ms. Tierny, a dentist, has been assigned a DEA number starting with the letter *A,* because she is a primary practitioner. A primary practitioner may write a prescription, in accordance with state regulations, for medications on Schedules II to V. The prescriber's last name starts with the letter *T,* which is the second letter in the DEA number. Using the checksum equation above, the DEA number can be validated:

$$6 + 7 + 2 = 15$$

$$3 + 9 + 4 = 16 \times 2 = 32$$

$$15 + 32 = 47$$

The last digit of the DEA number (1) does not match the last digit from the last step of the checksum equation (7). The DEA number is invalid.

TAKE NOTE

Schedule I drugs are not legally dispensed in the United States due to their high potential for abuse and addiction. Schedule II drugs are the most highly regulated, and sudden increases in usage in a particular pharmacy (or in prescriptions by a particular doctor) may cause the DEA to investigate. Schedule II drugs have no refills. Schedule III, IV, and V drugs have less potential for abuse and addiction than Schedule II drugs and have no limits on refills. See Table 3.1

© Paradigm Publishing, Inc.

TABLE 3.1 Drug Schedules under the Controlled Substances Act of 1970

Schedule	Manufacturer's Label	Abuse Potential	Accepted Medical Use	Examples
Schedule I	C-I	Highest potential for abuse and addiction	For research only; must have license to obtain; no accepted medical use in the United States	Heroin, lysergic acid diethylamide (LSD)
Schedule II	C-II	High potential for abuse, which can lead to severe psychological or physical dependence	Dispensing is severely restricted; cannot be prescribed by telephone except in an emergency; no refills on prescriptions	Morphine, oxycodone, meperidine, hydromorphone, fentanyl, methylphenidate, dextroamphetamine, hydrocodone with acetaminophen
Schedule III	C-III	Less potential for abuse and addiction than C-II	Prescriptions can be refilled up to five times within six months if authorized by physician	Codeine with aspirin, codeine with acetaminophen, anabolic steroids
Schedule IV	C-IV	Lower potential for abuse than C-II and C-III; associated with limited psychological or physical dependence	Same as for Schedule III	Benzodiazepines, meprobamate, phenobarbital
Schedule V	C-V	Lowest potential for abuse and addiction	Some sold without a prescription, depending on state law; if so, purchaser must be over 18 and is required to sign log and show driver's license	Liquid codeine combination cough preparations, diphenoxylate-atropine

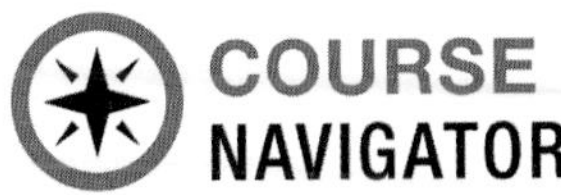

Access interactive chapter review exercises, practice activities, flash cards, and study games.

© Paradigm Publishing, Inc.

Name: ______________________________ Date: ______________

Lab 3 Validating DEA Numbers

Worksheet 3.1

Certify the DEA numbers below. If the number is valid, mark it as "Valid." If the number is invalid, mark it as "Invalid," and describe the corrections needed to make it a valid number.

Example:

Lisa Tierny, DDS AT6379241

____ Valid __X__ Invalid Corrections: The last digit should be 7.
6 + 7 + 2 = 15; 3 + 9 + 4 = 16 x 2 = 32; 15 + 32 = 47. Since the last digit of the checksum is 7, the last digit of the DEA number should be 7, not 1.

1. Floyd's Pharmacy FP1743263

   ____ Valid ____ Invalid Corrections: ______________________________

   ____

   ____

2. Michela Zuckerman, FNP AZ6321474

   ____ Valid ____ Invalid Corrections: ______________________________

   ____

   ____

3. Robert Montague, DPM FM4721362

   ____ Valid ____ Invalid Corrections: ______________________________

   ____

   ____

4. Albert Pickerman, MD BP3419202

   ____ Valid ____ Invalid Corrections: ______________________________

   ____

   ____

 © Paradigm Publishing, Inc.

5. Vivek Rajeev, PA MR1842005

____ Valid ____ Invalid Corrections: ________________________________

____

____

6. Kitty Corners Animal Hospital AK7249089

____ Valid ____ Invalid Corrections: ________________________________

____

____

7. Roberta Goodson, DDS FR1720617

____ Valid ____ Invalid Corrections: ________________________________

____

____

8. Jason van Alstyne, OD MV3621148

____ Valid ____ Invalid Corrections: ________________________________

____

____

9. Curtis Longbottom, MD FL6392423

____ Valid ____ Invalid Corrections: ________________________________

____

____

10. Silvia Romero, DO BR9007469

____ Valid ____ Invalid Corrections: ________________________________

____

____

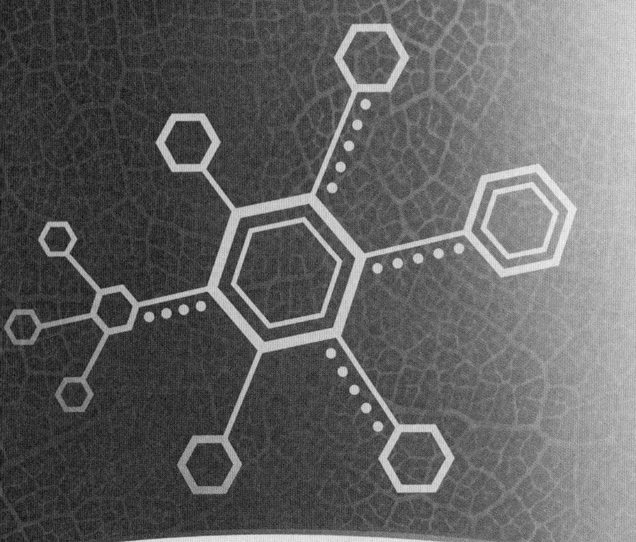

4 Inventory Management Procedures

Learning Objectives

1 Discover the process of basic inventory management in the retail and hospital pharmacy settings.

2 Describe the processes and procedures related to determining inventory levels, want listing, ordering, reconciling, and putting up pharmacy inventory.

3 Demonstrate proficiency in basic inventory management procedures.

Supplies

- Purchase order printout
- Tote filled with items identified on purchase order printout
- Tamperevident lock on filled tote (if available)
- Shipping invoice listing items in tote
- Pharmacy lab stocked with various prescription and over-the-counter (OTC) medications and supply items
- Want list log sheet

Access additional chapter resources.

The term **pharmacy inventory** refers to all the prescription drugs, over-the-counter (OTC) medications, supply items, **durable medical equipment (DME)** (reusable items such as wheelchairs, walkers, crutches, and bedpans), and **non-durable medical equipment (non-DME)** (disposable medical supply items such as needles, syringes, cholesterol checking supplies, and blood sugar testing supplies) that are stocked in the pharmacy. **Inventory management** refers to a set of activities or procedures that are completed by pharmacy personnel to ensure that medications and supply items are available when needed. Pharmacy personnel are also tasked with making sure pharmacy inventory is purchased in a manner that is within the constraints of the pharmacy budget and follows established policies with regard to the facility's wholesaler contracts and **formulary** (a list of approved drugs).

Inventory management is comprised of three primary functions: determining what is needed, purchasing medications and supplies from wholesalers or other vendors, and then receiving, reconciling, and stocking pharmacy inventory.

Most pharmacies contract their inventory purchases through a **pharmacy wholesaler.** Pharmacy wholesalers, sometimes referred to as *prime vendors*, maintain ample stock of thousands of the most widely used medications and supply items from a variety of manufacturers. Wholesalers provide secure, computerized ordering systems that may be fully or partially automated. The contract between the pharmacy and the pharmacy wholesaler will identify the responsibilities of each party and will also delineate the payment terms and delivery timeline expectations, which are often within 24 hours of when the pharmacy places the order. Wholesalers also play an important role in maintaining the safety of the drug supply by ensuring that all medications they stock are approved by the U.S. Food and Drug Administration (FDA) and by participating in recall procedures (as necessary). Working with a pharmacy wholesaler saves the pharmacy a great deal of time and money.

Most pharmacies and pharmacy wholesalers use a formulary system to control drug costs. Formularies are determined based on the types of drugs used by the pharmacy, treatment needs of the primary patient population served by the pharmacy, therapeutic equivalencies, cost, and contractual obligations to insurance companies or third-party payers. The vast majority of inventory items are purchased through a pharmacy wholesaler. Because of drug shortages or immediate need, some medications may be purchased directly from the manufacturer or from another pharmacy.

Inventory Management

All members of the pharmacy staff engage in some aspect of inventory management. Nearly all pharmacy settings use a **want list** to keep track of new items that need to be ordered or pharmacy items that are running low. The want list may also be referred to as a *want book*, *short list*, or *reorder list*. This is a log sheet where pharmacy personnel write down information that will be used when placing orders with the pharmacy's wholesaler. The information recorded on the want list varies between facilities, but it will generally include the date; a drug's name, strength, and form; and the quantity needed. Many facilities also provide a space on the form to add miscellaneous information that might be helpful to the person who orders pharmacy inventory from the wholesaler, who is often referred to as the **inventory technician**. For example, if multiple patients have recently been prescribed a drug that is very rarely used, that information would assist the inventory technician in determining how much of the drug to order. There is also a place on the log sheet to record the name or initials of the person who is writing the information on the want list. This is necessary should the inventory technician have questions about what was written on the list.

In addition to recording information on the want list, nearly all pharmacy personnel will participate in the process of **reconciling**, or checking in, the order. This may include prescription drugs, OTC medications, supply items, DME, and non-DME. This may also be referred to as the *purchase order* or *supply order*. When the order is received from the wholesaler, pharmacists or a narcotic technician will likely be responsible for entering controlled substances into the pharmacy

 © Paradigm Publishing, Inc.

Practice Tip

While some pharmacies may use designated technicians to work with narcotics, some pharmacies limit narcotic access to pharmacists only. Refer to your pharmacy's policy and procedures for pharmacy-specific requirements.

inventory and storing them under proper security. A **narcotic technician** is a technician who, depending on the size of the facility, may work either full-time with narcotics or on an as-needed basis. They will likely be responsible for entering controlled substances into the pharmacy inventory and storing them under proper security. All the technicians on duty will likely participate in putting the rest of the order away in the appropriate areas of the pharmacy.

There are many things that must be considered with regard to inventory management in the pharmacy. This includes following the facility's formulary, managing and negotiating contracts with wholesalers or other vendors, and operating within the pharmacy's established budget. Medication availability, turnover rate, and expiration dating must also be considered. Finally, both the pharmacy setting and the type of inventory system employed by the pharmacy significantly affect the inventory management process.

Point-of-Sale Systems

In the community pharmacy setting, determining what to order is most often accomplished through the use of **point-of-sale (POS) computer systems** that track every item ordered, received, sold, and dispensed by the pharmacy. In a POS system, nearly every aspect of inventory management is computerized. This is most often accomplished through the use of barcode technology, which allows pharmacy personnel to quickly scan items and efficiently place online orders with the pharmacy wholesaler. These systems may also be referred to as *point-of-service systems*. In general, POS systems automatically generate a list of items that need to be ordered from the wholesaler, and that list is then reviewed by pharmacy personnel who adjust the order by adding or deleting items and/or amounts based on the pharmacy's anticipated needs. The order is then transmitted to the wholesaler via their online ordering system.

Once the order is received from the wholesaler (usually within 24 to 72 hours), technicians are able to quickly scan the barcode of each item received, which efficiently adds the items into the pharmacy's inventory prior to the technician placing them in the proper storage area in the pharmacy. The POS system is an efficient inventory management method and is a form of **perpetual inventory**, because stock levels are consistently maintained: medications and supplies are automatically ordered based on predetermined reorder points, which are triggered by sales. Perpetual inventory is an inventory system where every pill or dose is tracked from the time it enters the pharmacy via delivery from the wholesaler, until the time it leaves the pharmacy to be taken by, or administered to, a patient. As medication leaves the store with patients, it is automatically deducted from the pharmacy's inventory, and replenishment is ordered as necessary.

POS systems also allow for easy generation of reports that assist with defining daily, weekly, and monthly inventory needs and reorder points. These reports also help determine quarterly and annual inventory levels and assist in setting budget parameters. In small or independent community pharmacy settings, the pharmacist in charge (PIC) will use these reports to assist with annual budget development and tax reporting. In larger chain pharmacies, the PIC, store manager, and district or regional manager may use these and other inventory-related reports to identify store and regional trends and set staffing levels. This information may be further used by company personnel at the regional, state, and national level to identify inventory trends, negotiate wholesaler contracts, determine staffing needs, and set personnel incentives.

© Paradigm Publishing, Inc.

Placing the Purchase Order

In the community pharmacy setting, there may be an experienced or lead pharmacy technician who has primary responsibility for placing the purchase order with the contract wholesaler. The order may also be placed by a pharmacist. The determination of what to order may be entirely computerized based on par levels or reorder points, or it may be done by a combination of POS tracking and direct entry of data into the wholesaler's website by pharmacy personnel. Once what needs to be ordered has been determined, the order is placed via computer with the wholesaler. The wholesaler will then automatically generate a purchase order number that identifies the order placed by the pharmacy. In general, the pharmacy technician who placed the order will print out the purchase order, which will be used to reconcile the shipment once it is received.

In the institutional pharmacy setting, there is often an **inventory technician** whose primary responsibility revolves around inventory management. Inventory technicians are generally experienced pharmacy technicians who have received special training in the processes and procedures required for their position. In addition to the primary inventory management activities, inventory technicians in institutional pharmacies may also participate in committees or activities such as the Pharmacy and Therapeutics committee or other groups or committees that work to develop and maintain the hospital formulary. A Pharmacy and Therapeutics committee determines which drugs will appear on the pharmacies' formulary based on cost, contracts with insurance companies, and therapeutic treatment needed for patients served. Other technicians will participate with inventory management by recording information on the want list, processing credits and returning reusable stock items to the shelves, rotating inventory, and stocking shelves when orders are received from the wholesaler.

In the institutional pharmacy setting, there may be a combination of methods used to order and track inventory. Inventory management in this setting can be a more complex process because bulk drug bottles are often repackaged into unit dose containers to be dispensed at a later date, and because pharmacy items may be stored in decentralized pharmacy satellites, dispensing robots, or automated drug storage and dispensing systems (ADSDS). Institutional pharmacy inventory management may require the use of barcode scanning devices, perpetual inventory logs, automatically generated or manually determined par levels or reorder points, and computer-generated reports from pharmacy robots or ADSDSs.

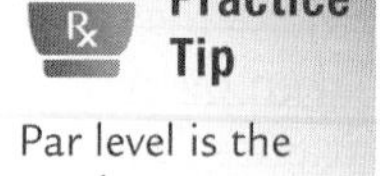

Par level is the total amount of a particular medication that the requesting unit keeps on hand when fully stocked. You will fill and check floor stock in lab 17.

Often, the inventory technician will use a barcode scanning device to "run the shelves" and determine how much of a medication or item is needed to bring it up to the **par level**. Pharmacies often set a predetermined reorder point, which is likely well below the par level, that triggers the inventory technician to order that item in sufficient time to keep it from running out.

The inventory technician will then upload the information from the scanner to the wholesaler's website or secure web portal. While on the wholesaler's website, the inventory technician will also order items that were identified on the want list or various computer-generated reports. Once the order is complete, the inventory technician will submit it electronically to the wholesaler and print out a receipt or purchase order that lists each item ordered.

Receiving and Reconciling the Order

A shipment of pharmacy items is received from the wholesaler in large plastic bins that are often referred to as *totes*. In order to deter theft and tampering, the

 © Paradigm Publishing, Inc.

wholesaler generally places a tamper-evident lock on each tote. If a tote is received without a tamper-evident lock or with a lock whose seal has been broken, the pharmacy technician receiving the order should immediately bring it to the attention of the person delivering the shipment to the pharmacy. If this discovery is not made until after the delivery person has departed the pharmacy, the pharmacy technician should immediately notify the pharmacist on duty and the PIC, and contact the wholesaler.

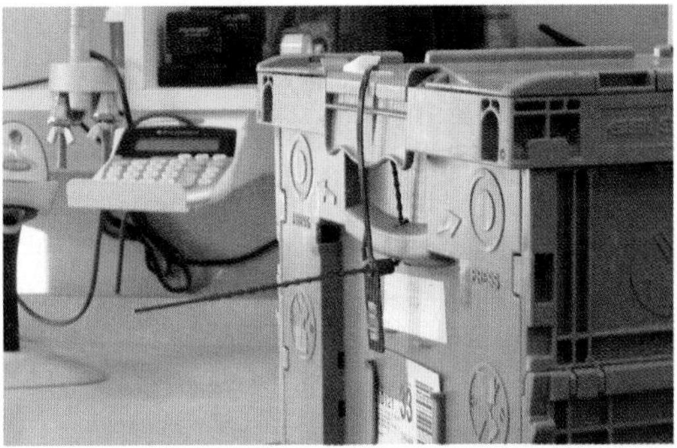

A tamper-evident lock ensures that the shipment has not been opened prior to it arriving in the pharmacy.

TAKE NOTE

The use of tamper-evident locks on totes of noncontrolled substance may vary between facilities. In practice, refer to your policies and procedures manual and your wholesaler's delivery policy to determine the proper procedure to follow in the event that a tote is received with a broken or missing lock.

Totes may come in several different colors, each denoting a particular type of item or a special handling or storage procedure required for the item. For example, blue or gray totes are often used for pharmaceuticals that do not require special handling or storage. Red, orange, yellow, or black totes will often be used to signify hazardous drugs, **investigational drugs** (drugs that are being studied in patient trials prior to approval by the FDA), or other items that require special handling or must be stored separately from other pharmacy stock.

TAKE NOTE

Hazardous drugs are shipped with a material safety data sheet (MSDS) for each item. The MSDS instructs pharmacy and other personnel in the special storage, handling, and use of hazardous drugs as well as the procedures that must be followed when there has been an accidental exposure to or spill of the hazardous material.

Items requiring refrigeration or freezer storage may arrive in specially labeled Styrofoam containers that use dry ice to maintain cold temperatures during transport. Items delivered in Styrofoam containers or otherwise identified as being temperature-sensitive should be opened, reconciled, and placed in the appropriate,

Practice Tip

Hazardous drugs have special shipping, handling, storage, and preparation requirements. In addition to the MSDS, you will need to refer to USP <800> *Hazardous Drugs –Handling in Healthcare Settings*, prior to performing inventory, or any other procedures using hazardous drugs.

temperature-controlled storage area as soon as possible after delivery (generally within 60 minutes). The shipping containers are only designed to maintain appropriate temperature levels through the time of delivery.

The person delivering the shipment will also produce a **shipping invoice**. This paperwork may also be referred to as a *shipping receipt* or *manifest*. The shipping invoice is used in the reconciliation process described later in this lab.

Controlled substances are generally shipped in a separate tote, which is secured with one or more tamper-evident lock devices. Because of problems with the theft and diversion of controlled substances, totes containing controlled substances should be opened and counted in the presence of the person delivering the shipment to the pharmacy. This requires the technician to verify the name, strength, form, package size, and quantity ordered for each item in the tote. Both the wholesaler's delivery person and the pharmacy technician receiving the controlled substances should then verify that the controlled substance shipping invoice exactly matches the controlled substance purchase order placed by the pharmacy. Both people should then sign and date the shipping invoice as evidence that the correct items and quantities were received by the pharmacy. The controlled substance tote should then be secured by pharmacy personnel while the other totes are being checked into the pharmacy.

TAKE NOTE

Upon completing the initial controlled substance reconciliation in front of the delivery driver, some pharmacies will place a new tamper-evident lock on the controlled substance tote until they have an opportunity to finish the process of scanning, entering into stock, and putting away the controlled substances in their secure location within the pharmacy. Refer to your facility's policies and procedures manual for specific information on handling, securing, and checking in controlled substances.

In most pharmacies, only the controlled substance tote is opened and reconciled in front of the delivery driver. All other totes in the shipment are counted without being opened. The shipping invoice is signed and dated by both the delivery driver and the person receiving the order. The items in the remaining totes will be fully reconciled once the totes are opened, just prior to putting them away. However, because of the busy pace of the pharmacy, the technicians often must wait until a slow period provides them with ample time to complete the reconciliation process and put away the order.

Once the order is received from the wholesaler, pharmacy technicians are generally responsible for reconciling the shipping invoice or receipt against the pharmacy's printed record of what was ordered online. The reconciliation process is a method of ensuring that the correct items were received in the correct quantities. When conducting the reconciliation process, it is best to begin at the top of the shipping invoice and proceed down line by line, verifying each item in the tote against what is listed on the shipping invoice. The reconciliation process also requires line-by-line comparison of the shipping invoice to the purchase

© Paradigm Publishing, Inc.

order printout. It is essential to confirm that what was received is exactly what was ordered.

Items that were received in error should be set aside for further action. Other items that should be set aside include any items *not* listed on the purchase order printout; items received in a strength, form, or quantity that does not exactly match the purchase order printout; and items that are broken, cracked, or otherwise in unsellable condition. If there are items on the purchase order printout that are either not listed on the shipping invoice or are listed as being out of stock, make a note of this on the purchase order printout.

In practice, the inventory technician or other designated pharmacy personnel will work with the wholesaler to return damaged stock and ensure that the pharmacy is given credit for the returned items. He or she will also follow up on any out of stock or unavailable items, to either attempt to order them directly from the drug's manufacturer (or another source) or refer the matter to a pharmacist who will contact the physician to determine if there is an alternative medication that the pharmacy has on hand that could be prescribed for the patient. However, for the purposes of this lab, you will not be required to engage in the process of handling returns with the wholesaler or securing alternate resources for out-of-stock items.

Once all the items in all the totes have been verified to be the correct drug, strength, form, and quantity, the shipping invoice and purchase order printout should be signed by pharmacy personnel who checked in the order, and given to the inventory technician, pharmacist, or other designated pharmacy personnel, who will later confirm that the prices charged for each item match what is on the contract with that wholesaler. This price is referred to as the **contract price**. Wholesalers are able to offer contract pricing, which is often significantly lower than off-contract pricing, because they deal in bulk and move large quantities of items that are on agreed formulary lists.

Prior to placing items from the totes onto the pharmacy shelves, they must be added into the pharmacy inventory. This is often done electronically by downloading the list of items from the shipping invoice directly into the pharmacy inventory via software that allows the pharmacy's inventory system to communicate with the wholesaler's system. In other pharmacies, each item must be individually scanned into the pharmacy's inventory system by means of a barcode scanning device. Although the overall process is essentially the same, the individual procedures for adding stock to the pharmacy inventory system vary significantly between facilities. Because of these variations, you will not engage in the process of adding stock to the pharmacy inventory system during this lab.

Putting Up Stock

Once the stock has been added to the pharmacy inventory system, the final step in the basic inventory management process is to put the stock away in the appropriate place in the pharmacy. This process is sometimes referred to as *putting up stock* or *stocking the shelves*. There are several things that must be considered when putting up stock. Care must be taken to ensure that the correct medication is placed in the correct place on the pharmacy shelf. Most medications are available in multiple strengths and forms. Because of the potential for medication error, it is essential that each medication be placed in the correct place for its strength and form.

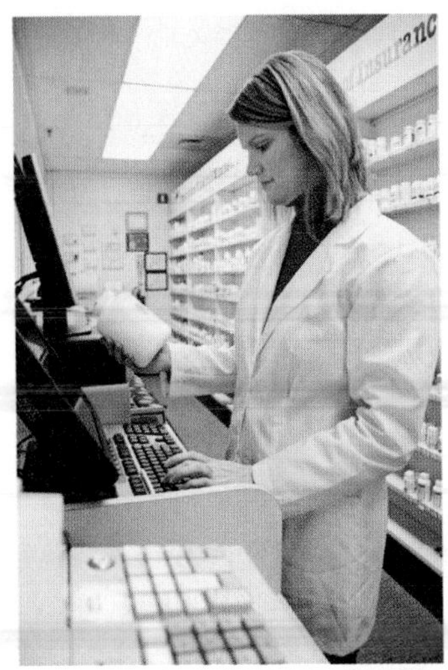

Pharmacy technicians should check a drug's expiration date prior to stocking it on the shelf.

Appropriate storage conditions must also be maintained, such as for items that must be refrigerated, kept frozen, be protected from light, or be placed in a medication warmer. Storage conditions are identified on the item's exterior packaging, on the container labeling, and in the package insert contained within the package for each medication.

In addition to properly placing and storing pharmacy stock it must be properly rotated to ensure that items do not expire prior to sale. Items that have expired or are about to expire cannot be sold and are not generally eligible for return to the wholesaler. Expired items end up as a loss to the pharmacy; therefore, **stock rotation** is an important aspect of inventory management and helps keep the pharmacy budget on track. Stock rotation is the process of placing items with the longest expiration dating which are generally the items that have just been ordered, behind the items that expire earlier. The latter are generally the items already on the pharmacy's shelf. This way, items with shorter expiration dating will be used or sold prior to items with longer expiration dating.

Your instructor may choose to make this lab experience more realistic by incorporating the use of barcode scanning devices, computer-generated reports, a POS system, or a simulated wholesale ordering system. If so, your instructor will provide additional equipment and instructions to supplement this lab.

In this lab, you will use a pharmacy purchase order printout and a shipping invoice to reconcile a tote filled with various pharmacy items. You will also put the items in the tote away in their appropriate locations in the pharmacy, based on their storage requirements, and use appropriate stock rotation procedures. Finally, you will use a want list to record information regarding medications that need to be ordered.

Procedure

1. Gather the filled and locked (if applicable) tote, purchase order receipt, and shipping invoice from your instructor.

2. Place the tote onto a tabletop or other suitable work surface.

3. If applicable, break open the tamper-evident lock, and remove it from the tote. Dispose of the lock in a waste receptacle.

4. Open the tote. Pick up the first item in the tote. Locate that item on the shipping invoice.

5. Compare the drug name, strength, and form listed on the exterior package of the first item to the item description on the shipping invoice. Once you have verified that this item is an exact match, put your initials on the shipping invoice next to that item.

© Paradigm Publishing, Inc.

6 Retrieve the purchase order printout. Compare the drug name, strength, and form listed on the exterior packaging of the first item to the item description on the purchase order printout. Once you have verified that this item is an exact match, put your initials on the purchase order printout next to that item.

7 Place the first item on the work surface, outside of the tote.

8 Pick up the next item from the tote. Locate that item on the shipping invoice.

9 Compare the drug name, strength, and form listed on the exterior package of the second item to the item description on the shipping invoice. Once you have verified that this item is an exact match, put your initials on the shipping invoice next to that item.

10 Return to the purchase order printout. Compare the drug name, strength, and form listed on the exterior packaging of the second item to the item description on the purchase order printout. Once you have verified that this item is an exact match, put your initials on the purchase order printout next to that item.

11 Place the second item on the work surface, outside of the tote.

12 Repeat Steps 8–11 until you have verified that each item in the tote matches both the shipping invoice and the purchase order printout.

13 Return to the purchase order printout. Determine if there are any items on the purchase order that you did not receive in the tote and were not on the shipping invoice.

14 Retrieve the want list. Put today's date in the first column of the want list.

15 Begin filling out each section of the want list with the information from the purchase order printout that identified the name, strength, form, and quantity of any items that were ordered but were not in the tote or on the corresponding shipping invoice.

16 In the Miscellaneous section of the want list, write the following: "Item listed as out of stock on shipping invoice."

17 In the last section of the want list, record your initials. Once all sections of the want list have been filled in, temporarily set it aside.

TAKE NOTE

An item listed as being out of stock will alert the inventory technician or other designated pharmacy personnel that they may need to find an alternative supplier for the out of stock item, or take steps to initiate pharmacist contact with the prescriber to determine if there is an alternate medication that the pharmacy has on hand and could be used in place of the medication that was not received.

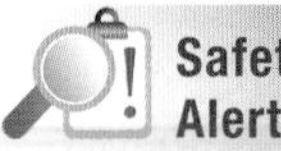

Special storage considerations may include refrigeration, protection from light, or storage in a medication warmer. Hazardous drugs, which must be specially packaged and shipped, must be stored in separate, specially labeled areas of the pharmacy.

18 Return to the shipping invoice. Verify that every item has been accounted for, that all received items have been verified and initialed, and that any items listed as being out of stock on the shipping invoice have been recorded on the want list.

19 Once the entire shipping invoice has been verified, legibly sign your name on it. Put today's date next to your name. Temporarily set the shipping invoice aside.

20 Return to the purchase order printout. Verify that every item has been accounted for, that all items have been verified and initialed, and that any items that were on the purchase order printout but were not in the tote have been recorded on the want list. Put your signature and today's date next to your printed name. Temporarily set the purchase order aside.

21 Return all the received and verified items to the tote. You will use the tote to carry the items to their various storage areas in the pharmacy.

TAKE NOTE

One of the advantages of POS, scanned barcode, or otherwise computerized inventory management systems is that the computer will automatically print out the specific location in the pharmacy where that item should be stored. Caution should be taken, as these locations may change over time based on a drug's usage or turnover rate.

22 Retrieve the first item from the tote. Read the exterior package information to determine if there are any special storage considerations for this item. If so, be sure to handle it according to the package directions. Consult your instructor for directions should you have any questions about special handling or storage procedures.

© Paradigm Publishing, Inc.

Practice Tip

The pharmacy is often divided into multiple sections based on the drug type, turnover rate, and storage requirements. Common pharmacy sections include fast movers, slow movers, topicals, ophthalmics, ear medications, nonformulary, refrigerated, investigational medications, and hazardous drugs.

23 Locate the area in the pharmacy where the item is to be stored, and proceed to that location with the item.

24 Verify that the item matches the drug name, strength, and form of the existing items on the shelf.

25 Examine each of the items currently stored on the shelf to determine their expiration dating.

26 Examine the item that you are going to be placing on the shelf to determine its expiration dating.

27 Place the items onto the shelf in chronological order so that the item with the longest expiration dating is located at the back, and the item with the shortest expiration dating is located at the front of the shelf.

28 Continue Steps 22–27 until the tote is empty.

29 Place the empty tote in the designated area of the pharmacy or pharmacy lab.

30 **Conclusion:** Gather the purchase order printout, shipping invoice, and want list, and give them to your instructor for grading. Then go to the Course Navigator, answer all questions in the Lab Review section, and submit your answers to your instructor.

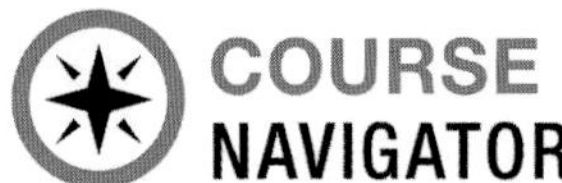

Access interactive chapter review exercises, practice activities, flash cards, and study games.

© Paradigm Publishing, Inc.

Name: ______________________ Date: ______________

Lab 4 Inventory Management Procedures

Inventory Want List

Today's Date	Drug Name	Drug Strength	Drug Form	Number to Dispense	Quantity Needed	Miscellaneous Information or Instructions	Your Initials

© Paradigm Publishing, Inc.

5

Reviewing a Patient Profile

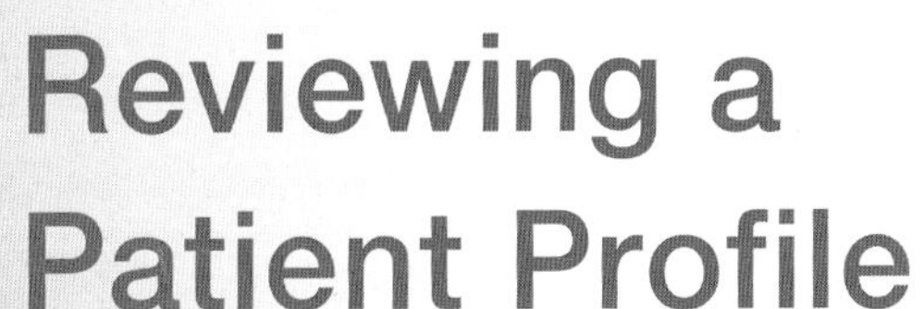

Learning Objectives

1 Demonstrate an understanding of the importance of a patient profile in pharmacy practice.

2 Gain skill in reviewing a patient profile form for completeness and accuracy of information.

3 Demonstrate an understanding of the types of problems that missing or inaccurate patient information can introduce to pharmacy practice.

4 Demonstrate strategies to resolve problems arising from incomplete patient profile forms.

Supplies

- None

Access additional chapter resources.

When patients first visit a pharmacy, they usually complete a physical copy of a patient profile form. This form establishes a patient record with the pharmacy. Once the form is signed and submitted to the pharmacy, the pharmacy technician is often responsible for **transcribing** the form—transferring information from the completed paper form to the electronic patient record in the pharmacy management software. The technician's transcription work plays an important role in ensuring and maintaining patient safety. You must be vigilant and verify that the information provided by the patient is both accurate and complete. If the patient profile is not complete, you may have the added responsibility of interviewing the patient to solicit further data.

The patient profile form itself is a simple document that includes basic demographic information, such as name, address, birth date, telephone numbers (home, work, and "other"), and e-mail address. The form requests other crucial information, including medications currently being taken, current or long-term health conditions, and allergies. All of this data has a direct impact on the patient's drug therapy, and some important cautions are in order. While it is not necessary to push for more than one phone number, it is a **best practice** (a technique designed to deliver the best results with little or no margin of error) to have multiple means of contacting a patient. You do need to record a street address for a patient, in case you must make contact in an emergency, and because state regulations may require one when you fill certain prescriptions (such as those for controlled substances). In addition, when a parent or guardian is providing information for a child, ensure that the information the adult writes down is, indeed, about the child. Dosage and review guidelines for a pediatric patient are of high importance, and accurate information is crucial to the child's safety.

While physicians have the knowledge to safely prescribe medications, having a complete and accurate patient record allows pharmacy staff to fully review a patient's prescriptions for safety. Pharmacy staff can screen the requested medications against the patient's current medications, check for errors caused by incorrect prescriptions, and respond competently if something undesired should result. Complete patient records provide a "big picture" view of a patient's medication program, enabling pharmacists and pharmacy technicians to serve patients well and to protect their welfare.

One final note regarding patient safety is to consider the use of two very similar phrases: "No Known Drug Allergies" (NKDA) and "No Known Allergies" (NKA). NKDA implies that the pharmacy staff has asked only about *drug* allergies and has specifically identified that the patient has no known allergies to drug products. NKA is a more broad claim, implying that the pharmacy has established that the patient has no known allergies whatsoever, in any allergy category (including drug allergies, food allergies, pet allergies, and plant allergies). As a pharmacy technician, you must ensure that you are using the proper phrase in the patient's pharmacy record.

As healthcare practitioners, pharmacy technicians are entrusted with personal data from each person receiving prescriptions and must protect that data. Always keep in mind the ethical implications of having access to confidential patient information and the necessity of not disclosing such information outside the pharmacy. The Health Insurance Portability and Accountability Act of 1996 (HIPAA) regulates the use and disclosure of protected health information (PHI). For example, consider this scenario:

> You are transcribing Miguel Esparza's profile (New Patient Profile 4) when you notice that he lives on the 7500 block of East 11th Street. Your Aunt Pamela lives on the 7600 block of the same street, so you strike up a conversation with the patient on how, according to your aunt, that neighborhood is slated for a street-paving project. You also notice that Miguel has come in for a prescription for Tamiflu and, later that night, call your Aunt Pamela to tell her that Miguel has a bad cold and that she should warn her friends that a cold or flu bug is circulating on East 11th Street.

 © Paradigm Publishing, Inc.

While it was not your intention, your actions constitute a breach of ethical conduct and are also a violation of HIPAA, which has potential legal implications. You have disclosed a patient's personal health information to a person not otherwise involved in his care and have violated the trust between you and your patient, Miguel. As a pharmacy technician, you must strictly respect your patients' privacy when handling their protected health information.

Procedure

Several patients have filled out new patient profile forms as shown in Figure 5.1 and New Patient Profiles 1 through 4. The form in Figure 5.1 is completely and accurately filled out, whereas those at the end of this lab may be incomplete. In this lab, you will check the new patient profile forms in New Patient Profiles 1 through 4 for completeness and accuracy.

As you proceed through the following steps, work thoughtfully, and consider questions such as the following: Are all blank areas filled in? What kind of information is missing? Is the missing information required or not? Are allergies noted? Is medical information present? Is the form signed? When you encounter missing or incorrect data that requires resolution, you should ask yourself how you would handle such circumstances if they arose at your pharmacy. Identify when it would be best to solicit the missing information from the patient, to discuss items that appear inaccurate, or to bring these issues to the pharmacist's attention. What would or should you do? What should you avoid doing or saying? If the question is quite personal, should you interview the patient at the pharmacy drop-off counter or pull the patient aside to the counseling window? How do you determine what a particular patient may consider "personal" information? Discuss all topics that you are unsure of with your instructor.

To complete the worksheets at the end of this lab, follow the steps outlined below to review each patient profile form for accuracy and completeness. Because this is a practice scenario, there is no patient present for you to speak with should you have questions about the profile form. Nonetheless, when a procedure step asks you to communicate with a patient, imagine that the patient is in front of you, and either whisper quietly to yourself (as if having that conversation) or imagine the patient's response. If your instructor permits it and time allows, you might also partner with another student to role-play these hypothetical pharmacy technician and patient conversations. Remember that not all information is required. Clearly circle all errors that you discover on each worksheet, and then describe the action you, as a pharmacy technician, would take to correct the error.

1. Carefully read over the completed, accurate profile (Figure 5.1) on the next page, noticing how the various sections are thoroughly and completely filled out.

© Paradigm Publishing, Inc.

FIGURE 5.1 Sample of a Fully Completed New Patient Profile

PATIENT PROFILE

Patient Name

Wilkins | Marquita | Middle Initial
Last | First |

6901 Westminster Chase
Street or PO Box

Providence | RI | 02908
City | State | ZIP

Date of Birth: 02/29/1984 (MM / DD / YYYY)
Gender: ☐ Male ☑ Female
Social Security No.: 000-00-0000
E-mail: marquita@email.com

Home Phone: (401) 555-1212
Work Phone: (401) 555-1313
Other Phone: ( )

☑ Yes, I would like medication dispensed in a child-resistant container.
☐ No, I do not want medication dispensed in a child-resistant container.

Medication Insurance: ☑ Yes ☐ No

Cardholder Name: ______

☑ Cardholder ☐ Child ☐ Disabled Dependent
☐ Spouse ☐ Dependent Parent ☐ Full-Time Student

(Please provide the pharmacy with your card.)

MEDICAL HISTORY

HEALTH		ALLERGIES AND DRUG REACTIONS
☐ No Known Medical Conditions	☐ Diabetes Mellitus	☐ No Known Drug Allergies
☐ Anemia	☐ Epilepsy	☐ Aspirin
☐ Arthritis	☐ Esophagitis	☐ Cephalosporins
☐ Asthma	☐ Generalized Anxiety Disorder	☐ Codeine
☐ Attention-Deficit Hyperactivity Disorder	☐ Heart Condition	☐ Erythromycin
☑ Blood Clotting Disorders	☐ Hypertension	☐ Iodine
☐ Cancer	☐ Kidney Disease	☑ Penicillin G Potassium
☐ Depression	☐ Liver Disease	☐ Sulfa
	☐ Lung Disease	☐ Tetracyclines
	☐ Ulcers	☐ Xanthines

ICD-10-CM for Checked Condition(s): D68.9

Details for Checked Allergy(ies): ______

Medication(s) Currently Being Taken: ______

Primary Care Physician: Geoff Taylor

Comments: ______

Health information changes periodically. Please notify the pharmacy of any new medications, allergies, drug reactions, or health conditions.

Signature: Marquita Wilkins Date: 4/9/19 ☐ I choose not to fill out this form.

2 Go to the profile in New Patient Profile 1. Read the patient name and verify the spelling, confirming that it is legible. Be aware of gender ambiguous names. In such cases, double-check the patient's gender by politely asking the patient if the prescription is for the patient or for someone else. You might also ask to see a driver's license and discreetly seek your answer there.

3 Review the street address, and verify spelling, city name, state, and ZIP code.

 © Paradigm Publishing, Inc.

4 Verify the patient's date of birth—especially the year.

5 If a Social Security number is required for patient identification, be sure to get the entire number and explain that the number is required for insurance purposes only. Due to increasing risk of identity theft, many patients are understandably hesitant to provide the number. Similarly, if the patient hesitates to provide an e-mail address, explain how and when your pharmacy plans to use that information.

6 Look over the phone number section, ensuring you have at least one contact number for the patient.

7 If the box for child-resistant containers is checked, verify that this is correct.

8 If the patient has prescription coverage, make sure the cardholder name is filled in and a relationship box is checked.

9 Ensure that the patient has indicated whether he or she has health conditions or allergies (medication allergies or other types). If the patient writes in "No Known Drug Allergies" or checks a box indicating NKDA, keep in mind that you will have to record this designation carefully when you get to the computerized profile data-entry stage (Lab 8).

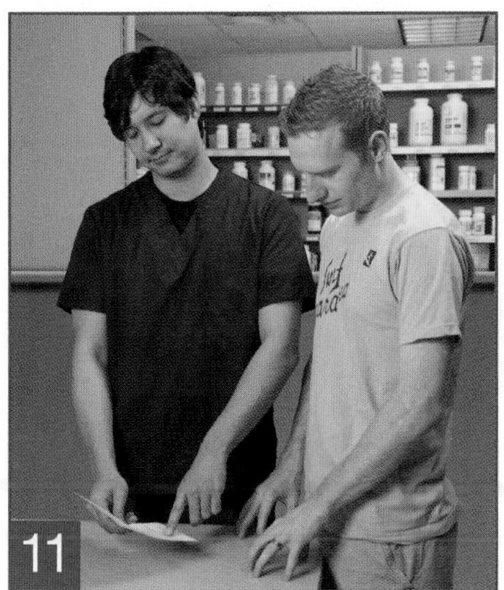

Pharmacy technician asking a customer to sign the patient profile form

10 Verify whether the patient has taken any prescription or over-the-counter (OTC) medications recently and whether he or she takes any on a regular basis.

11 Check that the patient has signed the form. If not, ask the patient to do so.

12 Repeat Steps 2 through 11 for the remaining worksheets, and complete New Patient Profiles 1 through 4. When you have completed all four worksheets, proceed to Step 13.

13 **Conclusion:** Verify that you have written your name and the date, circled all errors, and written in your explanations on all four worksheets. Tear out the worksheets, and turn them in to your instructor. Then go to the Course Navigator, answer all questions in the Lab Review section, and submit your answers to your instructor.

Access interactive chapter review exercises, practice activities, flash cards, and study games.

Name: ______________________________ Date: ________________

New Patient Profile 1

PATIENT PROFILE

Patient Name
DONALDSON | VANCE | ___
Last | First | Middle Initial

12 MAPLE LEAF TRAIL
Street or PO Box

ROUND ROCK | TX | 78644
City | State | ZIP

Date of Birth	Gender	Social Security No.	E-mail
MM / DD / YYYY	☒ Male ☐ Female	000-00-0000	VDONALDSON@EMAIL.COM

Home Phone	Work Phone	Other Phone
(512) 555-1212	(512) 555-1313	( )

☐ Yes, I would like medication dispensed in a child-resistant container.
☒ No, I do not want medication dispensed in a child-resistant container.

Medication Insurance: ☒ Yes ☐ No
Cardholder Name: SAME
☒ Cardholder ☐ Spouse ☐ Child ☐ Dependent Parent ☐ Disabled Dependent ☐ Full-Time Student
(Please provide the pharmacy with your card.)

MEDICAL HISTORY

HEALTH		ALLERGIES AND DRUG REACTIONS
☐ No Known Medical Conditions	☐ Diabetes Mellitus	☐ No Known Drug Allergies
☐ Anemia	☐ Epilepsy	☐ Aspirin
☐ Arthritis	☐ Esophagitis	☐ Cephalosporins
☐ Asthma	☐ Generalized Anxiety Disorder	☐ Codeine
☐ Attention-Deficit Hyperactivity Disorder	☐ Heart Condition	☐ Erythromycin
☐ Blood Clotting Disorders	☒ Hypertension	☐ Iodine
☐ Cancer	☐ Kidney Disease	☐ Penicillin G Potassium
☐ Depression	☐ Liver Disease	☐ Sulfa
	☐ Lung Disease	☐ Tetracyclines
	☐ Ulcers	☐ Xanthines

ICD-10-CM for Checked Condition(s): I10
Details for Checked Allergy(ies): ______

Medication(s) Currently Being Taken: ASPIRIN 81 MG, ACCUPRIL 10 MG

Primary Care Physician: ______

Comments: ______

Health information changes periodically. Please notify the pharmacy of any new medications, allergies, drug reactions, or health conditions.

Signature V. Donaldson Date 4/09/19 ☐ I choose not to fill out this form.

Circle the error(s) on this patient profile form.

Describe the action(s) you would take to correct the error(s):

____

____

© Paradigm Publishing, Inc.

Name: ______________________ Date: ______________

Lab 5 Reviewing a Patient Profile

New Patient Profile 2

PATIENT PROFILE

Patient Name
Gupta | Amala | ___
Last | First | Middle Initial

5473 W. 10th Street
Street or PO Box

Cedar Rapids | IA | 52401
City | State | ZIP

Date of Birth: 08/24/1961 (MM / DD / YYYY)
Gender: ☐ Male ☑ Female
Social Security No.: 000-00-0000
E-mail: gupta.amala@email.com

Home Phone: (401) 555-1212
Work Phone: (401) 555-1313
Other Phone: ( )

☐ Yes, I would like medication dispensed in a child-resistant container.
☑ No, I do not want medication dispensed in a child-resistant container.

Medication Insurance: ☑ Yes ☐ No

Cardholder Name: same
☑ Cardholder ☐ Child ☐ Disabled Dependent
☑ Spouse ☐ Dependent Parent ☐ Full-Time Student
(Please provide the pharmacy with your card.)

MEDICAL HISTORY

HEALTH
☑ No Known Medical Conditions
☐ Anemia
☐ Arthritis
☐ Asthma
☐ Attention-Deficit Hyperactivity Disorder
☐ Blood Clotting Disorders
☐ Cancer
☐ Depression
☐ Diabetes Mellitus
☐ Epilepsy
☐ Esophagitis
☐ Generalized Anxiety Disorder
☐ Heart Condition
☐ Hypertension
☐ Kidney Disease
☐ Liver Disease
☐ Lung Disease
☐ Ulcers

ALLERGIES AND DRUG REACTIONS
☑ No Known Drug Allergies
☐ Aspirin
☐ Cephalosporins
☐ Codeine
☐ Erythromycin
☐ Iodine
☐ Penicillin G Potassium
☐ Sulfa
☐ Tetracyclines
☐ Xanthines

ICD-10-CM for Checked Condition(s): ______
Details for Checked Allergy(ies): ______

Medication(s) Currently Being Taken: ______

Primary Care Physician: Sunjiter Patel

Comments: ______

Health information changes periodically. Please notify the pharmacy of any new medications, allergies, drug reactions, or health conditions.

Signature: Amala Gupta Date: 04/19/19 ☐ I choose not to fill out this form.

Circle the error(s) on this patient profile form.

Describe the action(s) you would take to correct the error(s):

____

____

© Paradigm Publishing, Inc.

Name: ______________________ Date: ______________

Lab 5 Reviewing a Patient Profile

New Patient Profile 3

PATIENT PROFILE

Patient Name

Riley — Last
Cas — First
Middle Initial

72650 Okade Court
Street or PO Box

Orlando — City
FL — State
32810 — ZIP

Date of Birth: 01/22/2010 (MM/DD/YYYY)
Gender: ☑ Male ☐ Female
Social Security No.: 000-00-0000
E-mail: cast@email.com

Home Phone: (407) 555-1212
Work Phone: ( )
Other Phone: ( )

☑ Yes, I would like medication dispensed in a child-resistant container.
☐ No, I do not want medication dispensed in a child-resistant container.

Medication Insurance: ☑ Yes ☐ No
Cardholder Name: Molly Riley
☐ Cardholder ☐ Spouse ☑ Child ☐ Dependent Parent ☐ Disabled Dependent ☐ Full-Time Student
(Please provide the pharmacy with your card.)

MEDICAL HISTORY

HEALTH
☐ No Known Medical Conditions
☐ Anemia
☐ Arthritis
☐ Asthma
☑ Attention-Deficit Hyperactivity Disorder
☐ Blood Clotting Disorders
☐ Cancer
☐ Depression
☐ Diabetes Mellitus
☐ Epilepsy
☐ Esophagitis
☐ Generalized Anxiety Disorder
☐ Heart Condition
☐ Hypertension
☐ Kidney Disease
☐ Liver Disease
☐ Lung Disease
☐ Ulcers

ALLERGIES AND DRUG REACTIONS
☐ No Known Drug Allergies
☐ Aspirin
☐ Cephalosporins
☐ Codeine
☐ Erythromycin
☐ Iodine
☐ Penicillin G Potassium
☐ Sulfa
☐ Tetracyclines
☐ Xanthines

ICD-10-CM for Checked Condition(s): F90.9
Details for Checked Allergy(ies):

Medication(s) Currently Being Taken: Rotalin 10 mg

Primary Care Physician: Philip Fleming

Comments:

Health information changes periodically. Please notify the pharmacy of any new medications, allergies, drug reactions, or health conditions.

Signature: Molly Riley Date: 4/9/19 ☐ I choose not to fill out this form.

Circle the error(s) on this patient profile form.

Describe the action(s) you would take to correct the error(s):

____

____

© Paradigm Publishing, Inc.

Name: ______________________________ Date: ________________

Lab 5 Reviewing a Patient Profile

New Patient Profile 4

PATIENT PROFILE

Patient Name
Esparza (Last) Miguel (First) ____ (Middle Initial)

7583 E. 11th Street
Street or PO Box

Austin (City) TX (State) 78705 (ZIP)

Date of Birth: 09/12/1965 (MM / DD / YYYY)
Gender: [X] Male [ ] Female
Social Security No.: 000-00-000
E-mail: ____

Home Phone: (512) 555-1212
Work Phone: ( ) ____
Other Phone: ( ) ____

[X] Yes, I would like medication dispensed in a child-resistant container.
[X] No, I do not want medication dispensed in a child-resistant container.

Medication Insurance: [X] Yes [ ] No

Cardholder Name: ____
[X] Cardholder [ ] Spouse [ ] Child [ ] Dependent Parent [ ] Disabled Dependent [ ] Full-Time Student
(Please provide the pharmacy with your card.)

MEDICAL HISTORY

HEALTH
- [ ] No Known Medical Conditions
- [ ] Anemia
- [ ] Arthritis
- [ ] Asthma
- [ ] Attention-Deficit Hyperactivity Disorder
- [ ] Blood Clotting Disorders
- [ ] Cancer
- [ ] Depression
- [X] Diabetes Mellitus
- [ ] Epilepsy
- [ ] Esophagitis
- [ ] Generalized Anxiety Disorder
- [ ] Heart Condition
- [ ] Hypertension
- [ ] Kidney Disease
- [ ] Liver Disease
- [ ] Lung Disease
- [ ] Ulcers

ALLERGIES AND DRUG REACTIONS
- [ ] No Known Drug Allergies
- [ ] Aspirin
- [ ] Cephalosporins
- [ ] Codeine
- [ ] Erythromycin
- [ ] Iodine
- [X] Penicillin G Potassium
- [ ] Sulfa
- [ ] Tetracyclines
- [ ] Xanthines

ICD-10-CM for Checked Condition(s): Z13.1

Details for Checked Allergy(ies): ____

Medication(s) Currently Being Taken: ____

Primary Care Physician: ____

Comments: ____

Health information changes periodically. Please notify the pharmacy of any new medications, allergies, drug reactions, or health conditions.

Signature: Miguel Esparza Date: 4/9/19 [ ] I choose not to fill out this form.

Circle the error(s) on this patient profile form.

Describe the action(s) you would take to correct the error(s):

____

____

 © Paradigm Publishing, Inc.

6

Reviewing a Prescription Form

Learning Objectives

1 Evaluate unprocessed prescriptions for completeness and accuracy.

2 Learn the additional steps for reviewing controlled substance prescriptions.

Supplies

- None

Access additional chapter resources.

A written prescription is the primary form of communication between a prescribing healthcare provider and pharmacy staff in community pharmacies. Hospitals and institutional pharmacies tend to use medication orders instead of written prescriptions. A prescription establishes the appropriate therapy protocol in an effort to relieve the patient of symptoms or illness.

A pharmacy technician's first responsibility is to process prescriptions—from receiving them from patients at the drop-off counter, to interpreting the data, to labeling the bottles. Prescription data is presented in the form of a **signa**, a series of abbreviations that begins with an action verb and communicates dispensing and patient directions in this order: dose, quantity, route of administration, time interval, and additional information. As a pharmacy technician, you will notice that prescriptions arrive in a variety of ways. As technology in healthcare advances, many prescribers and pharmacies opt to transmit and receive prescriptions electronically using a highly secure method of transmitting prescription amongst service providers. Handwritten and computer-generated physical prescriptions are still very common today as e-prescribing can be very expensive. The use of fax machines to send and receive information regarding prescriptions is still also prevalent in pharmacies as well.

Accurate filling of a prescription begins with a careful review of the form. Thus, paying attention to detail is imperative. You must develop

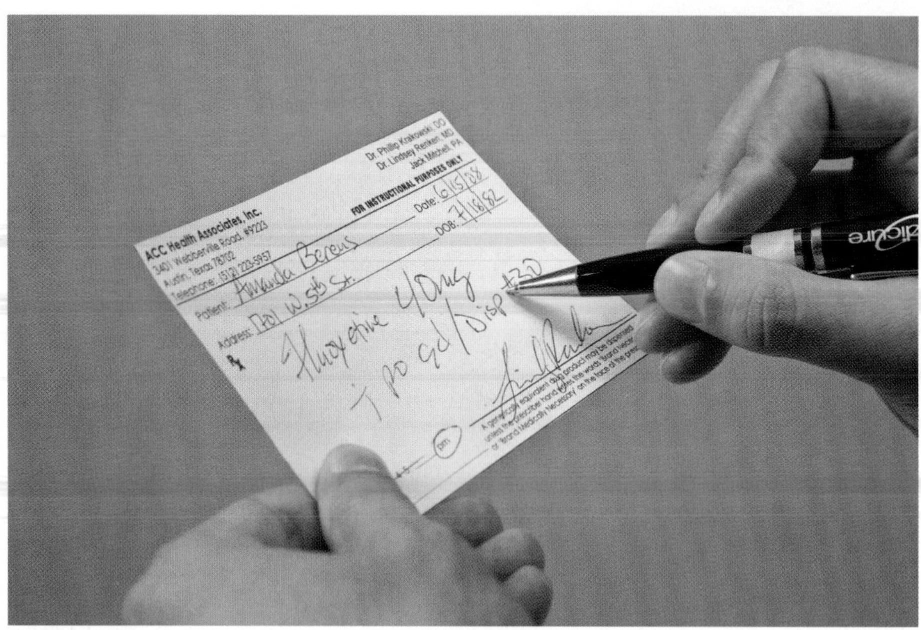

Pharmacy technician verifying information on a prescription form

expertise in reviewing prescriptions for complete and accurate components including the patient, physician, and pharmacy data; the signa; and the DEA number.

A **DEA number** is a unique identifier assigned by the US Drug Enforcement Administration to track the prescribing, preparation, and dispensing of controlled substances. (For more information on DEA numbers, refer to Lab 3). You must also check adherence to additional state regulations for prescription drugs and controlled substances, and you must verify any data specific to electronic prescriptions, which currently require information about the receiving pharmacy and a transmit date.

When preparing prescriptions, it is always a best practice to be mindful of the type of prescription that you are filling. When filling a prescription for a controlled substance, use added caution because regulations governing the preparation and dispensing of controlled substances are much stricter than

TAKE NOTE

The laws regulating pharmacy practice and filling of prescriptions vary from state to state. Check with your instructor regarding any special exceptions concerning laws, rules, and regulations discussed in this text. Prescriptions for noncontrolled substances are valid for one year, while those for controlled substances are valid for six months. Prescriptions for noncontrolled substances can be refilled for up to one year, while those for controlled substances can be refilled only five times in a six-month period.

 © Paradigm Publishing, Inc.

are those for noncontrolled substances (due to the potential for abuse). The quantity prescribed must be written in *both* numeral form and word form (e.g., "30, thirty") to prevent alteration of a prescribed quantity. If one of the two forms is missing, alert the pharmacist, and contact the prescriber's office to verify the prescription. Also, federal regulations limit the quantity of refills on most controlled substances to five, for a maximum of six total fills in six months (180 days). Lastly, be sure that a *valid* DEA number is on the prescription. See Lab 3 for more information on validating DEA numbers.

Procedure

This lab helps you develop your skills in reviewing prescriptions for completeness and accuracy. The worksheets at the end of the lab contain forms for unprocessed prescriptions. Using your current knowledge of pharmacy practice, information from this textbook, and the instructions in the steps below, you will evaluate and comment on each prescription to ensure that the required information is included.

As you proceed through the numbered steps, you will use Checklist A for each worksheet prescription form. However, be aware that there may be more information to verify on some of the forms. In cases where the prescription was sent electronically, you must also take the additional steps listed in Checklist B. In cases where the prescription is for a controlled substance, you must also take the additional steps listed in Checklist C. In some cases, you may need to use all three checklists. It is your responsibility to determine which checklists to consult for each prescription form. Checklists A, B, and C follow Step 6.

1. Carefully read over the prescription form and the scenario included below the form.

2. On each worksheet, verify the information in Checklist A. If you find any errors or questionable components, mark them by clearly circling them on the prescription form itself.

3. In the space provided under the prescription form, explain the error(s) or issue(s) and the best practice to correct the error(s) or resolve the issue(s).

4. If the prescription was sent electronically, also check the items in Checklist B. As you did for Checklist A, mark the errors clearly on the prescriptions, and write your explanations on the blank lines provided.

5. If the prescription is for a controlled substance, also check the items in Checklist C. As you did for Checklist A, mark the errors clearly on the prescriptions, and write your explanations on the blank lines provided.

6 **Conclusion**: Tear out and turn in the completed worksheets to your instructor. Then go to the Course Navigator, answer all questions in the Lab Review section, and submit your answers to your instructor.

Checklist A, for all prescriptions on the worksheets:

- Check the physician information: name, address, phone number, and handwritten signature.
- Check the patient information: date of birth, name, and address.
- Check the prescription information: date written, drug name, strength, quantity, and refill information.
- Check the directions to the patient (the signa): dose quantity, route of administration, time interval, and additional information.

Checklist B, for electronic prescriptions on the worksheets:

- Check the receiving pharmacy information for your pharmacy's name, address, and phone number.
- Check whether the transmit date is different from the written date. If it is, you may need to call to verify the prescription's validity.
- Check that an electronic signature is on file.
- Check whether this electronic prescription is for a controlled substance. If it is, verify with your instructor whether your state allows electronic transmission for such prescriptions, and respond accordingly on the worksheet.

Checklist C, for controlled substance (Schedules III and IV) prescriptions on the worksheets:

- Check that today's date, as presented in the scenario, is within six months (180 days) of when the prescription was written.
- Check the validity of the DEA number.
- Check that the quantity is written in both numeral form and word form.
- Check that the maximum number of refills is no greater than five.
- Check the quantity, verify with your instructor whether your state places limitations on this substance, and respond accordingly on the worksheet.
- C-V prescriptions have no federal limit; be sure to check the regulations in your state.

© Paradigm Publishing, Inc.

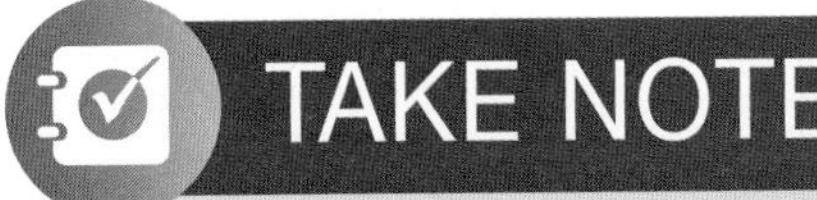

Because each state regulates the prescribing and dispensing of prescription drugs (especially C-II medications) differently, be sure to ask your instructor how these prescriptions are prepared and regulated in your state.

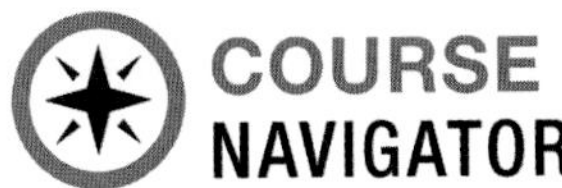

Access interactive chapter review exercises, practice activities, flash cards, and study games.

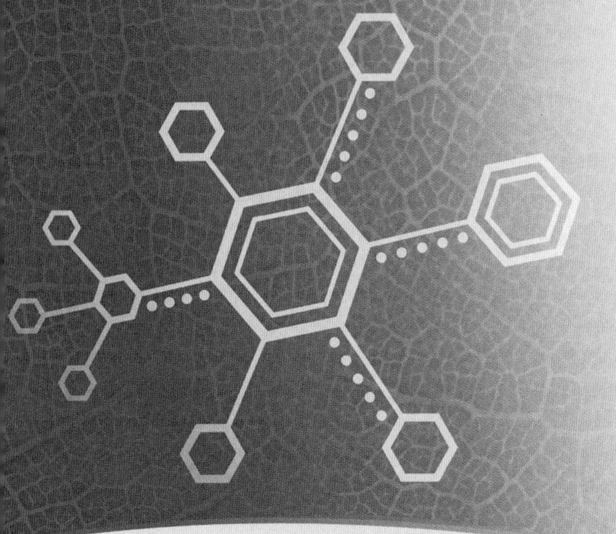

7

Reviewing a Filled Prescription

Learning Objectives

1 Gain the skills necessary to compare a processed prescription with a printed label for completeness and accuracy.

2 Identify practices to correct errors on printed labels generated from prescriptions.

Supplies

- None

Access additional chapter resources.

The prescription is the primary means by which a prescriber communicates with pharmacy staff. The accurate interpretation of prescriptions is crucial in your work as a pharmacy technician. Patient safety is the primary concern of any healthcare provider. As a pharmacy technician, your work directly affects the health and welfare of those you serve. According to the US Food and Drug Administration (FDA), prescription errors cause over 7,000 deaths each year; in your role as a pharmacy technician, you can help reduce this number through the careful handling and preparation of prescriptions.

During the filling process, the prescription must be frequently reviewed to ensure that it is properly interpreted and the information is accurately transcribed from the prescription to the patient profile in the computer system. Although the pharmacist is ultimately accountable for any prescription dispensed to a patient, many states also hold pharmacy technicians responsible for errors made on prescriptions. Therefore, it is important that whenever you are presented with a prescription—no matter what stage of the filling process you are focused on—you review the prescription for accuracy.

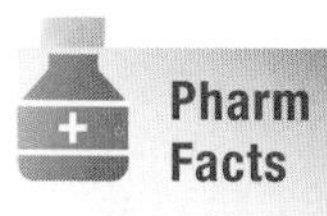

Pharm Facts

Similar to the DEA number, an identifier of prescribers of controlled substances, the National Provider Identifier (NPI) number, is a unique 10-digit identification number issued to healthcare providers in the United States by the Centers for Medicare and Medicaid Services (CMS).

The **9-point check** is a systematic approach to verifying prescription data during the filing process. It is often done first by a pharmacy technician and again by a pharmacist. Special attention is given to the following items:

1. Patient name
2. Patient date of birth
3. Date the prescription was written
4. Prescription drug name
5. Prescription drug strength
6. Prescription drug quantity
7. Label instructions
8. Prescriber information (name, DEA number, NPI number, etc.)
9. Refill information

When a prescription is first received, the staff member accepting it at the drop-off window reviews it for accuracy and completeness using the 9-point check. After the prescription is transcribed, it should be reviewed again. Next, after the label is generated, the technician filling the prescription should focus on comparing the information on the prescription with the information on the label.

The **filling technician** plays a vital role in prescription processing, because he or she is the last person to see the prescription prior to final verification and dispensing by the pharmacist. The filling technician is the pharmacy technician responsible for prescription counting or pouring, packaging, and labeling during the filling process. Before filling the prescription, the filling technician, should closely examine the prescription and compare it with the printed label for accuracy. If a mistake is caught, the incorrect information must be circled or highlighted and brought to the attention of the technician who prepared the label. That technician must correct the error, or if that original technician is unavailable or unable to correct the error at that time, the filling technician should correct the information and print a new label.

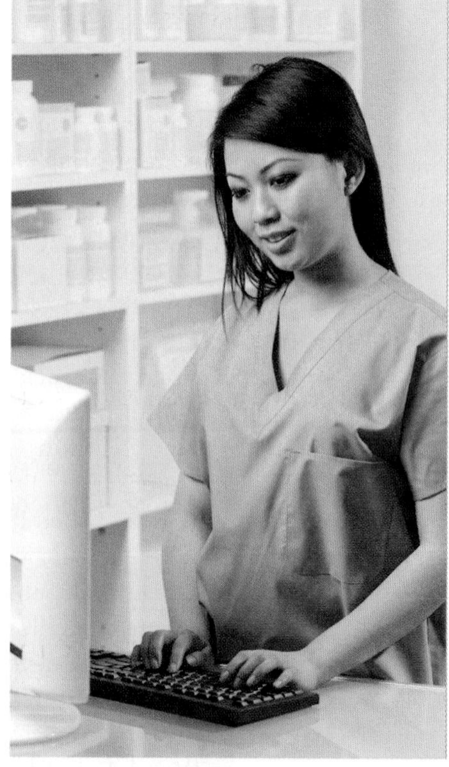

The filling technician is the last person to see the prescription prior to final verification and dispensing.

© Paradigm Publishing, Inc.

TAKE NOTE

The number of refills on prescriptions is legally regulated. According to federal law, Schedule II controlled substances can never be refilled without a new prescription (except in emergency situations, when a pharmacist must handle the situation). Controlled substances on Schedules III and IV may have up to five refills within a six-month period. Noncontrolled prescriptions and controlled substances on Schedule V have no limitation on refills (stated as "PRN"), provided the prescription is not expired. Note that with both controlled and noncontrolled medications, the prescriber can choose to prohibit refills or stipulate a maximum number of refills. You may have additional regulations in your state.

The filling technician then verifies that the corrected label is accurate, fills the prescription, and passes it on to the pharmacist for final verification.

When you review prescriptions for controlled substances, remember that they have special characteristics that you must verify, including a DEA number and restrictions on refills, dates, and how the quantity is indicated.

Keep in mind that the more people assigned to verify a prescription, the less likely it is that an error will occur.

Procedure

In this lab, you will review a series of prescriptions and printed labels grouped together at the end of this lab. Your task is to verify that the information on the printed label corresponds to the information on the prescription. This textbook is written with federal regulations in mind. However, you should ask your instructor about standards and regulations in your state prior to completing the following steps.

1 Perform the 9-point check by comparing the printed label with the prescription for each of these nine items:

1. Patient name
2. Patient date of birth
3. Date the prescription was written
4. Prescription drug name
5. Prescription drug strength
6. Prescription drug quantity
7. Label instructions
8. Prescriber information (name, DEA number, NPI number, etc.)
9. Refill information

2 If an error is present on the label, circle the error, and clearly write in the correct information on the blank lines provided.

3 **Conclusion:** When you are satisfied that you have verified the prescriptions and have noted corrections for all label errors on the blank lines of the worksheets, tear out the worksheet pages and submit them to your instructor. Then go to the Course Navigator, answer all questions in the Lab Review section, and submit your answers to your instructor.

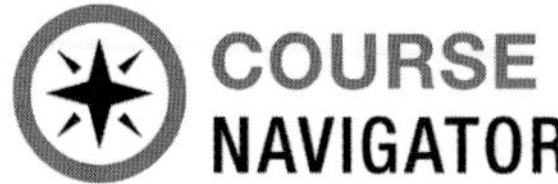

Access interactive chapter review exercises, practice activities, flash cards, and study games.

© Paradigm Publishing, Inc.

8

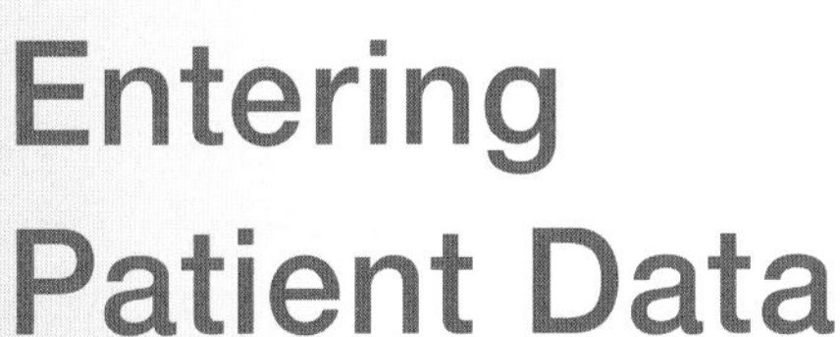

Entering Patient Data

Learning Objectives

1 Begin using the Course Navigator to complete Lab tutorials and assessments.

2 Become more familiar with the patient profile as a means of recording patients' personal and health information for access by pharmacy staff.

3 Learn to navigate efficiently within a model patient profile software system.

4 Increase skills in identifying standard patient profile information and evaluating profiles for completeness and accuracy.

Supplies

- NRx-based tutorial and assessments, available on the Course Navigator

Access additional chapter resources.

The patient profile is the first bit of information a pharmacy collects. As one of the chief means of recording patient information in the pharmacy, the profile is initiated when patients first patronize a pharmacy and complete a paper form. Because you will work with patients to establish their profiles on paper, remember to be as empathetic as possible. New patients must divulge information that is private and very personal.

Like the file in a doctor's office, the computerized profile contains all of a patient's medical information. The pharmacy must always have easy access to view or update the profile, particularly when patients wish to update their information, such as by listing new allergies or changing their address or insurance information. The computerized profile provides such access at your fingertips. Your role in entering and keeping accurate, up-to-date computerized patient profiles is vital to helping the pharmacy manage patients' medication therapy.

This lab is the first of seven that will simulate use of the NRx pharmacy management software produced by QS/1. Your textbook includes access to a a simulation of the NRx software, which closely resembles the programs that you are likely to encounter in your pharmacy work. The purpose of these electronic labs is to familiarize you with the essential steps leading up to and including prescription preparation, which is an electronic or computer-based process in most pharmacies. The principles of practice on which pharmacy management software programs operate are generally the same. However, several brands of software programs are used in pharmacy practice and will differ from pharmacy to pharmacy. Therefore, your focus is not to master any particular software system. Instead, your goal is to master the *principles* of using software to serve your patients effectively and accurately.

Procedure

In order to complete this lab and the remaining labs (Labs 9–14) in the Community Pharmacy Practice unit, you must first go to the Course Navigator and launch the interactive tutorial.

For entering your first patient profile in this lab, imagine that Vance Donaldson has just moved into the neighborhood and would like to have his prescriptions filled at your pharmacy. Vance has given you his completed profile, his insurance card, and a new prescription to fill. Using his profile and insurance card (see Figure 8.1) and the steps below, you will add the patient's information in the NRx system tutorial via the Course Navigator. When you reach the end of the tutorial, you will complete the assessments, repeating the main steps taught in the tutorial for additional patients.

The assessments represent the different patients you will be processing throughout the lab procedures. Most labs present several assessments for processing; however, some labs have only one assessment.

1 Launch the Course Navigator learning management system. Click on Lab 8 in the left navigation pane, and then click Tutorial 8.

2 The tutorial will launch in your browser, and you will be able to follow the steps online or in this lab manual. After you have completed the tutorial, you can complete the assessments, located under Assessments, for Lab 8.2, Lab 8.3, Lab 8.4, and so on.

3 When the NRx Security screen appears, log in to the NRx-based training software as the Primary User by typing STUDENT as the Login ID and PRACTICE as the Password. Click Log In.

 © Paradigm Publishing, Inc.

NRx Security

NRx

Login ID: Password:

Primary User: STUDENT **********

Secondary User:

Log In Cancel

3 191.0.26

4 On the Rx Processing Tasks menu, click Search or press F3 in the F-Key menu presented in NRx (see the Take Note feature on the next page).

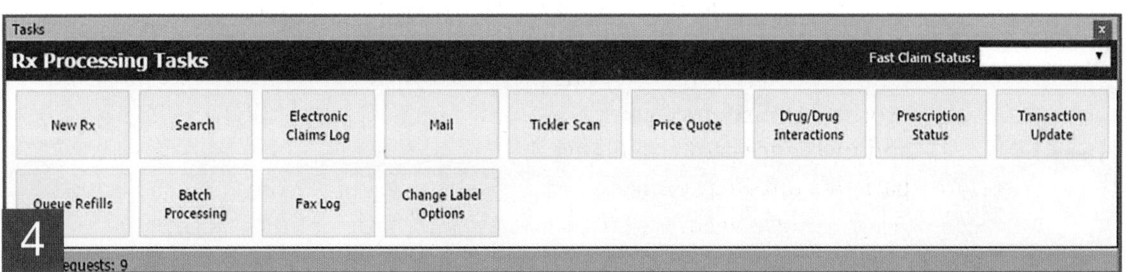

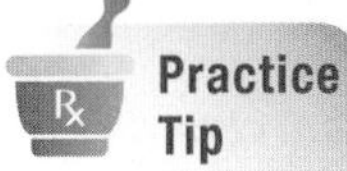

Practice Tip

Some pharmacy management software systems are case sensitive, and in your pharmacy work you will need to be careful about using uppercase (capital) or lowercase letters when typing in patient names and other data. However, for the purposes of Labs 8–14, you will not have to be concerned about case sensitivity.

5 When the Rx/Patient Search screen appears, type the patient's name in Lastname, Firstname format in the Search Criteria field (for the tutorial, you will use Figure 8.1 and enter Donaldson, Vance). Click Find or press Enter.

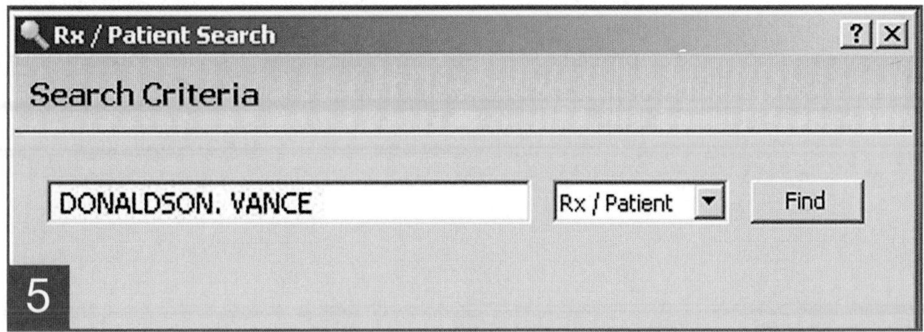

6 The Patient Scan screen will appear. Because this is the only patient with this name and the patient is new to the pharmacy, no names will appear in the search results. Click the New Patient icon on the top toolbar to begin the process of adding this patient.

7 Continue using Figure 8.1 to enter into the NRx system the following categories of Mr. Donaldson's personal data, in order: Last Name, First Name, full and *exact* Address, Phone Number(s), Birth Date, and E-mail, pressing Tab to move between fields. After entering the final item—the E-mail, or the Birth Date, if the patient has no E-mail—press Tab.

8 To add the primary care physician, click the double arrows to the right of the Doctor field. When the Prescriber Record Scan screen appears, look for the desired physician's name. If it is listed, double-click it or press the corresponding function key (or F-key, as explained in the following Take Note). If the physician's name is not listed, type it into the Search Criteria field in Lastname, Firstname format, and click Find or press Enter. When the desired physician's name appears, double-click it or press the corresponding F-key.

The Patient Information screen will appear. Compare the information on-screen with the information on the Patient Profile form. When you are satisfied that the new electronic profile is complete and accurate, click Save on the top toolbar.

TAKE NOTE

As you work with tutorials and assessments of the NRx pharmacy software and with the pharmacy software program at your job, you will often have the option of using function keys, or F-keys. On your keyboard, the F-keys are F1, F2, F3, and so on, and are usually found along the top row of your keyboard. However, in the NRx tutorials and assessments, if you wish to use F-keys, you must click the F-key button located on the toolbar. From there, you can click on the simulated F-keys—F2, F3, F4, and F7—to complete tasks. In pharmacy practice, using F-keys can speed up your process quite a bit. However, accuracy should always be your first priority.

© Paradigm Publishing, Inc.

FIGURE 8.1
Patient Profile and Insurance Card

PATIENT PROFILE

Patient Name

Donaldson | Vance |
Last | First | Middle Initial

12 Maple Leaf Trail
Street or PO Box

Round Rock | TX | 78664
City | State | ZIP

Date of Birth: 05/15/1987 (MM / DD / YYYY)
Gender: ☑ Male ☐ Female
Social Security No.: 000-00-0000
E-mail: vdonaldson@email.com

Home Phone: (512) 555-1212
Work Phone: (512) 555-1313
Other Phone: ( )

☐ Yes, I would like medication dispensed in a child-resistant container.
☑ No, I do not want medication dispensed in a child-resistant container.

Medication Insurance: ☑ Yes ☐ No

Cardholder Name: same
☑ Cardholder ☐ Spouse ☐ Child ☐ Dependent Parent ☐ Disabled Dependent ☐ Full-Time Student
(*Please provide the pharmacy with your card.*)

MEDICAL HISTORY

HEALTH
☐ No Known Medical Conditions
☐ Anemia
☐ Arthritis
☐ Asthma
☐ Attention-Deficit Hyperactivity Disorder
☐ Blood Clotting Disorders
☐ Cancer
☐ Depression
☐ Diabetes Mellitus
☐ Epilepsy
☐ Esophagitis
☐ Generalized Anxiety Disorder
☐ Heart Condition
☑ Hypertension
☐ Kidney Disease
☐ Liver Disease
☐ Lung Disease
☐ Ulcers

ALLERGIES AND DRUG REACTIONS
☐ No Known Drug Allergies
☐ Aspirin
☐ Cephalosporins
☐ Codeine
☐ Erythromycin
☐ Iodine
☑ Penicillin G Potassium
☐ Sulfa
☐ Tetracyclines
☐ Xanthines

ICD-10-CM for Checked Condition(s): I10

Details for Checked Allergy(ies):

Medication(s) Currently Being Taken: aspirin 81 mg, Accupril 10 mg

Primary Care Physician: Gregory Smythe

Comments:

Health information changes periodically. Please notify the pharmacy of any new medications, allergies, drug reactions, or health conditions.

Signature: Vance Donaldson Date: 4/9/19 ☐ I choose not to fill out this form.

Cobalt Care
Insurance card

VANCE DONALDSON
BIN: 00123
ID: ZVD996274638

GROUP: 11770
RELATIONSHIP: 01, CARDHOLDER

MEMBER SERVICES: 1-800-555-3232
CLAIMS/INQUIRIES: 1-800-555-6363

As you gain experience on the job, you will become familiar with the most common allergies and the abbreviations used to designate some of them. For example, common allergies include penicillin (PCN), aspirin (ASA), acetaminophen (APAP), codeine (no standard abbreviation), and sulfonamides (no standard abbreviation).

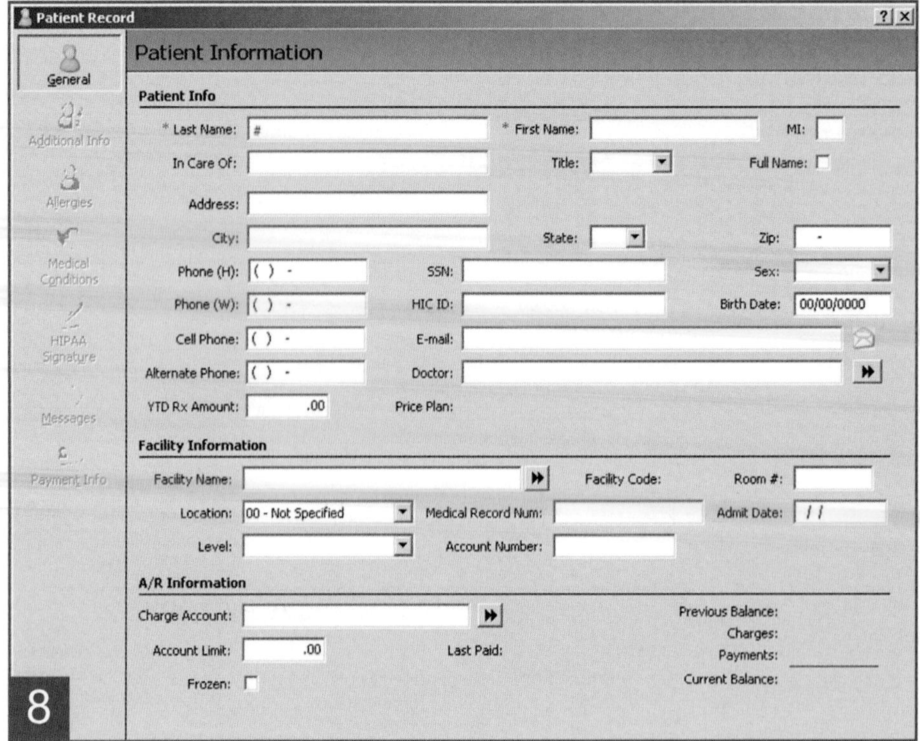

9 Click the Allergies button on the left menu bar. In cases where the patient has indicated having no known drug allergies, you would type in the exact phrase "No Known Drug Allergies," press Enter, and proceed to Step 10. However, because Mr. Donaldson *does* have allergies, you will do the following for him and all patients declaring allergies on their forms. In the Search for Allergy field, type in the exact word or words following the checked box under ALLERGIES AND DRUG REACTIONS. Press Enter. If the allergy does not appear, check your spelling and revise as needed.

TAKE NOTE

Your textbook provides you with a simulation of the NRx software. However, because it is only a simulation, it does not fully replicate all functions of the software itself. When you are working with a fully operational software system at the pharmacy, you will notice that when typing into a field, you will often need to type only the first few letters of the phrase or word you are entering. To save you time, the software will pull up a complete phrase or word matching the first few characters you have entered, and after verifying that what is filled in is exactly what you want, you will simply press Enter to complete your task without having to type all the characters.

 © Paradigm Publishing, Inc.

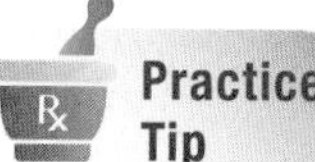

At the pharmacy, if you encounter patients listing more than one allergy on their forms, you would need to repeat Steps 10 and 11 as necessary to enter all listed allergies.

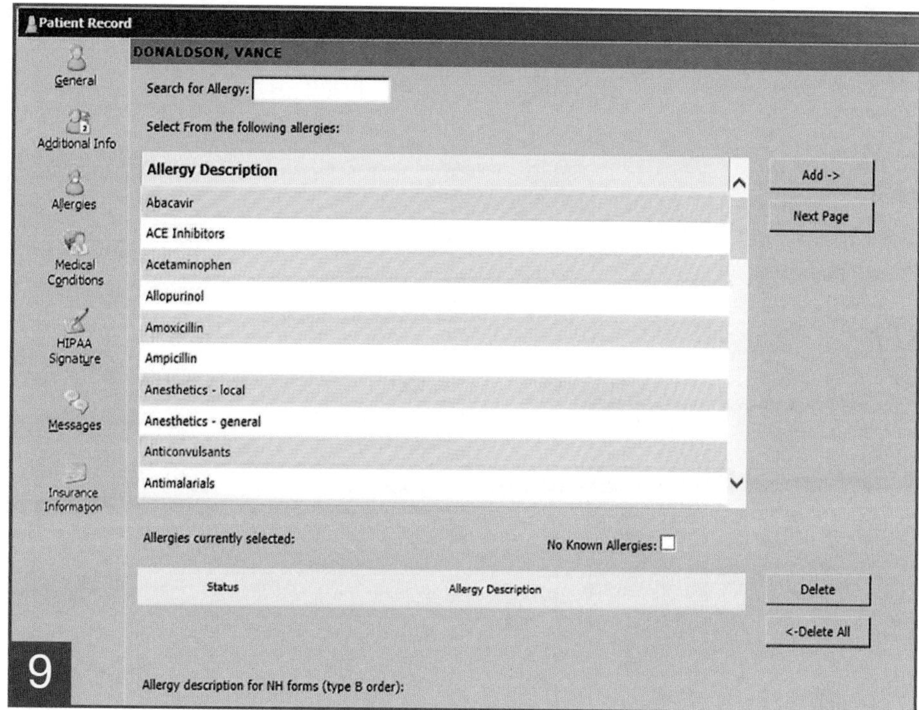

In the actual NRx software, if an incorrect allergy were still present at this point, you would have one more chance to remove it and replace it with the correct allergy. For the purposes of this lab, you have only one chance to verify allergy spelling and correctness, which you did in Step 10.

10 When the Allergy Description field appears, either click the correct allergy name (using any additional Patient Profile form details provided below the checked box) or click the phrase "NO KNOWN DRUG ALLERGIES," as is appropriate for the patient. Click Add.

11 Cross-check that the allergies on the Patient Profile form are the same as those now listed on-screen in the Allergies currently selected field. Click Save on the top toolbar.

12 Click the Medical Conditions button on the left menu bar. In the Search for ICD-10 or Medical Condition field, type the name of the patient's condition or the *exact* phrase "No Known Medical Conditions" if the patient has checked that item on the Patient Profile form. Press Enter. If the condition does not appear, check your spelling and revise as needed.

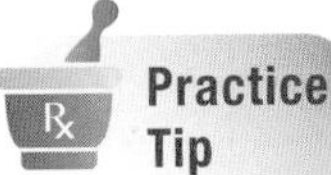

Practice Tip

If more than one entry appears on-screen for the same medical condition, compare the ICD-10 code on the Patient Profile form with the on-screen ICD-10 codes, and select the correct condition based on the code.

13 When the appropriate medical condition appears in the Select from the following medical conditions field, click the correct phrase or condition name, and click Add.

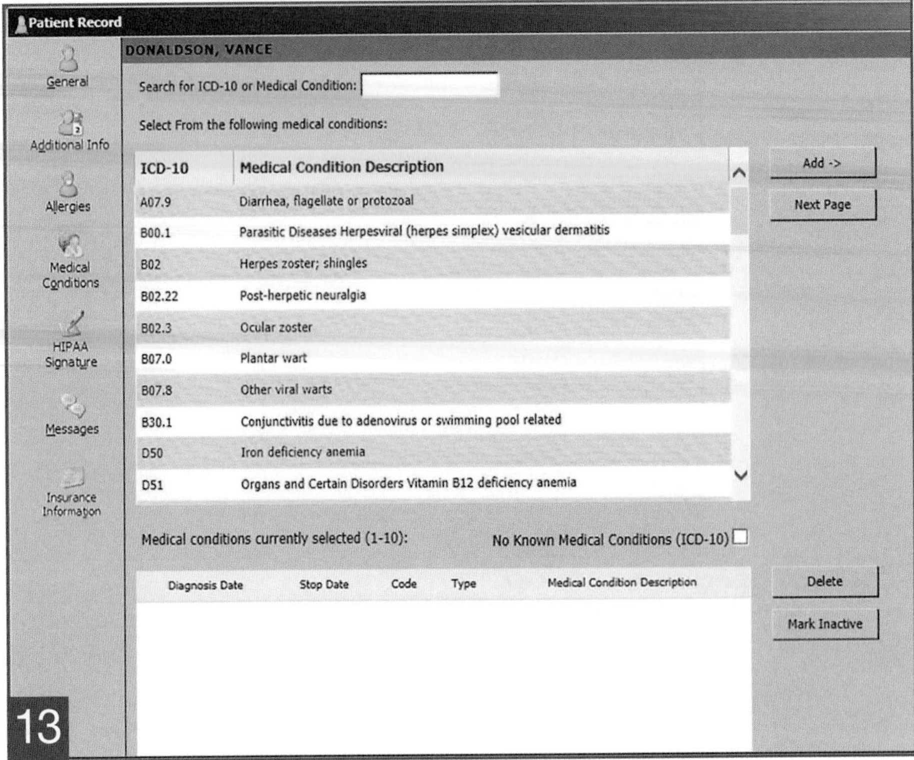

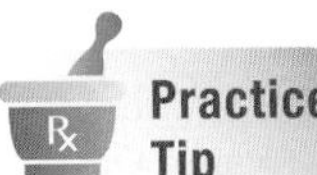

Practice Tip

In the actual NRx software, if an incorrect medical condition were still present at this point, you would have one more chance to remove it and replace it with the correct condition. For the purposes of this lab, you have only one chance to verify condition spelling and correctness, which you did in Step 13.

14 Cross-check the reported medical conditions on the Patient Profile form with those listed on-screen in the Medical Conditions currently selected field. When you are satisfied that it is complete, click Save on the top toolbar.

15 To add payment information to the patient's record, you will need to have the patient's insurance card, which is provided to the patient by the insurance carrier. (See Figure 8.1 for an example of what an insurance card may look like; for the purposes of this lab, the payment plan name appears above the words "Insurance card.") Click the Payment Info button on the left menu bar. Click New on the top toolbar, and a blank Patient Insurance Record will appear. Click the double arrows to the right of the Payment Plan field for a list of available price plans.

© Paradigm Publishing, Inc.

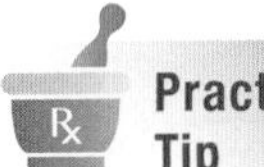

Practice Tip

Be aware that not all insurance cards will look alike. Also note that not all patients will have an insurance card; some may pay the cash price (covered in Step 17).

16 In the Price Plan Scan screen, select the desired price plan by double-clicking the plan name. If the desired price plan is not shown in the alphabetical list currently on-screen, you may search within the available plans by typing the full plan name (or the word "cash" for cash plan patients) in the blank Search Criteria field. Leave Description in the adjacent drop-down menu, and click Find or press Enter. When your choices appear, double-click the correct plan name (or the Cash Pricing category).

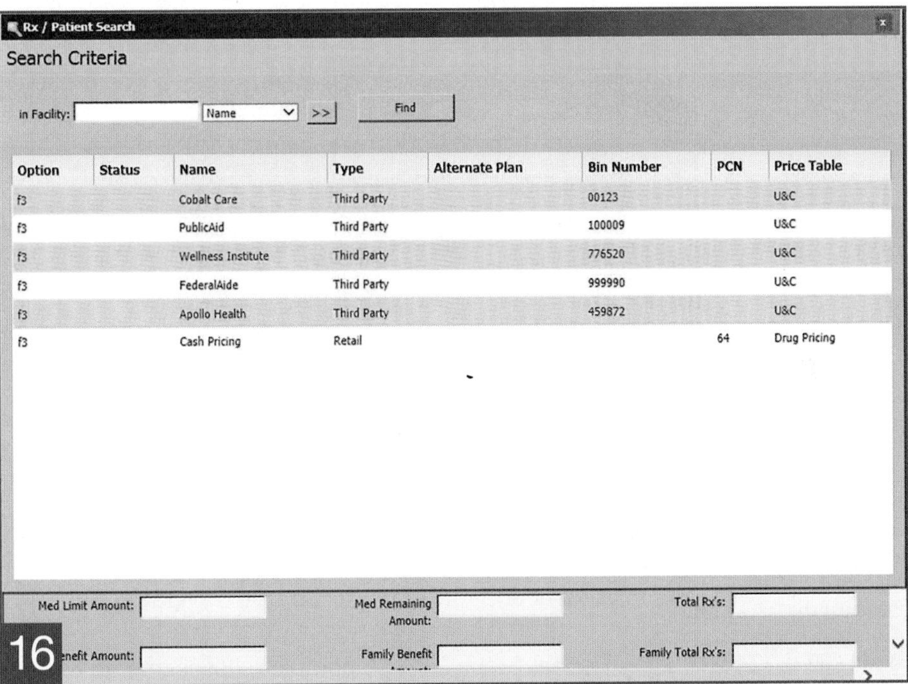

Rx / Patient Search

Search Criteria

In Facility: [ ] Name >> Find

Option	Status	Name	Type	Alternate Plan	Bin Number	PCN	Price Table
f3		Cobalt Care	Third Party		00123		U&C
f3		PublicAid	Third Party		100009		U&C
f3		Wellness Institute	Third Party		776520		U&C
f3		FederalAide	Third Party		999990		U&C
f3		Apollo Health	Third Party		459872		U&C
f3		Cash Pricing	Retail			64	Drug Pricing

Med Limit Amount: Med Remaining Amount: Total Rx's:

16 ...nefit Amount: Family Benefit ... Family Total Rx's:

Practice Tip

Many pharmacy management software systems will also allow you to search for the price plan by entering the bank identification number (BIN) located on the insurance card (see Figure 8.1 for an example of a card with a BIN). For the purposes of this lab, however, you may search only by entering the plan name.

17 The Patient Insurance Record screen will return, and you will enter three additional items from the patient's insurance card (Figures 8.1 through 8.12). However, if you are processing a cash plan patient and selected Cash Pricing in the previous step, you should simply click Save on the top toolbar, and proceed to Step 18. For all other patients, first click in the Policy ID Number field, type in the ID number, and press Tab. Next, type the group name or number in the Group Number field and press Tab (unless the insurance card indicates "None" for the group, in which case you should leave the Group Number field blank). Then, for the Relationship data, click on the Relationship drop-down menu and select the corresponding code number and name (if the Relationship on the insurance card is "00-Not Specified," leave the field as is). Click Save on the top toolbar.

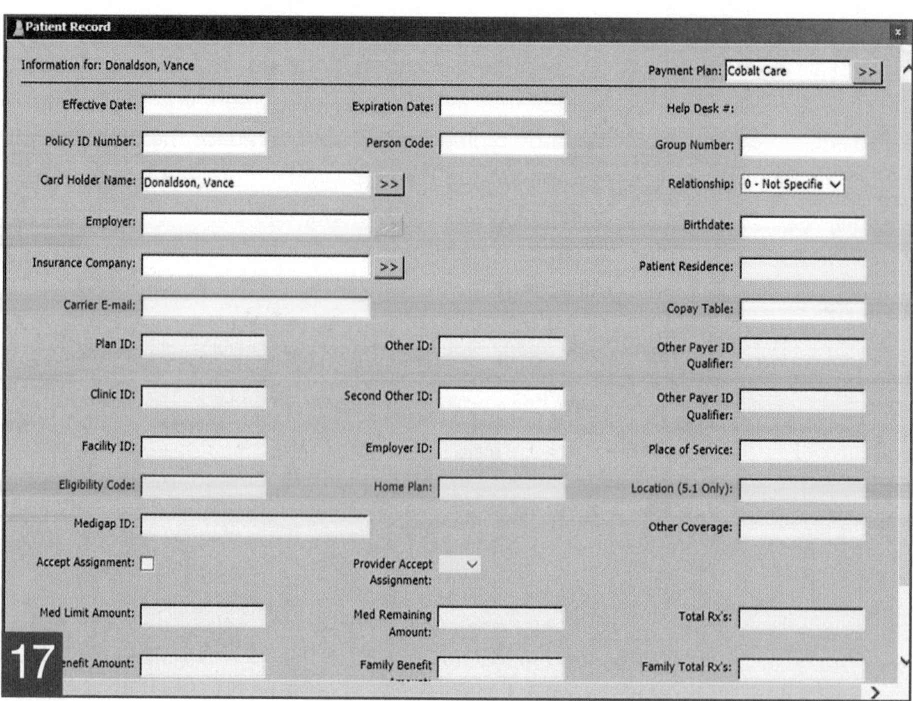

Practice Tip

Be careful! Do *not* click the large red "X" found in the upper-right corner of the lab window. Doing so will (always) close the entire lab and your work will be lost.

18 The patient's record is now complete. Press Esc or click the small black "X" in the upper-right corner of the Insurance Record screen.

19 The Patient Payment Information screen and the newly added plan will be briefly displayed. The tutorial will end. Click Close to close the tutorial and return to the Course Navigator.

20 Repeat Steps 2–19 to complete assessments 8.2–8.12. As you complete the procedure steps for those profiles, you should ignore the initial references to Vance Donaldson and substitute the name and data from each subsequent patient profile. You will click the Submit button once you are satisfied you have completed all the lab steps for each of the assessments. Clicking Submit will submit your assessment to your instructor, and will bring you back to the Course Navigator, where you will be able to see your score.

21 **Conclusion:** Complete the tutorial and assessments 8.1–8.12. Then go to the Course Navigator, answer all questions in the Lab Review section, and submit your answers to your instructor.

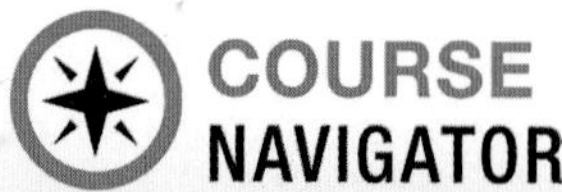

COURSE NAVIGATOR

Access interactive chapter review exercises, practice activities, flash cards, and study games.

© Paradigm Publishing, Inc.

FIGURE 8.2
Patient Profile and Insurance Card

PATIENT PROFILE

Patient Name

Gupta | Amala | ______
Last | First | Middle Initial

5473 W 10th Street
Street or PO Box

Cedar Rapids | IA | 52401
City | State | ZIP

Date of Birth	Gender	Social Security No.	E-mail
08/24/1961 MM / DD / YYYY	☐ Male ☑ Female	000-00-0000	guptaamala@email.com

Home Phone	Work Phone	Other Phone
(319) 555-1212	( )	( )

☐ Yes, I would like medication dispensed in a child-resistant container.
☑ No, I do not want medication dispensed in a child-resistant container.

Medication Insurance
☑ Yes
☐ No

Cardholder Name same
☑ Cardholder ☐ Child ☐ Disabled Dependent
☐ Spouse ☐ Dependent Parent ☐ Full-Time Student
(Please provide the pharmacy with your card.)

MEDICAL HISTORY

HEALTH
- ☑ No Known Medical Conditions
- ☐ Anemia
- ☐ Arthritis
- ☐ Asthma
- ☐ Attention-Deficit Hyperactivity Disorder
- ☐ Blood Clotting Disorders
- ☐ Cancer
- ☐ Depression
- ☐ Diabetes Mellitus
- ☐ Epilepsy
- ☐ Esophagitis
- ☐ Generalized Anxiety Disorder
- ☐ Heart Condition
- ☐ Hypertension
- ☐ Kidney Disease
- ☐ Liver Disease
- ☐ Lung Disease
- ☐ Ulcers

ALLERGIES AND DRUG REACTIONS
- ☑ No Known Drug Allergies
- ☐ Aspirin
- ☐ Cephalosporins
- ☐ Codeine
- ☐ Erythromycin
- ☐ Iodine
- ☐ Penicillin G Potassium
- ☐ Sulfa
- ☐ Tetracyclines
- ☐ Xanthines

ICD-10-CM for Checked Condition(s): ______

Details for Checked Allergy(ies): ______

Medication(s) Currently Being Taken: ______

Primary Care Physician: Sunjita Patel

Comments: ______

Health information changes periodically. Please notify the pharmacy of any new medications, allergies, drug reactions, or health conditions.

Signature Amala Gupta Date 4/14/19 ☐ I choose not to fill out this form.

PublicAid
Insurance card

AMALA GUPTA
BIN: 100009
ID: 778342987

GROUP: NONE
RELATIONSHIP: 01, CARDHOLDER

MEMBER SERVICES: 1-800-555-3232
CLAIMS/INQUIRIES: 1-800-555-6363

© Paradigm Publishing, Inc.

FIGURE 8.3
Patient Profile and Insurance Card

PATIENT PROFILE

Patient Name

Klein — Last
Jeffrey — First
Middle Initial

1157 North Plaza Ave — Street or PO Box

Cedar Rapids — City
IA — State
52411 — ZIP

Date of Birth: 10/18/1991 (MM / DD / YYYY)
Gender: ☑ Male ☐ Female
Social Security No.: 000-00-0000
E-mail: kleinj@email.com

Home Phone: (319) 555-1212
Work Phone: (319) 555-1313
Other Phone: ( )

☐ Yes, I would like medication dispensed in a child-resistant container.
☑ No, I do not want medication dispensed in a child-resistant container.

Medication Insurance: ☑ Yes ☐ No
Cardholder Name: Katja Klein
☐ Cardholder ☑ Spouse ☐ Child ☐ Dependent Parent ☐ Disabled Dependent ☐ Full-Time Student
(Please provide the pharmacy with your card.)

MEDICAL HISTORY

HEALTH

☐ No Known Medical Conditions
☐ Anemia
☐ Arthritis
☐ Asthma
☐ Attention-Deficit Hyperactivity Disorder
☐ Blood Clotting Disorders
☐ Cancer
☑ Depression
☐ Diabetes Mellitus
☐ Epilepsy
☐ Esophagitis
☐ Generalized Anxiety Disorder
☐ Heart Condition
☐ Hypertension
☐ Kidney Disease
☐ Liver Disease
☐ Lung Disease
☐ Ulcers

ALLERGIES AND DRUG REACTIONS

☐ No Known Drug Allergies
☐ Aspirin
☐ Cephalosporins
☑ Codeine
☐ Erythromycin
☐ Iodine
☐ Penicillin G Potassium
☐ Sulfa
☐ Tetracyclines
☐ Xanthines

ICD-10-CM for Checked Condition(s): F43.21

Details for Checked Allergy(ies):

Medication(s) Currently Being Taken:

Primary Care Physician: Ethel Jacobson

Comments:

Health information changes periodically. Please notify the pharmacy of any new medications, allergies, drug reactions, or health conditions.

Signature: Jeffrey Klein Date: 4/17/19 ☐ I choose not to fill out this form.

ApolloHealth
Insurance card

JEFFREY KLEIN
BIN: 459872
ID: 882646507

GROUP: NONE
RELATIONSHIP: 02, SPOUSE

MEMBER SERVICES: 1-800-555-3232
CLAIMS/INQUIRIES: 1-800-555-6363

© Paradigm Publishing, Inc.

FIGURE 8.4
Patient Profile and Insurance Card

PATIENT PROFILE

Patient Name

Nguyen | Lily | ______
Last | First | Middle Initial

2934 Anderson Lane
Street or PO Box

Boise | ID | 83722
City | State | ZIP

Date of Birth: 10/18/1990 (MM / DD / YYYY)
Gender: ☐ Male ☑ Female
Social Security No.: 000-00-0000
E-mail: lilyflower@email.com

Home Phone: (208) 555-1212
Work Phone: (208) 555-1313
Other Phone: ( ) ______

☐ Yes, I would like medication dispensed in a child-resistant container.
☑ No, I do not want medication dispensed in a child-resistant container.

Medication Insurance
☐ Yes
☑ No

Cardholder Name ______
☐ Cardholder
☐ Spouse
☐ Child
☐ Dependent Parent
☐ Disabled Dependent
☐ Full-Time Student
(Please provide the pharmacy with your card.)

MEDICAL HISTORY

HEALTH
☐ No Known Medical Conditions
☐ Anemia
☐ Arthritis
☐ Asthma
☐ Attention-Deficit Hyperactivity Disorder
☐ Blood Clotting Disorders
☐ Cancer
☐ Depression
☐ Diabetes Mellitus
☐ Epilepsy
☐ Esophagitis
☑ Generalized Anxiety Disorder
☐ Heart Condition
☐ Hypertension
☐ Kidney Disease
☐ Liver Disease
☐ Lung Disease
☐ Ulcers

ALLERGIES AND DRUG REACTIONS
☑ No Known Drug Allergies
☐ Aspirin
☐ Cephalosporins
☐ Codeine
☐ Erythromycin
☐ Iodine
☐ Penicillin G Potassium
☐ Sulfa
☐ Tetracyclines
☐ Xanthines

ICD-10-CM for Checked Condition(s): F41.1

Details for Checked Allergy(ies): ______

Medication(s) Currently Being Taken: ______

Primary Care Physician: Todd Jackson

Comments: ______

Health information changes periodically. Please notify the pharmacy of any new medications, allergies, drug reactions, or health conditions.

Signature: Lily Nguyen   Date: 4/10/19   ☐ I choose not to fill out this form.

No insurance card presented; patient on cash plan.

© Paradigm Publishing, Inc.

FIGURE 8.5
Patient Profile and Insurance Card

PATIENT PROFILE

Patient Name

Riley | Cas |
Last | First | Middle Initial

72650 Okade Court
Street or PO Box

Orlando | FL | 32810
City | State | ZIP

Date of Birth: 01/22/2010 (MM / DD / YYYY)
Gender: ☑ Male ☐ Female
Social Security No.: 000-00-0000
E-mail: casr@email.com

Home Phone: 407 555-1212
Work Phone: ( )
Other Phone: ( )

☑ Yes, I would like medication dispensed in a child-resistant container.
☐ No, I do not want medication dispensed in a child-resistant container.

Medication Insurance
☑ Yes
☐ No

Cardholder Name: Molly Riley
☐ Cardholder
☐ Spouse
☑ Child
☐ Dependent Parent
☐ Disabled Dependent
☐ Full-Time Student
(Please provide the pharmacy with your card.)

MEDICAL HISTORY

HEALTH
☐ No Known Medical Conditions
☐ Anemia
☐ Arthritis
☐ Asthma
☑ Attention-Deficit Hyperactivity Disorder
☐ Blood Clotting Disorders
☐ Cancer
☐ Depression
☐ Diabetes Mellitus
☐ Epilepsy
☐ Esophagitis
☐ Generalized Anxiety Disorder
☐ Heart Condition
☐ Hypertension
☐ Kidney Disease
☐ Liver Disease
☐ Lung Disease
☐ Ulcers

ALLERGIES AND DRUG REACTIONS
☐ No Known Drug Allergies
☐ Aspirin
☐ Cephalosporins
☐ Codeine
☐ Erythromycin
☐ Iodine
☐ Penicillin G Potassium
☑ Sulfa
☐ Tetracyclines
☐ Xanthines

ICD-10-CM for Checked Condition(s): F90.9

Details for Checked Allergy(ies): Sulfa (Sulfonamides)

Medication(s) Currently Being Taken: Ritalin 10mg

Primary Care Physician: Philip Fleming

Comments:

Health information changes periodically. Please notify the pharmacy of any new medications, allergies, drug reactions, or health conditions.

Signature: Molly Riley Date: 3/31/19 ☐ I choose not to fill out this form.

Wellness Institute
Insurance card

CAS RILEY
BIN: 776520
ID: YPJ75113

GROUP: RXCare
RELATIONSHIP: 03, CHILD

MEMBER SERVICES: 1-800-555-3232
CLAIMS/INQUIRIES: 1-800-555-6363

© Paradigm Publishing, Inc.

FIGURE 8.6
Patient Profile and Insurance Card

PATIENT PROFILE

Patient Name

Esparza (Last) | Miguel (First) | ______ (Middle Initial)

7583 E 11th St. (Street or PO Box)

Austin (City) | TX (State) | 78705 (ZIP)

Date of Birth: 09/12/1965 (MM / DD / YYYY)

Gender: ☑ Male ☐ Female

Social Security No.: 000-00-0000

E-mail: ______

Home Phone: (512) 555-1212

Work Phone: ( ) ______

Other Phone: ( ) ______

☑ Yes, I would like medication dispensed in a child-resistant container.
☐ No, I do not want medication dispensed in a child-resistant container.

Medication Insurance
☑ Yes
☐ No

Cardholder Name: same
☑ Cardholder
☐ Spouse
☐ Child
☐ Dependent Parent
☐ Disabled Dependent
☐ Full-Time Student
(Please provide the pharmacy with your card.)

MEDICAL HISTORY

HEALTH
☐ No Known Medical Conditions
☐ Anemia
☐ Arthritis
☐ Asthma
☐ Attention-Deficit Hyperactivity Disorder
☐ Blood Clotting Disorders
☐ Cancer
☐ Depression
☑ Diabetes Mellitus
☐ Epilepsy
☐ Esophagitis
☐ Generalized Anxiety Disorder
☐ Heart Condition
☐ Hypertension
☐ Kidney Disease
☐ Liver Disease
☐ Lung Disease
☐ Ulcers

ALLERGIES AND DRUG REACTIONS
☑ No Known Drug Allergies
☐ Aspirin
☐ Cephalosporins
☐ Codeine
☐ Erythromycin
☐ Iodine
☐ Penicillin G Potassium
☐ Sulfa
☐ Tetracyclines
☐ Xanthines

ICD-10-CM for Checked Condition(s): E10.9

Details for Checked Allergy(ies): ______

Medication(s) Currently Being Taken: ______

Primary Care Physician: Simona Brushfield

Comments: ______

Health information changes periodically. Please notify the pharmacy of any new medications, allergies, drug reactions, or health conditions.

Signature: Miguel Esparza Date: 3/14/19 ☐ I choose not to fill out this form.

FederalAide
Insurance card

MIGUEL ESPARZA
BIN: 999990
ID: 119875639

GROUP: B
RELATIONSHIP: 00, NOT SPECIFIED

MEMBER SERVICES: 1-800-555-3232
CLAIMS/INQUIRIES: 1-800-555-6363

© Paradigm Publishing, Inc.

FIGURE 8.7
Patient Profile and Insurance Card

PATIENT PROFILE

Patient Name

Jackson (Last) | Kimberly (First) | Middle Initial

4590 Settling Glen Dr
Street or PO Box

Boston (City) | MA (State) | 02109 (ZIP)

Date of Birth: 06/23/2000 (MM / DD / YYYY)
Gender: ☐ Male ☑ Female
Social Security No.: 000-00-0000
E-mail: jacksok@email.com

Home Phone: (617) 555-1212
Work Phone: (617) 555-1313
Other Phone: ( )

☐ Yes, I would like medication dispensed in a child-resistant container.
☑ No, I do not want medication dispensed in a child-resistant container.

Medication Insurance: ☑ Yes ☐ No
Cardholder Name: Chris Redcedar
☐ Cardholder ☑ Spouse ☐ Child ☐ Dependent Parent ☐ Disabled Dependent ☐ Full-Time Student
(Please provide the pharmacy with your card.)

MEDICAL HISTORY

HEALTH
- ☐ No Known Medical Conditions
- ☐ Anemia
- ☐ Arthritis
- ☐ Asthma
- ☐ Attention-Deficit Hyperactivity Disorder
- ☐ Blood Clotting Disorders
- ☐ Cancer
- ☐ Depression
- ☐ Diabetes Mellitus
- ☐ Epilepsy
- ☑ Esophagitis
- ☐ Generalized Anxiety Disorder
- ☐ Heart Condition
- ☐ Hypertension
- ☐ Kidney Disease
- ☐ Liver Disease
- ☐ Lung Disease
- ☐ Ulcers

ALLERGIES AND DRUG REACTIONS
- ☐ No Known Drug Allergies
- ☑ Aspirin
- ☐ Cephalosporins
- ☐ Codeine
- ☐ Erythromycin
- ☐ Iodine
- ☐ Penicillin G Potassium
- ☐ Sulfa
- ☐ Tetracyclines
- ☐ Xanthines

ICD-10-CM for Checked Condition(s): K20.9

Details for Checked Allergy(ies):

Medication(s) Currently Being Taken:

Primary Care Physician: Frieda Nadal

Comments:

Health information changes periodically. Please notify the pharmacy of any new medications, allergies, drug reactions, or health conditions.

Signature: Kimberly Jackson Date: 4/17/19 ☐ I choose not to fill out this form.

PublicAid
Insurance card

KIMBERLY JACKSON
BIN: 100009
ID: 711937589

GROUP: NONE
RELATIONSHIP: 02, SPOUSE

MEMBER SERVICES: 1-800-555-3232
CLAIMS/INQUIRIES: 1-800-555-6363

© Paradigm Publishing, Inc.

FIGURE 8.8
Patient Profile and Insurance Card

PATIENT PROFILE

Patient Name

Wilkins | Marquita |
Last | First | Middle Initial

6901 Westminster Chase
Street or PO Box

Providence | RI | 02908
City | State | ZIP

Date of Birth: 02/29/1996 (MM / DD / YYYY)

Gender: ☐ Male ☑ Female

Social Security No.: 000-00-0000

E-mail: marquita@email.com

Home Phone: (401) 555-1212

Work Phone: (401) 555-1313

Other Phone: ( )

☑ Yes, I would like medication dispensed in a child-resistant container.
☐ No, I do not want medication dispensed in a child-resistant container.

Medication Insurance
☑ Yes
☐ No

Cardholder Name: same
☑ Cardholder
☐ Spouse
☐ Child
☐ Dependent Parent
☐ Disabled Dependent
☐ Full-Time Student
(Please provide the pharmacy with your card.)

MEDICAL HISTORY

HEALTH
☑ No Known Medical Conditions
☐ Anemia
☐ Arthritis
☐ Asthma
☐ Attention-Deficit Hyperactivity Disorder
☐ Blood Clotting Disorders
☐ Cancer
☐ Depression
☐ Diabetes Mellitus
☐ Epilepsy
☐ Esophagitis
☐ Generalized Anxiety Disorder
☐ Heart Condition
☐ Hypertension
☐ Kidney Disease
☐ Liver Disease
☐ Lung Disease
☐ Ulcers

ALLERGIES AND DRUG REACTIONS
☐ No Known Drug Allergies
☐ Aspirin
☐ Cephalosporins
☐ Codeine
☐ Erythromycin
☐ Iodine
☑ Penicillin G Potassium
☐ Sulfa
☐ Tetracyclines
☐ Xanthines

ICD-10-CM for Checked Condition(s): ____________

Details for Checked Allergy(ies): ____________

Medication(s) Currently Being Taken: ____________

Primary Care Physician: Geoff Taylor

Comments: ____________

Health information changes periodically. Please notify the pharmacy of any new medications, allergies, drug reactions, or health conditions.

Signature: Marquita Wilkins   Date: 4/15/19   ☐ I choose not to fill out this form.

Wellness Institute
Insurance card

MARQUITA WILKINS
BIN: 776520
ID: GHT88729

GROUP: RXCare
RELATIONSHIP: 01, CARDHOLDER

MEMBER SERVICES: 1-800-555-3232
CLAIMS/INQUIRIES: 1-800-555-6363

© Paradigm Publishing, Inc.

FIGURE 8.9
Patient Profile and Insurance Card

PATIENT PROFILE

Patient Name

Acosta | Lisa | M
Last | First | Middle Initial

3369 Cedar Springs Road
Street or PO Box

Dallas | TX | 75219
City | State | ZIP

Date of Birth: 08/01/1983 (MM / DD / YYYY)
Gender: ☐ Male ☑ Female
Social Security No.: 000-00-0000
E-mail: l.acosta@email.com

Home Phone: (214) 555-0005
Work Phone: (214) 555-0350
Other Phone: (   )

☐ Yes, I would like medication dispensed in a child-resistant container.
☑ No, I do not want medication dispensed in a child-resistant container.

Medication Insurance: ☑ Yes ☐ No

Cardholder Name: Self
☑ Cardholder ☐ Spouse ☐ Child ☐ Dependent Parent ☐ Disabled Dependent ☐ Full-Time Student
(*Please provide the pharmacy with your card.*)

MEDICAL HISTORY

HEALTH

☑ No Known Medical Conditions
☐ Anemia
☐ Arthritis
☐ Asthma
☐ Attention-Deficit Hyperactivity Disorder
☐ Blood Clotting Disorders
☐ Cancer
☐ Depression
☐ Diabetes Mellitus
☐ Epilepsy
☐ Esophagitis
☐ Generalized Anxiety Disorder
☐ Heart Condition
☐ Hypertension
☐ Kidney Disease
☐ Liver Disease
☐ Lung Disease
☐ Ulcers

ALLERGIES AND DRUG REACTIONS

☑ No Known Drug Allergies
☐ Aspirin
☐ Cephalosporins
☐ Codeine
☐ Erythromycin
☐ Iodine
☐ Penicillin G Potassium
☐ Sulfa
☐ Tetracyclines
☐ Xanthines

ICD-10-CM for Checked Condition(s): ______

Details for Checked Allergy(ies): ______

Medication(s) Currently Being Taken: ______

Primary Care Physician: Mason Jacskon

Comments: ______

Health information changes periodically. Please notify the pharmacy of any new medications, allergies, drug reactions, or health conditions.

Signature: Lisa Acosta Date: 4/19/19 ☐ I choose not to fill out this form.

ApolloHealth
Insurance card

LISA ACOSTA
BIN: 459844
ID: 774652970

GROUP: NONE
RELATIONSHIP: 01, CARDHOLDER

MEMBER SERVICES: 1-800-555-3232
CLAIMS/INQUIRIES: 1-800-555-6363

© Paradigm Publishing, Inc.

FIGURE 8.10
Patient Profile and Insurance Card

PATIENT PROFILE

Patient Name

Richardson — Last | Zack — First | T — Middle Initial

4142 Ohlen Road — Street or PO Box

Colorado Springs — City | CO — State | 89119 — ZIP

Date of Birth: 05/20/1969 (MM / DD / YYYY)

Gender: ☑ Male ☐ Female

Social Security No.: 000-00-0000

E-mail: z.richardson@email.com

Home Phone: (719) 555-8884

Work Phone: (719) 555-2312

Other Phone: ( )

☑ Yes, I would like medication dispensed in a child-resistant container.
☐ No, I do not want medication dispensed in a child-resistant container.

Medication Insurance: ☐ Yes ☑ No

Cardholder Name: ____

☐ Cardholder ☐ Spouse ☐ Child ☐ Dependent Parent ☐ Disabled Dependent ☐ Full-Time Student

(Please provide the pharmacy with your card.)

MEDICAL HISTORY

HEALTH

☐ No Known Medical Conditions
☐ Anemia
☐ Arthritis
☐ Asthma
☐ Attention-Deficit Hyperactivity Disorder
☐ Blood Clotting Disorders
☐ Cancer
☑ Depression
☐ Diabetes Mellitus
☐ Epilepsy
☐ Esophagitis
☐ Generalized Anxiety Disorder
☐ Heart Condition
☐ Hypertension
☐ Kidney Disease
☐ Liver Disease
☐ Lung Disease
☐ Ulcers

ALLERGIES AND DRUG REACTIONS

☐ No Known Drug Allergies
☐ Aspirin
☐ Cephalosporins
☐ Codeine
☐ Erythromycin
☐ Iodine
☑ Penicillin G Potassium
☐ Sulfa
☐ Tetracyclines
☐ Xanthines

ICD-10-CM for Checked Condition(s): F32.1

Details for Checked Allergy(ies): ____

Medication(s) Currently Being Taken: ____

Primary Care Physician: Michael Knotts

Comments: ____

Health information changes periodically. Please notify the pharmacy of any new medications, allergies, drug reactions, or health conditions.

Signature: Z. Richardson Date: 4/20/19 ☐ I choose not to fill out this form.

No insurance card presented; patient on cash plan.

FIGURE 8.11
Patient Profile and Insurance Card

PATIENT PROFILE

Patient Name

Askew — Zeina — O
Last — First — Middle Initial

3201 South Eads Street
Street or PO Box

Arlington — VA — 22204
City — State — ZIP

Date of Birth: 01/22/1975 (MM / DD / YYYY)
Gender: ☐ Male ☑ Female
Social Security No.: 000-00-0000
E-mail: z.askew@email.com

Home Phone: (571) 555-0047
Work Phone: (703) 555-3087
Other Phone: ( )

☐ Yes, I would like medication dispensed in a child-resistant container.
☑ No, I do not want medication dispensed in a child-resistant container.

Medication Insurance: ☑ Yes ☐ No

Cardholder Name: Self
☑ Cardholder ☐ Spouse ☐ Child ☐ Dependent Parent ☐ Disabled Dependent ☐ Full-Time Student
(Please provide the pharmacy with your card.)

MEDICAL HISTORY

HEALTH
☐ No Known Medical Conditions
☐ Anemia
☐ Arthritis
☐ Asthma
☐ Attention-Deficit Hyperactivity Disorder
☐ Blood Clotting Disorders
☐ Cancer
☐ Depression
☐ Diabetes Mellitus
☐ Epilepsy
☐ Esophagitis
☐ Generalized Anxiety Disorder
☑ Heart Condition
☐ Hypertension
☐ Kidney Disease
☐ Liver Disease
☐ Lung Disease
☐ Ulcers

ALLERGIES AND DRUG REACTIONS
☐ No Known Drug Allergies
☐ Aspirin
☐ Cephalosporins
☐ Codeine
☐ Erythromycin
☐ Iodine
☑ Penicillin G Potassium
☐ Sulfa
☐ Tetracyclines
☐ Xanthines

ICD-10-CM for Checked Condition(s): I50.3

Details for Checked Allergy(ies):

Medication(s) Currently Being Taken:

Primary Care Physician: Carter Stein

Comments:

Health information changes periodically. Please notify the pharmacy of any new medications, allergies, drug reactions, or health conditions.

Signature: Zeina Askew — Date: 4/21/19 — ☐ I choose not to fill out this form.

ContinuumRx
Insurance card

ZEINA ASKEW
BIN: 49287
ID: THL9X6G

GROUP: FED37
RELATIONSHIP: 01, CARDHOLDER

MEMBER SERVICES: 1-800-555-3232
CLAIMS/INQUIRIES: 1-800-555-6363

© Paradigm Publishing, Inc.

FIGURE 8.12
Patient Profile and Insurance Card

PATIENT PROFILE

Patient Name

Green	Derek	X
Last	First	Middle Initial

873 Broad Way
Street or PO Box

Memphis	TN	38104
City	State	ZIP

Date of Birth	Gender	Social Security No.	E-mail
02/27/1988 MM / DD / YYYY	☑ Male ☐ Female	000-00-0000	derek.green@email.com

Home Phone	Work Phone	Other Phone
(901) 555-0047	(901) 555-8700	( )

☐ Yes, I would like medication dispensed in a child-resistant container.
☑ No, I do not want medication dispensed in a child-resistant container.

Medication Insurance
☑ Yes
☐ No

Cardholder Name Julia Green
☐ Cardholder ☐ Child ☐ Disabled Dependent
☑ Spouse ☐ Dependent Parent ☐ Full-Time Student
(Please provide the pharmacy with your card.)

MEDICAL HISTORY

HEALTH
- ☐ No Known Medical Conditions
- ☐ Anemia
- ☐ Arthritis
- ☐ Asthma
- ☐ Attention-Deficit Hyperactivity Disorder
- ☑ Blood Clotting Disorders
- ☐ Cancer
- ☐ Depression
- ☐ Diabetes Mellitus
- ☐ Epilepsy
- ☐ Esophagitis
- ☐ Generalized Anxiety Disorder
- ☐ Heart Condition
- ☐ Hypertension
- ☐ Kidney Disease
- ☐ Liver Disease
- ☐ Lung Disease
- ☐ Ulcers

ALLERGIES AND DRUG REACTIONS
- ☐ No Known Drug Allergies
- ☐ Aspirin
- ☐ Cephalosporins
- ☐ Codeine
- ☐ Erythromycin
- ☑ Iodine
- ☐ Penicillin G Potassium
- ☐ Sulfa
- ☐ Tetracyclines
- ☐ Xanthines

ICD-10-CM for Checked Condition(s): E78.2

Details for Checked Allergy(ies):

Medication(s) Currently Being Taken:

Primary Care Physician: Gabrielle Nelson

Comments:

Health information changes periodically. Please notify the pharmacy of any new medications, allergies, drug reactions, or health conditions.

Signature Derek Green Date 4/22/19 ☐ I choose not to fill out this form.

Cobalt Care
Insurance card

DERERK GREEN
BIN: 10132
ID: 774652970

GROUP: NONE
RELATIONSHIP: 02, SPOUSE

MEMBER SERVICES: 1-800-555-3232
CLAIMS/INQUIRIES: 1-800-555-6363

9

Processing a Prescription

Learning Objectives

1 Accurately process patient prescriptions.

2 Accurately process serialized prescription forms used in prescription monitoring programs.

3 Practice using pharmacy management software for prescriptions and monitored prescriptions.

Supplies

- NRx-based tutorials and assessments, available on the Course Navigator

Access additional chapter resources.

One of the primary duties of pharmacy technicians is prescription processing. To be successful, you must accurately interpret and process prescriptions so that the patient receives the proper medication in the correct dosage form and strength, accompanied by the appropriate instructions. Knowing how to transcribe information accurately, including interpreting signa abbreviations and keeping current on legal requirements for prescriptions in your state, is fundamental to your pharmacy technician work. **Signa abbreviations** are a series of abbreviations used to communicate prescriptions and patient directions. Signa abbreviations follow a specific order, always beginning with an action verb and continuing through dose quantity, route of administration, time interval, and additional information.

Also key to your career success is familiarity with pharmacy software. As technology and computer software (such as pharmacy management systems) are further integrated into pharmacy practice, pharmacy technicians must become more technologically savvy. Pharmacies use pharmacy management software products (such as NRx) in the daily practice of serving patients. Gaining experience with such systems is important, and this lab will build your general awareness of pharmacy software systems.

However, because pharmacies can choose from numerous software products, once in the field you will need to gain expertise with the specific functions of your workplace software.

Regardless of the particular software system at your pharmacy, some prescriptions will require careful, close monitoring. In response to the increase in prescription drug abuse, many states have adopted regulations known as prescription monitoring programs (PMPs) for monitoring prescribed controlled substances. These programs were originally designed to monitor Schedule II (C-II) prescriptions through mandatory reporting of specific information, including prescriber, pharmacy, and patient information; drug name, strength, quantity, and National Drug Code (NDC); and number of days supplied. In recent years, however, many states have expanded these programs to include specific drug classes (such as benzodiazepines) or specific drug products (such as carisoprodol and tramadol). In addition, some states have expanded these programs to require mandatory reporting on *all* controlled substance prescriptions (Schedules II–IV).

To monitor such prescriptions more accurately, several states (including Texas and New York) require that each monitored prescription be written on a specially designed, tamper proof prescription pads. The pads' blanks are serialized, or individually numbered, with a specific **control number**, a unique number assigned to any monitored prescription for management and tracking purposes. The control number must also be entered into the pharmacy management software, which occurs at different points for different software systems. For tracking purposes, the number is then electronically reported—along with specific prescriber, pharmacy, patient, and prescription information—to the state regulatory agency enforcing controlled substance monitoring. The agency responsible for these state-level programs is typically a law enforcement agency (such as the Department of Public Safety in Texas or the Department of Health in New York), rather than the state's board of pharmacy.

When filling prescriptions, you may process them in one of two ways. For most prescriptions, whether for controlled or noncontrolled substances, you may either fill them immediately—the most common practice—or you may add them to the profile and place them "on hold" to be filled at a later date. When you fill a prescription for immediate use, the label will print with a "last filled" date and monograph, which will then be passed on to the next station for counting and pouring, either by you or another technician. When the patient simply wants to add the prescription to his or her profile for later use, a label will still print. However, the "last filled" date and the monograph will not print, indicating that the prescription is not being dispensed but simply being placed on file for filling at another time.

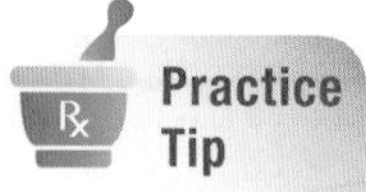

While this lab reflects the process for partially filling a non controlled drug, the process for doing a partial fill on a controlled substance can can differ from pharmacy to pharmacy and state to state.

In your pharmacy practice, you will at times be asked to partially fill a prescription. A partial fill might be necessary when a pharmacy does not have enough of the medication in stock or when a patient does not have enough money to pay for the entire prescription. Should such an event occur, the pharmacy may fill only a few days' or a week's worth of medication. The patient would return to pick up the remaining fill quantity at a later date—when the pharmacy has acquired the rest of the stock or when

 © Paradigm Publishing, Inc.

the patient is able to pay for the rest of the prescription. Pharmacy management software systems, such as the NRx system, enable pharmacies to account for partial fills.

Procedure

In the previous lab, you set up a computer profile for a new patient, Vance Donaldson. After his profile was created, Mr. Donaldson gave you his prescription to fill. Using the following steps, fill his prescription (Figure 9.1, corresponding to tutorial 9.1 in the software), and continue practicing by filling the prescriptions included for other patients (Figures 9.2–9.17, corresponding to assessments 9.2–9.17 in the software). When you encounter a monitored prescription, you must enter the control number. For the NRx-based training software, control number entry occurs at the end of the filling process.

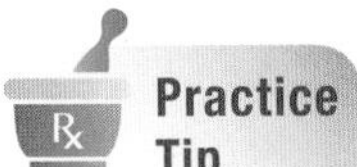

Practice Tip

The assessments represent the different patients you will be processing through the lab procedures. Most labs present several assessments for processing; however, some labs have only one assessment.

This lab provides you with practice processing prescriptions using a particular feature of the NRx software system: short codes. This NRx feature, found in many similar software products, allows you to enter prescription directions using a shorthand system. Short codes are designed to ensure that spelling is consistent and directions are standardized within the pharmacy, from prescription to prescription and patient to patient. Short codes also save pharmacy technicians considerable time, because entering prescription directions with short codes is quicker than typing each full word of the entire set of directions. Imagine typing "take 1 to 2 tablets by mouth every 4 to 6 hours as needed for pain" multiple times a day when, instead, you could use short codes and simply type "t 1-2 tab po q 4-6h prn fp". Short codes alleviate the burden of lengthy repetition and also save time. In Step 7 of this lab, you will be directed to use the short codes found in Appendix A of this textbook to enter prescription directions into the software.

1. Log in to the Course Navigator, and select Lab 9 from the left navigation pane. Then select NRx Tutorials and Assessments.

2. When the menu for all available labs appears, click the tutorial or assessment you wish to perform, beginning with Tutorial 9.1.

3. When the NRx Security screen appears, log in to the NRx-based training software as the Primary User by typing STUDENT as the Login ID and PRACTICE as the Password. Click Log In.

4. On the Rx Processing Tasks menu, click New Rx. When the New Prescription screen appears, type the patient's name in the Patient field in Lastname, Firstname format, and press Tab. The patient's payment information (either third party or cash) and primary prescriber will appear in the appropriate fields.

FIGURE 9.1

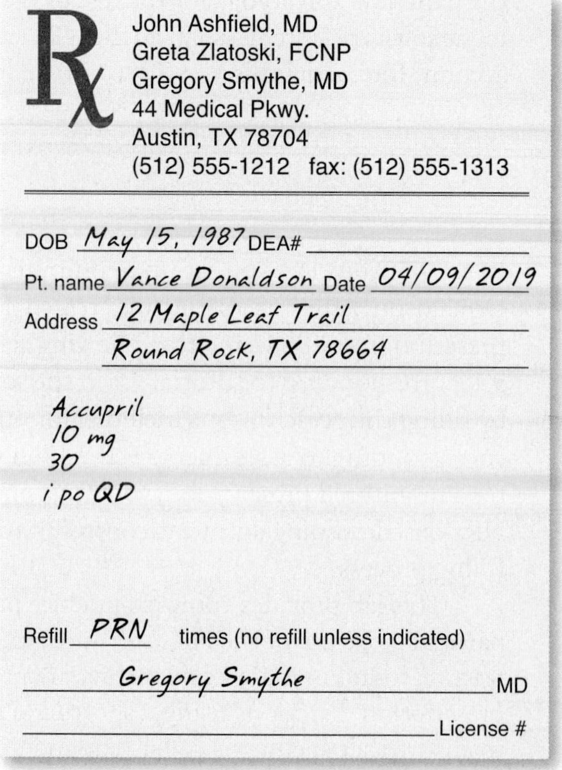
John Ashfield, MD
Greta Zlatoski, FCNP
Gregory Smythe, MD
44 Medical Pkwy.
Austin, TX 78704
(512) 555-1212 fax: (512) 555-1313

DOB May 15, 1987 DEA# ______
Pt. name Vance Donaldson Date 04/09/2019
Address 12 Maple Leaf Trail
Round Rock, TX 78664

Accupril
10 mg
30
i po QD

Refill PRN times (no refill unless indicated)
Gregory Smythe MD
______ License #

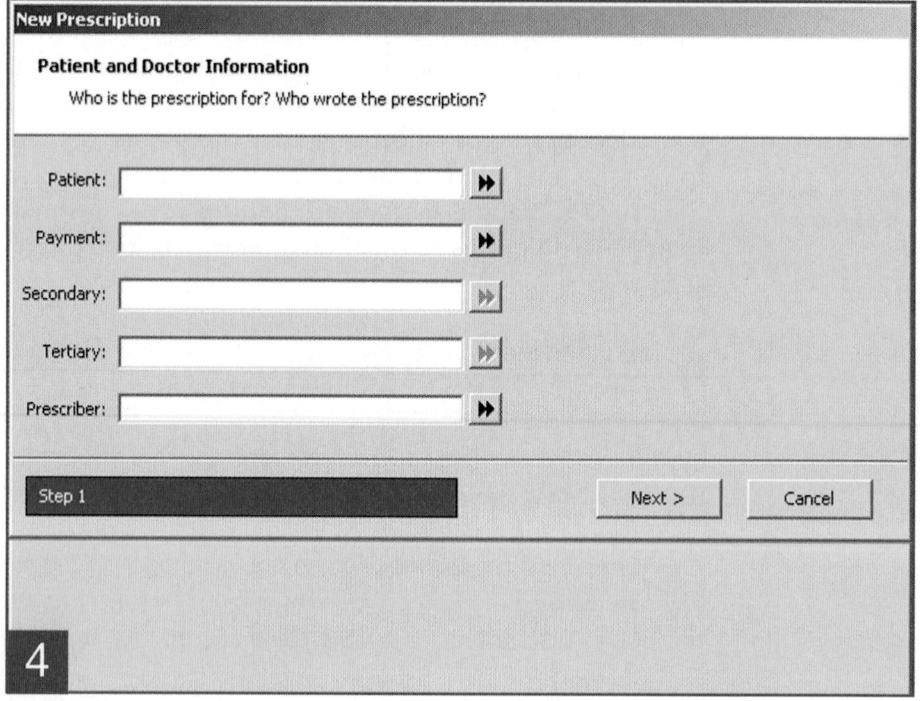

5 Verify that the physician's name, as it appears in the Prescriber field, is correct. Click Next.

 © Paradigm Publishing, Inc.

6 The Drug and Dosage Information screen now appears. Type the drug name in the Drug field, and press Tab. If the system finds an exact match to the drug name, it adds the drug strength and form to the name in the Drug field. In this case, you may proceed to Step 7. However, if the system does *not* find an exact match, a Drug Record Scan list appears with the closest matches. Select the correct drug from the list by double-clicking it.

TAKE NOTE

Your textbook provides you with a simulation of the NRx software. However, because it is only a simulation it does not fully replicate all functions of the software itself. When you are working with a fully operational software system at the pharmacy, you will notice that when typing into a field, you will often need to type only the first few letters of the phrase or word you are entering. To save you time, the software will pull up a complete phrase or word matching the first few characters you have entered, and after verifying that what is filled in is exactly what you want, you will simply press Enter to complete your task without having to type all the characters.

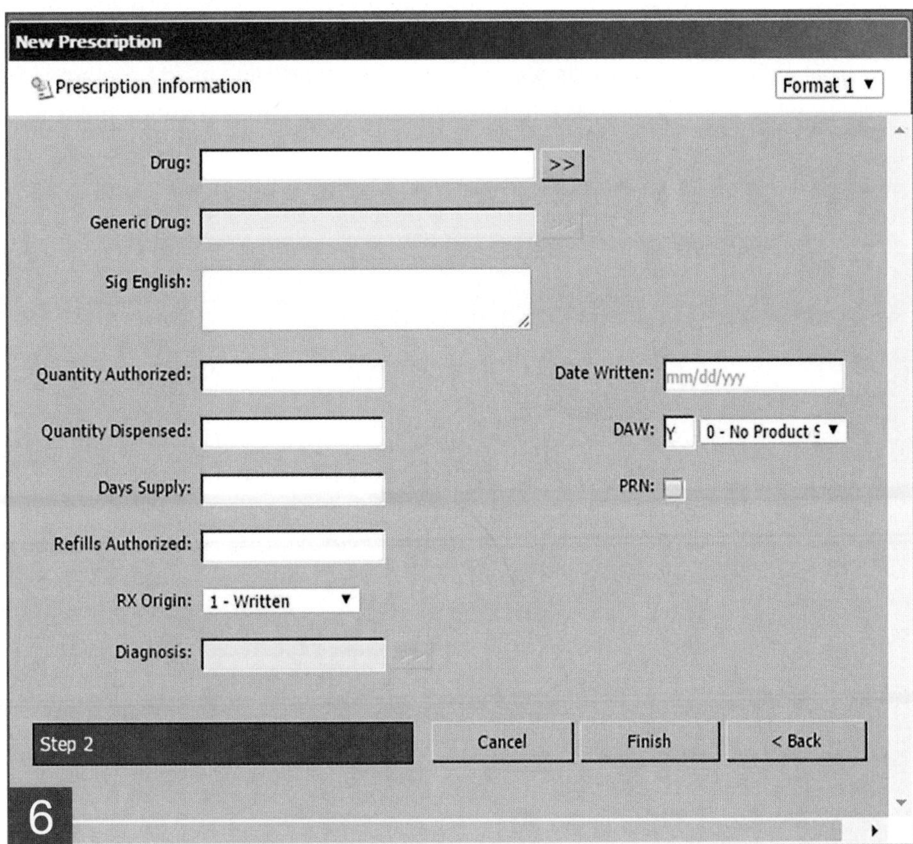

Practice Tip

If you need assistance translating the signa into short codes, ask your instructor for help. You might also take a moment to write out the full sentence translation of the signa on the prescription forms represented in Figures 9.1–9.17. Then use your sentences and Appendix A to determine the short codes you should type into the Sig field on screen.

7 Refer to the prescriber's signa and to Appendix A, and enter the short codes into the Sig field, beginning with the action verb short code and leaving a space between each of the six short code elements as you type. Press Tab. The software will translate your short codes into clear patient instructions, which will appear in the Sig field and also be printed on the prescription label at the end of the lab.

8 Type the quantity into the Quantity Authorized field, and press Tab. Note that the same number automatically appears in the Quantity Dispensed field (and may also appear in the Days Supply field). When working in the pharmacy, you would change the Quantity Dispensed number only if you were going to fill the prescription partially rather than completely. For the purposes of this lab, you are completely filling all prescriptions, so leave the Quantity Dispensed field as is.

9 To decide what to enter in the Days Supply field, use the signa as your guide to calculate the number of days this prescription will last. If the field has already been populated with a number, verify that the quantity is correct according to your calculations, and proceed to Step 10. If there is no number in the Days Supply field, type in the quantity you have calculated, and press Tab.

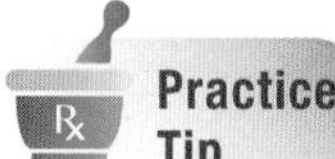

Practice Tip

If you have not yet practiced calculating a day's supply, ask your instructor to demonstrate the process.

10 To enter the number of refills, you have two choices. If the physician has authorized a specific number of refills (including "0"), enter that numeral in the Refills Authorized field, and press Tab. However, if PRN refills are authorized, instead click inside the small field, or box, next to the term PRN, which will cause a check mark to appear.

TAKE NOTE

The number of refills on prescriptions is legally regulated. According to federal law, controlled Schedule II substances can never be refilled without a new prescription (except in emergency situations, when a pharmacist must handle the situation). Substances controlled on Schedules III and IV may have up to five refills within a six-month period. Noncontrolled prescriptions and controlled substances on Schedule V have no limitation on refills (stated as "PRN"), provided the prescription is not 365 days old and expired. Note that with both controlled and noncontrolled medications, the prescriber can choose to prohibit refills or stipulate a maximum number of refills. You may have additional regulations in your state.

 © Paradigm Publishing, Inc.

11 Just above the PRN box is the Dispense as Written (DAW) field. When working in the pharmacy, you would need to look closely at the prescription to determine whether the prescriber has authorized a generic substitution or has mandated that the brand be dispensed. You would then type either "Y" (Yes) or "N" (No) into the DAW field. Although state laws vary, assume for the purposes of this lab that substitution is permitted. Notice that "Y" (Yes) is already present by default in the DAW field, and leave it as is.

TAKE NOTE

Dispense as Written (DAW) code terminology may vary among different pharmacy software systems. However, some common DAW codes include the following: 0—Selection permitted; 1—Physician requests brand; and 2—Patient requests brand.

Practice Tip

For the purposes of this lab, use only numerals to enter the date and use two digits for the month. For example, January would be "01," February would be "02," and so on.

12 Just above the DAW field, click your cursor in the Date Written field. Using numerals only, enter the date the prescription was written, and press Tab.

13 The Rx Summary/General Information screen will appear, and you should verify that all information is entered correctly. Review the patient, the prescriber, and all prescription information. If there are no errors, simply click Save. (Notice that the question marks in the Rx number are updated and the prescription now has an assigned Rx number.)

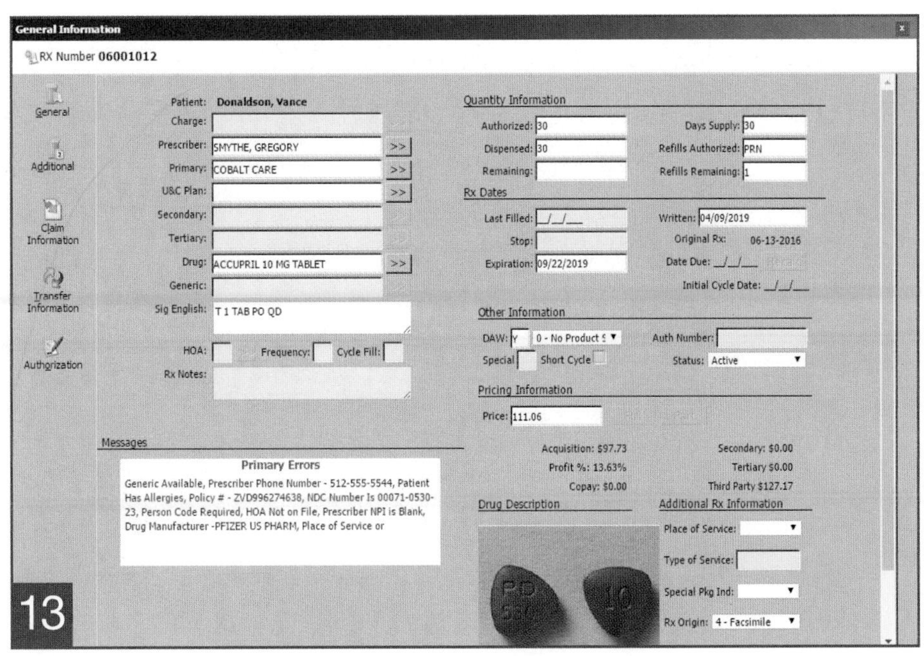

TAKE NOTE

While you might not have access to a stock bottle in your particular educational facility or pharmacy course lab, be aware that in pharmacy practice, verification of the stock bottle NDC number is a best practice and may also be required by law. Thus, when filling a prescription in pharmacy practice, you would look to the Messages field at the bottom left to note the NDC number and verify that it matches the NDC number on the stock bottle.

Practice Tip

When working at the pharmacy, if you want to place the prescription into the patient profile but not fill it right away, you would click Profile Only on the top toolbar to be done with the patient's prescription for the time being.

14 On this same screen, select your filling option. Mr. Donaldson wants his prescription filled immediately rather than placed on hold, so click Fill on the top toolbar. For the purposes of this lab, assume that all other patients want their prescriptions filled at this time, and when you reach this step for those patients, click Fill for each of them.

15 A Filling Options dialog box will pop up and ask how many labels you would like to print. The default quantity appears automatically and is set to "01." On the job, you might choose to change the print quantity. For the purposes of this lab, leave the quantity as is, and click Fill.

16 If the prescription is for a noncontrolled drug, proceed to Step 17. If the prescription is for a C-II drug, the Controlled Substance Editing dialog box will appear and require you to enter the control number and Doctor State License number. Transcribe this information from the face of the prescription into those two fields, and click Continue. Then proceed to Step 17.

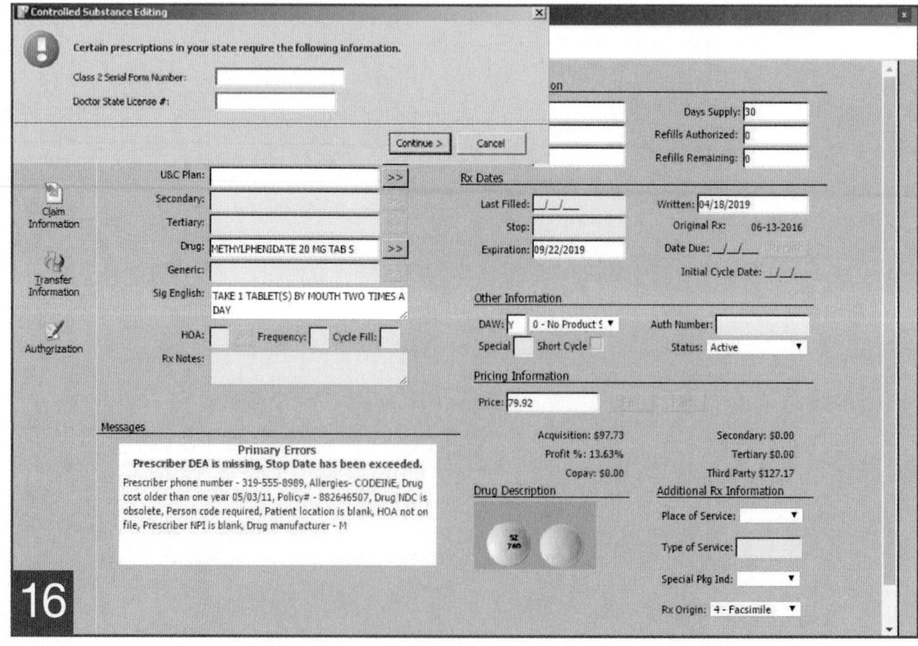

© Paradigm Publishing, Inc.

17 If a Clinical Checking dialog box appears on the screen, you would have to alert the pharmacist while on the job, because possible adverse effects or contraindications may be present for this prescription. The pharmacist would inform you of the next steps to take. For the purposes of this lab, alert your instructor about the box, click Bypass on the top toolbar, and proceed to Step 18.

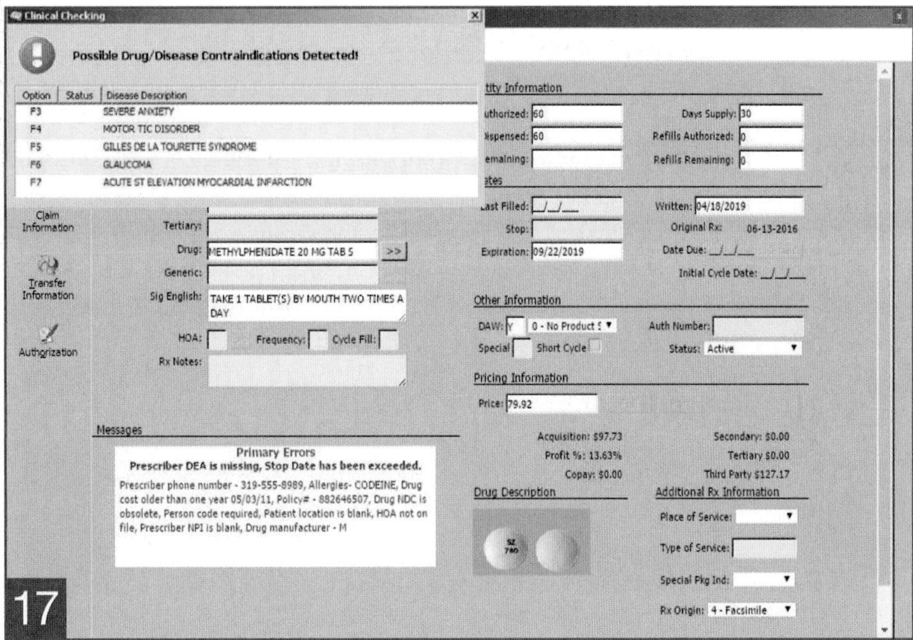

18 A window previewing the prescription label is now on screen. To print this prescription label at your local printer, click Print this screen in the upper-right corner. (A small window associated with your local printer options will appear. Make the necessary selections for the printer you wish to use, and click as required to print the label.) Retrieve the printed prescription label, and set it aside for your instructor to evaluate at the end of the lab.

19 Click Next at the bottom of the print preview window. The tutorial will end. Click Close to close the tutorial and return to the Course Navigator.

20 Repeat Steps 4–19 to complete assessments 9.2–9.17, setting aside all printed prescription labels in a stack. When you have processed all 17 prescriptions, proceed to Step 21 to conclude the lab.

© Paradigm Publishing, Inc.

TAKE NOTE

According to your instructor's preference and the available lab time and capacity, you might now have the chance to prepare the prescription itself—not just process the data associated with the prescription—and label a bottle including contents. Consult your instructor for additional supplies and materials needed to prepare the prescription in laboratory practice.

21 **Conclusion:** Complete the tutorial and assessments 9.2–9.17. Turn in the stack of printed prescription labels and results screens to your instructor. Then go to the Course Navigator, answer all questions in the Lab Review section, and submit your answers to your instructor.

Access interactive chapter review exercises, practice activities, flash cards, and study games.

© Paradigm Publishing, Inc.

FIGURE 9.2

℞ Sunjita Patel, MD
7612 N. HWY 27
Cedar Rapids, IA 52404
(319) 555-1212 fax: (319) 555-1313

DOB *Aug 24, 1961* DEA# *AP4756687*
Pt. name *Amala Gupta* Date *04/14/2019*
Address *5473 W 10th Street*
Cedar Rapids, IA 52401

Lorazepam
0.5 mg
120 (one hundred twenty)
i po q4–6 h prn anxiety

Refill *5* times (no refill unless indicated)

Sunjita Patel, MD MD

License #

FIGURE 9.3

℞ Todd Jackson, MD
Anita Johnson, MD
Kunal Gupta, MSN, FCNP
5730 Congress Avenue
Boise, ID 83702
(208) 555-1212 fax: (208) 555-1313

DOB *Oct 18, 1990* DEA# *FJ1234563*
Pt. name *Lily Nguyen* Date *04/10/2019*
Address *2934 Anderson Lane*
Boise, ID 83722

Alprazolam
2 mg
120 (one hundred twenty)
i po q6 h prn anxiety

Refill *5* times (no refill unless indicated)

Todd Jackson MD

License #

FIGURE 9.4

℞ Randal Binder, MD
Philip Fleming, MD
Terrence McDowell, MD
5874 Kempston Dr.
Orlando, FL 32812
(407) 555-1212 fax: (407) 555-1313

DOB *Jan 22, 2010* DEA#
Pt. name *Cas Riley* Date *03/31/2019*
Address *72650 Okade Court*
Orlando, FL 32810

Ciprofloxacin
250 mg
28
i po bid x 14D

Refill *0* times (no refill unless indicated)

Philip Fleming MD

License #

FIGURE 9.5

℞ Simona Brushfield, MD
2222 IH-35 South
Austin, TX 78703
(512) 555-1212 fax: (512) 555-1313

DOB *Sep 12, 1965* DEA#
Pt. name *Miguel Esparza* Date *03/13/2019*
Address *7583 E 11th St.*
Austin, TX 78705

Humalog
100 Units/mL Vial
1 vial
12 units subQ qAM;
18 units subQ qPM pc

Refill *PRN* times (no refill unless indicated)

Simona Brushfield, MD MD

License #

FIGURE 9.6

Rx

Frieda Nadal, MD
67 Savin Hill Ave
Boston, MA 02109
(617) 555-1212 fax: (617) 555-1313

DOB *Jun 23, 2000* DEA# ____________

Pt. name *Kimberly Jackson* Date *04/17/2019*

Address *4590 Settling Glen Dr*
Boston, MA 02109

Amoxicillin
250 mg/5 mL
150 mL
1 tsp po TID x 10D

Refill *0* times (no refill unless indicated)

Frieda Nadal MD

____________ License #

FIGURE 9.7

Rx

Geoff Taylor, MD
67 Whitford Avenue
Providence, RI 02908
(401) 555-1212 fax: (401) 555-1313

DOB *Feb 29, 1996* DEA# ____________

Pt. name *Marquita Wilkins* Date *04/17/2019*

Address *6901 Westminster Chase*
Providence, RI 02908

Patanol
5 mL
i–ii gtts ou BID

Refill *0* times (no refill unless indicated)

Geoff Taylor MD

____________ License #

FIGURE 9.8

```
------------------------------------------------------------------------
!!! -- START SECURED ELECTRONIC PRESCRIPTION TRANSMISSION -- !!!
------------------------------------------------------------------------
FROM THE OFFICES OF PHIL JACKSON, MD; ETHEL JACOBSON, MD;
                    PETER JARKOWSKI, PA; EUGENE JOHNSON, DO

OFFICE ADDRESS:        67 EAST ELM
                       CEDAR RAPIDS, IA 52411
OFFICE TELEPHONE:      (319) 555-1212   TRANSMIT DATE: 04/18/2019
OFFICE FAX:            (319) 555-1313   WRITTEN DATE:  04/18/2019
------------------------------------------------------------------------
TRANSMITTED TO         THE CORNER DRUG STORE
PHARMACY ADDRESS:      875 PARADIGM WAY
                       CEDAR RAPIDS, IA 52410
PHARMACY TELEPHONE:    (319) 555-1414
------------------------------------------------------------------------
PATIENT NAME:          JEFFREY KLEIN     D.O.B.: OCT 18, 1991
PATIENT ADDRESS:       1157 NORTH PLAZA AVE
                       CEDAR RAPIDS, IA 52411
------------------------------------------------------------------------
PRESCRIBED MEDICATION: FLUOXETINE 20 MG
SIGNA:                 i PO QD
DISPENSE QUANTITY:     30
REFILL(S):             PRN
------------------------------------------------------------------------
PHYSICIAN SIGNATURE:   [[ ELECTRONIC SIGNATURE ON FILE ]]
                       [[ FOR DR. ETHEL JACOBSON ]]
------------------------------------------------------------------------
!!! -- END SECURED ELECTRONIC PRESCRIPTION TRANSMISSION -- !!!
------------------------------------------------------------------------
```

 © Paradigm Publishing, Inc.

FIGURE 9.9

State License # J76839 DEA # MJ1234563

Ethel Jacobson, MD
MONITORED PRESCRIPTION FORM
67 EAST ELM
CEDAR RAPIDS, IA 52411
PHONE: (319) 555-1212 FAX: (319) 555-1313

CTRL # 678290463718

Name *Jeffrey Klein*

Address *1157 North Plaza Avenue, Cedar Rapids, IA 52411*

Age or DOB *October 18, 1991* Date *04/17/2019*

SECURITY FEATURES ON BACK

℞ *Methylphenidate*
20 mg
60 (sixty)
i po BID, 30 min a breakfast,
second dose a 6PM

Ethel Jacobson, MD

Practitioner Signature–Indicate if "Brand Medically Necessary"

Pharmacist Signature	
Rx Number	Date Filled

FIGURE 9.10

℞
Jack Mason, MD
Peter Albrecht, DO
Jason Matson, MD
15 Medical Parkway
Salt Lake City, UT 84106
(801) 555-2121 fax: (801) 555-2323

DOB Nov 20, 1980 DEA# ______

Pt. name Marco Domingo Date 04/09/2019

Address 869 Blythe Street
Salt Lake City, UT 84106

Zocor
20mg
30 (Thirty)
i po qd

Refill 5 times (no refill unless indicated)

Jack Mason MD

______ License #

FIGURE 9.11

℞
Amber Matheson, MD
Andrew Matthews, MD
Doris Franklin, FNCP
45 Pavilion Ave
Missoula, MT 59802
(406) 555-2121 fax: (406) 555-2323

DOB Aug 01, 1988 DEA# M123456

Pt. name Felicity Wruck Date 04/09/2019

Address 506 Washington Drive
Missoula, MT 59802

Z-pak 250mg
1 package (6 tabs)
ii po qd day 1,
i po qd days 2-5

Refill 0 times (no refill unless indicated)

Amber Matheson MD

______ License #

FIGURE 9.12

℞
Rebeka Patterson, MD
11830 Research Blvd
Irvine, CA 92614
(657) 555-2121 fax: (657) 555-2323

DOB Oct 28, 1975 DEA# ______

Pt. name Allison Sutter Date 04/09/2019

Address 5672 Paso Robles Way
Irvine, CA 92614

Prozac
20mg
30 (Thirty)
i po qd

Refill 5 times (no refill unless indicated)

Rebeka Patterson MD

______ License #

FIGURE 9.13

℞
Meredith Hawke, MD
1002 Caduceus Ave
Atlanta, GA 30317
(678) 555-2121 fax: (658) 555-2323

DOB Feb 27, 1947 DEA# ______

Pt. name Brenda Kreuger Date 04/09/2019

Address 67430 Hartsfield Avenue
Atlanta, GA 30317

Xalatan
2.5mL
i gtts os qhs

Refill 2 times (no refill unless indicated)

Meredith Hawke MD

______ License #

© Paradigm Publishing, Inc.

FIGURE 9.14

State License # R1404 DEA # T123456

David Townsend, MD
MONITORED PRESCRIPTION FORM
3785 MEDICAL ARTS AVENUE
CHEYENNE, WY 82001
PHONE: (307) 555-2121 FAX: (307) 555-2323

CTRL # 758862314059

Name *Brian Koch*

Address *14562 Saddleback Pass, Cheyenne, WY 82001*

Age or DOB *April 04, 1979* Date *04/09/2019*

SECURITY FEATURES ON BACK

℞ *Vicodin 5*
30 (Thirty)
i–ii po q46h prn pain. Not to exceed 8 tabs qd

Refills: 1

David Townsend, MD
Practitioner Signature–Indicate if "Brand Medically Necessary"

Pharmacist Signature

Rx Number Date Filled

© Paradigm Publishing, Inc.

FIGURE 9.15

State License # V55870 DEA # D123456

Frank Davis, MD
MONITORED PRESCRIPTION FORM
4475 MEDICAL DRIVE
WASILLA, AK 99629
PHONE: (907) 555-2121 FAX: (907) 555-2323
CTRL # 021456378415

Name Bradley Malloy

Address 20 Guarded Pass, Wasilla, AK 99629

Age or DOB March 20, 1989 Date 04/09/2019

SECURITY FEATURES ON BACK

℞ promethazine c codeine syrup
180 (One Hundred and Eighty)
i tsp po q4-6h prn cough

Refills: 1

Frank Davis, MD

Practitioner Signature–Indicate if "Brand Medically Necessary"

Pharmacist Signature

Rx Number Date Filled

 © Paradigm Publishing, Inc.

FIGURE 9.16

Robert Margerison, MD
Peter Blankenship, MD
Richard Burgraff, MN
Cassandra Poll, MD
7658 Apollo Str. Washington, DC 20001
(202) 555-2121 fax: (202) 555-2323

DOB Sept 03, 1994 DEA#

Pt. name Kade Frost Date 04/09/2019

Address 573 K Street NW
Washington, DC 20001

Truvada
30 (Thirty)
i po qid

Refill 1 times (no refill unless indicated)

Robert Margerison MD

License #

FIGURE 9.17

Simona Brushfield, MD
2222 IH-35
South Austin, TX 78703
(512) 555-1212 fax: (512) 555-1313

DOB 1/22/1993 DEA#

Pt. name Kait Seegmiller Date 04/09/2019

Address 4239 Calara Road
Austin, TX 78703

Prednisone 2
40 (Forty)
i po qid for 10 days for inflammation

Refill 1 times (no refill unless indicated)

Simona Brushfield MD

License #

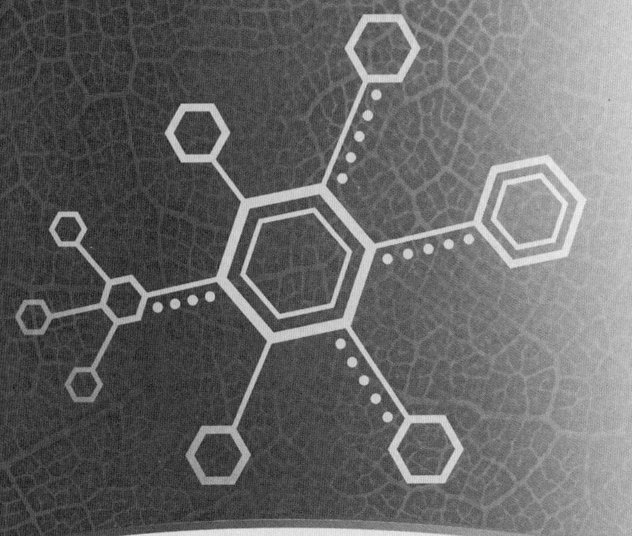

10

Processing a Refill

Learning Objectives

1 Demonstrate proficiency in the use of pharmacy management software for processing prescription refills.

Supplies

- NRx-based tutorial and assessments, available on the Course Navigator

Access additional chapter resources.

While many patients take prescription medications to cure symptoms and diseases, many more take them to treat chronic and ongoing medical conditions such as diabetes, hypertension, and depression. By definition, ongoing and **chronic conditions** (health concerns that recur frequently or last for a long time) require treatment over an extended period of time, and patients with such conditions will likely have prescriptions that need long-term refilling. A significant part of your work time as a pharmacy technician includes processing refill requests, often for such medical conditions. In fact, you will probably find that you process refill requests just as frequently as you process new prescription requests. Thus, knowing how to accurately and quickly process refills is critical to your pharmacy practice.

Accurate processing of refill requests requires that you build awareness and skills beyond those necessary to process and fill new prescriptions. Always verify refill regulations for the state in which you practice. At the federal level, there are particular restrictions on refilling the various prescription categories. Knowledge of these restrictions will eventually become second nature to you in your pharmacy work. Start to learn these rules, and eventually integrate them into your practice:

- Substances controlled on Schedule II can *never be refilled* and require a new prescription (except in an emergency, when a pharmacist must handle the situation).

- Substances controlled on Schedules III and IV may have *up to five refills* within a six-month period.
- Noncontrolled prescriptions and controlled substances on Schedule V have *no limitation* on refills (stated as "PRN"), provided the prescription is not 365 days old and has not expired. Note that the prescriber can choose to prohibit refills or stipulate a maximum number of refills for both controlled and noncontrolled medications.

Also be aware that in the NRx pharmacy management software system, but not necessarily in all similar programs, the prescription profile is color coded for easy reference. Pharmacy staff can take advantage of color coding to easily and quickly distinguish active prescriptions from prescriptions that are expired or have been placed on hold. (Note that an unfilled prescription can remain on hold for an unspecified period of time, but if it is not filled, it can still expire per legal limitations.) You will find the following color coding in the NRx system:

Black: Prescription is valid and has refills remaining.
Red: No refills remain, or the prescription has expired.
Purple: Prescription was placed into profile and has not been filled.

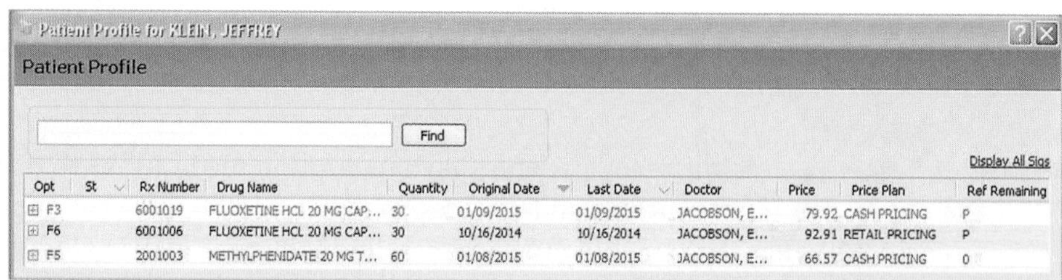

Patient Profile for KLEIN, JEFFREY

Patient Profile

Find

Display All Sigs

Opt	St	Rx Number	Drug Name	Quantity	Original Date	Last Date	Doctor	Price	Price Plan	Ref Remaining
F3		6001019	FLUOXETINE HCL 20 MG CAP...	30	01/09/2015	01/09/2015	JACOBSON, E...	79.92	CASH PRICING	P
F6		6001006	FLUOXETINE HCL 20 MG CAP...	30	10/16/2014	10/16/2014	JACOBSON, E...	92.91	RETAIL PRICING	P
F5		2001003	METHYLPHENIDATE 20 MG T...	60	01/08/2015	01/08/2015	JACOBSON, E...	66.57	CASH PRICING	0

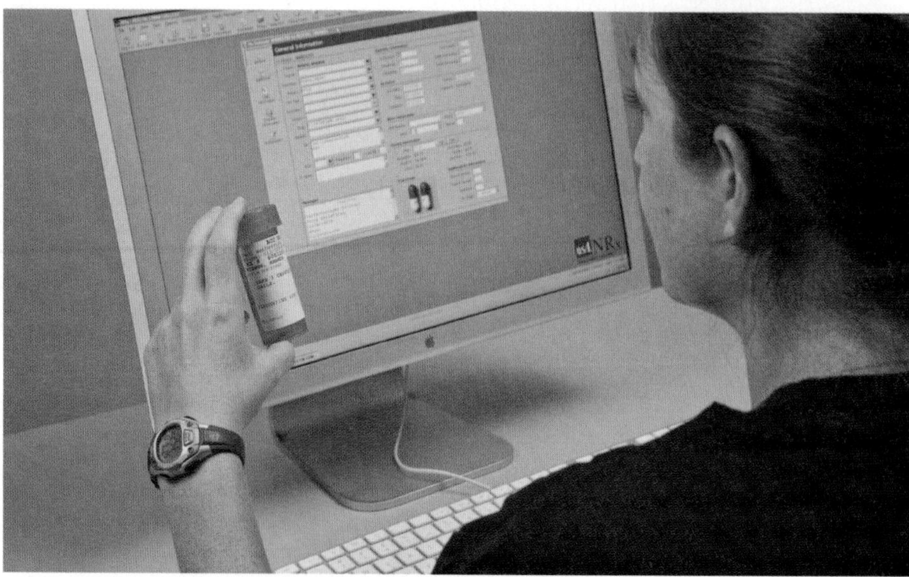

Pharmacy technician using patient's prescription bottle to process a refill request

© Paradigm Publishing, Inc.

When patients telephone or come into the pharmacy seeking refills, some might have their prescription bottle in hand, some might simply have the prescription number or medication name written on a piece of paper, and others might know only the drug name or what the medication is supposed to treat. Knowing how to access and read a patient profile and understanding medications' uses will help you to serve patients and provide them with the correct medication at the proper time. If you ever have a question about which medication to fill, ask your pharmacist before proceeding.

Procedure

In this lab, you will practice using the NRx-based tutorial and assessments to process refill requests for prescriptions filled in earlier labs. You will find the refill request data on the end-of-lab worksheet. Use the data to enter the requests into the software system. When you reach Step 5, you will be guided through filling out the Result column for each worksheet entry. For example, consider this scenario:

> Several of your regular patients have either phoned in requests or brought their used prescription bottles into the pharmacy and are requesting refills. You will encounter one of two conditions as you work through these refill requests: either patients will request a refill and have their prescription number on hand, or patients will request a refill but not have their prescription number with them.

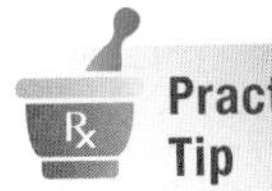

Practice Tip

The assessments represent the different patients you will be processing through the lab procedures. Most labs present several assessments for processing; however, some labs have only one assessment.

As you follow the steps to practice processing refills and complete the worksheet, pay special attention to Step 4 and Step 5. At Step 4, you will need to choose either Step 4a or 4b for each refill request, based on whether the patient presents a prescription number. At Step 5, you will need to choose either Step 5a or 5b for each refill request, based on how the software responds to your request.

1 Launch the Course Navigator learning management system and select Lab 10 in the left navigation pane. Then select NRx Tutorial and Assessments. When the menu for all available labs appears, click the tutorial or assessment you wish to perform, beginning with Tutorial 10.1.

2 The tutorial will launch in your browser, and you will be able to follow the steps online or in this lab manual. After you have completed the tutorial, you can complete the assessments, located under Assessments, for Lab 10.2, Lab 10.3, and so on.

3 When the NRx Security screen appears, log in to the NRx-based training software as the Primary User by typing STUDENT as the Login ID and PRACTICE as the Password. Click Log In.

© Paradigm Publishing, Inc.

4 At this point, you will choose to follow either Step 4a or 4b, depending on whether the patient has brought in a prescription number with the refill request. If the patient brought in the number, it is listed under the Rx Number, Prescription column of the worksheet.

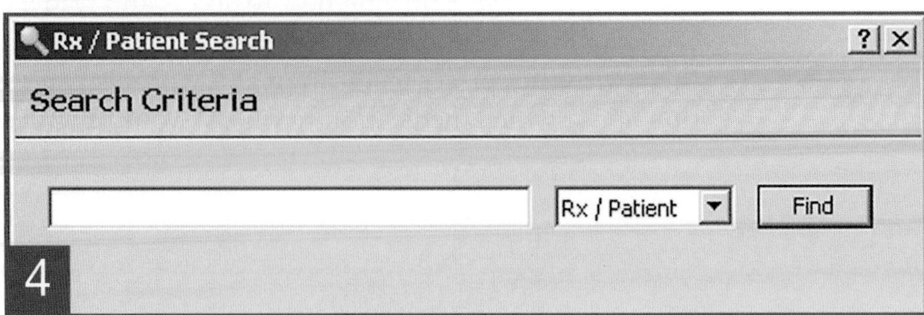

4a If the patient requests a refill *with* a prescription number, do the following:

- From the Rx Processing Tasks menu, click Search.
- Type the patient's prescription number into the search field, and click Find.
- Proceed to Step 5.

4b If the patient requests a refill *without* a prescription number, do the following:

- From the Rx Processing Tasks menu, click Search.
- Type the patient's name (in Lastname, Firstname format) in the empty field, and click Find.
- When the Patient Information screen appears, click the Rx Profile icon on the top toolbar.
- When the Patient Profile screen appears, find and double-click the requested prescription.
- Proceed to Step 5.

5 At this point, the Rx Summary screen should appear. However, one of two things will occur. Either the Rx Summary screen will appear in full view (Step 5a), or that screen will appear with the Refill Request Options dialogue box popped up over it, signifying that you must take further action because the prescription is no longer valid (Step 5b). According to what your screen displays, follow the associated step below for each refill request. When you have completed Step 5a or 5b for all of the refill requests and indicated each result on the worksheet, proceed to the final step, Step 6, which is the conclusion of this lab.

 © Paradigm Publishing, Inc.

5a If the Rx Summary screen appears, you *may* be able to process the refill request without incident. But first, verify patient name and medication name, and compare the on-screen Last Filled date and Days Supply quantity with the Refill Request date on the worksheet.

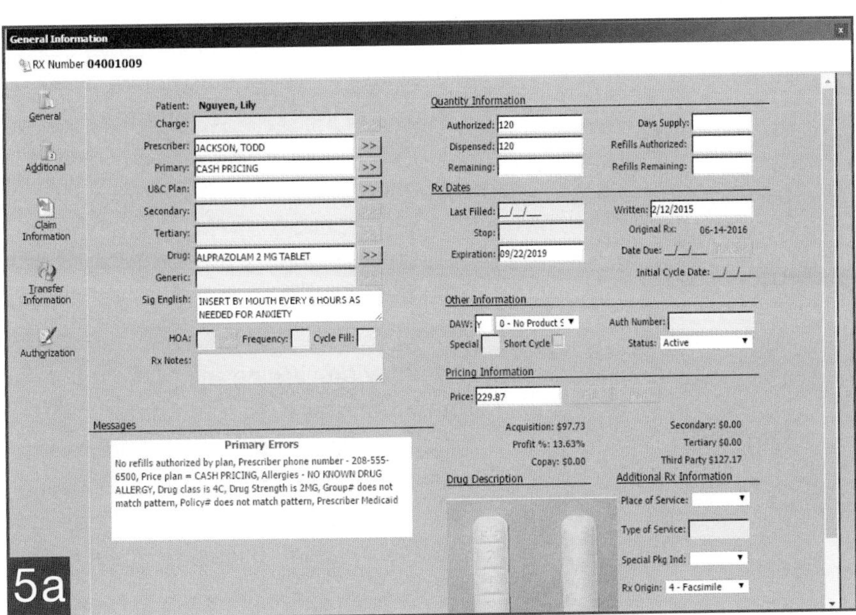

According to how the Last Filled date and Days Supply quantity compare with the Refill Request date, proceed with one of the following two bulleted "If" sections:

If too little time has passed since the Last Filled date for what the Days Supply had provided, you are in a situation known as "refill too soon," and the patient's insurance plan might not cover the prescription. You will be *unable* to process this prescription during this lab.

- Complete the worksheet entry for this refill request by circling Refill Too Soon in the Result column and writing the number of days since the last fill date on the blank line provided.
- Be aware that in the next lab, Lab 11, you will learn about seeking authorization and filling expired prescriptions. At this time, stop the refill request process for this particular prescription by pressing Esc.

© Paradigm Publishing, Inc.

- When you return to the Course Navigator, you may process the next refill request by clicking on the next assessment. First, double-check that you have marked the worksheet Result column for the patient you have just finished processing. Then, progress in numerical order down the worksheet by returning to Step 4a or 4b, according to the next patient's situation.

If the Refill Request date is just a day or two before the supply is intended to run out or if the date exceeds the time span covered by the days supply, you *will* be able to fill the prescription.

- Click the Fill icon on the top toolbar, and a Filling Options dialogue box will appear. Verify that the Print Label box is checked, and then click Fill.
- A window previewing the prescription label is now on screen. To print this label at your printer, click Print this screen in the upper-right corner. A small window associated with your printer options will appear. Make the necessary selections for the printer you wish to use, and click as required to print the label. Retrieve the printed label, and set it aside to turn in at the end of the lab.
- Complete the worksheet entry for this refill request by circling Refill Processed in the Result column.
- Click Next at the bottom of the print-preview window. The tutorial will end. Click Close to close the tutorial and return to the Course Navigator.
- When you return to the Course Navigator, you may process the next refill request by clicking on the next assessment. First, double-check that you have marked the worksheet Result column for the patient you have just finished processing. Then, progress in numerical order down the worksheet by returning to Step 4a or 4b, according to the next patient's situation.

5b If the Refill Request Options dialogue box pops up (alerting you that the prescription is no longer valid), you will be *unable* to process this prescription during this lab. For this refill request, do the following:

- Complete the worksheet entry for this refill request by circling Invalid Prescription in the Result column.
- Be aware that in the next lab, Lab 11, you will learn about seeking authorization and refilling expired prescriptions. At this time, do not click anything in the Refill Request Options dialogue box. Stop the refill request process for this particular prescription by pressing Esc.

© Paradigm Publishing, Inc.

- When you return to the Course Navigator, you may process the next refill request by clicking on the next assessment. First, double-check that you have marked the worksheet Result column for the patient you have just finished processing. Then, progress in numerical order down the worksheet by returning to Step 4a or 4b, according to the next patient's situation.

TAKE NOTE

Controlled substances should never be refilled early. When the prescription is for a controlled substance, check the last fill date and the proper day's supply against today's date. Refills must be delayed until after the supply is depleted or until the pharmacy receives permission after contacting the physician. If you encounter a request for the early refill of a controlled substance, ask the pharmacist to intervene.

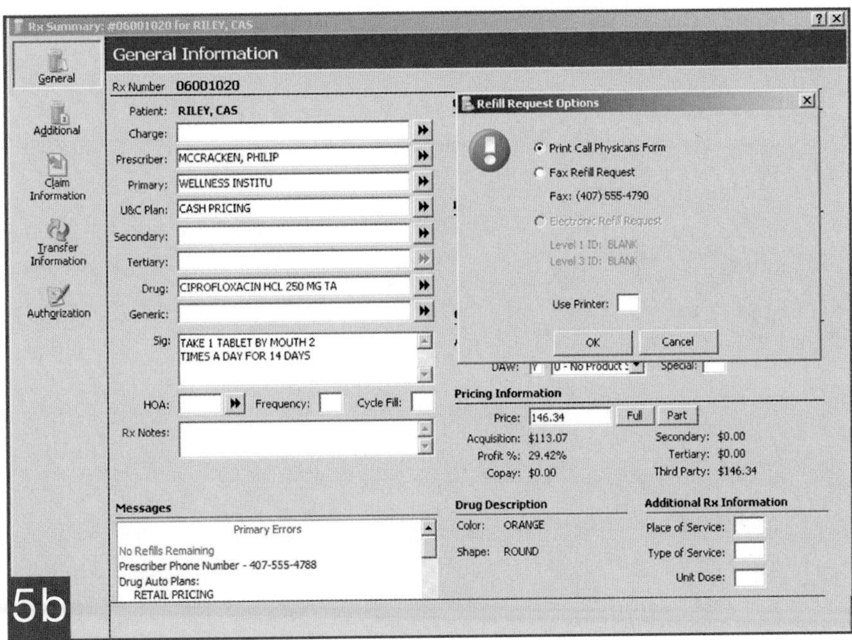

6 **Conclusion:** Complete the tutorial and assessments 10.1 through 10.11. Double-check that you have completed the Result column for all entries on the worksheet before concluding. Write your name and the date on the worksheet, and tear it out. Attach all printed labels to the worksheet, and turn in the whole set to your instructor. Then go to the Course Navigator, answer all questions in the Lab Review section, and submit your answers to your instructor.

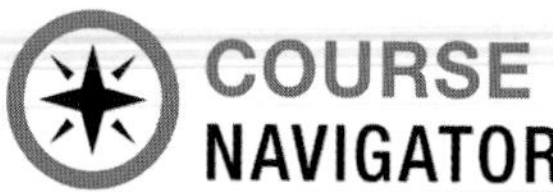

Access interactive chapter review exercises, practice activities, flash cards, and study games.

© Paradigm Publishing, Inc.

Name: ______________________ Date: ______________

Lab 10 Processing a Refill

Worksheet for Refill Request Processing

Assessment /Tutorial Number	Refill Request Date	Patient Name, Birth Date	Rx Number, Prescription	Result (Circle one/Fill blank if needed)
10.1	03/15/2019	Donaldson, Vance, 05/15/1987	6001012, Accupril 10 mg	• Refill Too Soon: Last fill __ days ago • Invalid Prescription • Refill Processed
10.2	03/03/2019	Gupta, Amala, 08/24/1961	Lorazepam 0.5 mg	• Refill Too Soon: Last fill __ days ago • Invalid Prescription • Refill Processed
10.3	03/17/2019	Nguyen, Lily, 10/18/1990	4001009, Alprazolam 2 mg	• Refill Too Soon: Last fill __ days ago • Invalid Prescription • Refill Processed
10.4	05/19/2019	Riley, Cas, 01/22/2010	6001020, Ciprofloxacin 250 mg	• Refill Too Soon: Last fill __ days ago • Invalid Prescription • Refill Processed
10.5	02/18/2019	Esparza, Miguel, 09/12/1965	Humalog Insulin	• Refill Too Soon: Last fill __ days ago • Invalid Prescription • Refill Processed
10.6	07/24/2019	Jackson, Kimberly, 06/23/2000	Amoxicillin 250mg/5mL	• Refill Too Soon: Last fill __ days ago • Invalid Prescription • Refill Processed
10.7	03/28/2019	Wilkins, Marquita, 02/29/1996	Patanol	• Refill Too Soon: Last fill __ days ago • Invalid Prescription • Refill Processed
10.8	02/21/2019	Klein, Jeffrey, 10/18/1991	Fluoxetine 20 mg	• Refill Too Soon: Last fill __ days ago • Invalid Prescription • Refill Processed
10.9	04/17/2019	Malloy, Bradley, 03/20/1989	Promethazine codeine syrup 180 mg	• Refill Too Soon: Last fill __ days ago • Invalid Prescription • Refill Processed
10.10	04/19/2019	Kreuger, Brenda, 02/27/1947	Xalatan 2.5 mL	• Refill Too Soon: Last fill __ days ago • Invalid Prescription • Refill Processed
10.11	04/10/2019	Frost, Kade, 09/03/1994	Truvada 30 mg	• Refill Too Soon: Last fill __ days ago • Invalid Prescription • Refill Processed

© Paradigm Publishing, Inc.

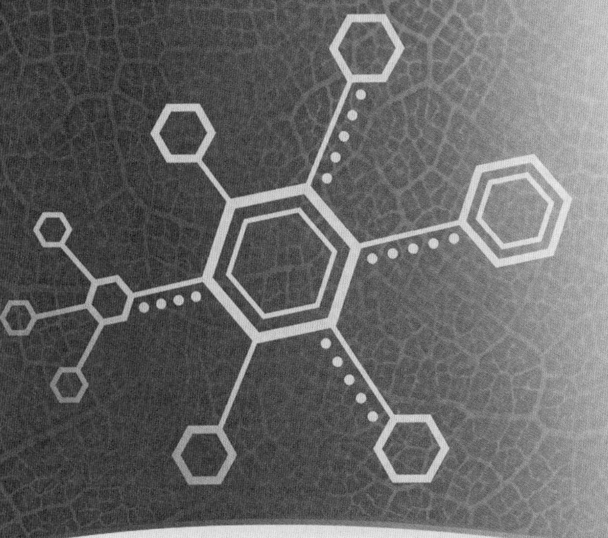

11

Obtaining Refill Authorization

Learning Objectives

1 Learn strategies for resolving problems associated with expired prescriptions.

2 Demonstrate proficiency in using pharmacy management software for prescription refill authorization.

3 Practice securing authorization for prescription refills via paper forms.

4 Learn protocol for communicating refill authorizations through simulated telephone conversations with prescribers.

Supplies

- NRx-based tutorial and assessments, available on the Course Navigator

Access additional chapter resources.

Frequently, a patient will come into or telephone the pharmacy with a prescription that you cannot fill because the prescription has expired. A prescription expires when all refills have been exhausted or when the final date to fill the prescription has passed. Because state laws differ regarding prescription refills, you must be aware of your state's regulations. According to federal regulations, prescriptions may be refilled if authorized by the prescriber.

To secure authorization for refills of an expired prescription, the pharmacy technician may—in many states—contact the prescriber. However, in some states, pharmacy technicians are *not permitted* to perform this duty, and only the pharmacist may legally obtain authorization. Determine what the law is in your state. If your state allows pharmacy technicians to process refill requests, this lab is accurate as written. However, if your state prohibits pharmacy technicians from processing refill requests, replace the term "pharmacy technician" or "technician" with "pharmacist" throughout the remainder of this lab. For the same prohibitive reason, your instructor may have you skip this lab.

Precise restrictions are in place at the federal level to regulate refilling the various prescription categories. Knowledge of these restrictions will eventually become second nature to you in your pharmacy work. Start to learn these rules and integrate them into your practice:

- Substances controlled on Schedule II can *never be refilled* and require a new prescription (except in emergency situations, when a pharmacist must handle the situation).
- Substances controlled on Schedules III and IV may have *up to five refills* within a six-month period.
- Noncontrolled prescriptions and controlled substances on Schedule V have *no limitation* on refills (stated as "PRN"), provided the prescription is not 365 days old and has not expired. Note that the prescriber can choose to prohibit refills or stipulate a maximum number of refills for both controlled and noncontrolled prescriptions.

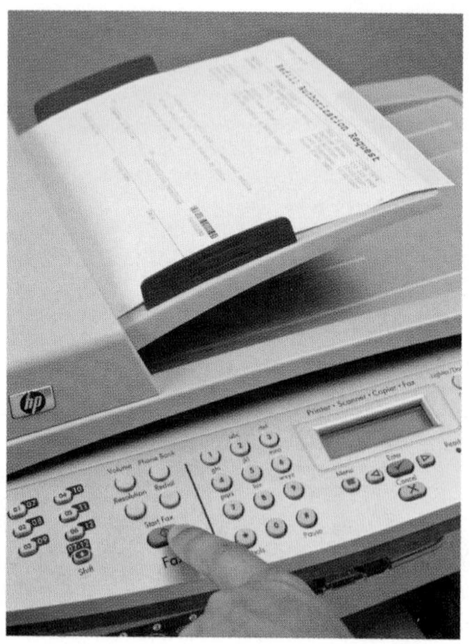

Pharmacy technician faxing a refill authorization request to prescriber's office

Pharmacy technicians must follow a clear-cut process to refill an expired prescription. First, a technician must generate a refill authorization request form using the pharmacy's software program. Information on this form is then phoned in, faxed, or electronically transmitted to the prescriber's office for authorization. Some prescriber offices will require you to send the request via fax so that they will possess a hard copy. However, in some cases the request can be phoned in by providing a specific set of patient and prescription information. You will be guided through the phoning-in process for refill requests during this lab.

Once the prescriber's office receives the refill request, it can either deny the request or approve it and designate a certain number of refills. When responding to the refill request, the prescriber may also communicate special instructions for the patient. For example, the patient may be required to obtain additional lab work or return for an office visit before receiving further refills. If the prescriber denies the request, a pharmacy technician must make a note of this decision and then notify the patient of the denial, relaying any special instructions given by the prescriber's office to the patient. If the prescriber approves the request, a pharmacy technician can generate a new prescription according to the prescriber's stipulations.

Procedure

In this lab, you will continue gaining skills with the NRx-based simulation by processing refill requests for prescriptions filled in earlier labs. For the purposes of this lab, however, those prescriptions will have

 © Paradigm Publishing, Inc.

expired. As in the previous lab, some patients will present a prescription number, and others will not. Figures 11.1–11.7, located at the end of this lab, represent prescription labels brought in by patients and sticky notes jotted by pharmacy staff when patients have called in a refill request.

Because all of these prescriptions have expired, you must use the data from the figures to request and successfully obtain refill authorization before you can fill the patients' prescriptions. In Part I, following the steps below, you will practice generating a Refill Authorization Request form by using the NRx-based software accessed through the Course Navigator.

You will then spend class time off the computer to complete Parts II and III. In Part II, you will communicate the authorization request to the prescriber by role-playing telephone conversations with a partner. Such role-play enables you to practice medical terminology, pronunciation, professionalism, and communication skills while guided by your instructor. In Part III, you will participate in a class discussion about the evolving roles of the pharmacy technician and the pharmacist when seeking refill authorization, the skills required to successfully perform those roles, and the varied state-based regulations regarding those roles.

Part I: Generating a Refill Authorization Request Form

You will perform this part of the procedure for each of the seven patients requesting refills as presented in Figures 11.1–11.7 at the end of the lab. Once all seven patient requests have been processed through Step 9, you will move on to Part II, beginning with Step 10.

1 Launch the Course Navigator learning management system. Click on Lab 11 in the left navigation pane, and then click Tutorials and Assessments. When the menu for all available labs appears, click the tutorial or assessment you wish to perform, beginning with Tutorial 11.1.

2 The tutorial will launch in your browser, and you will be able to follow the steps online or in this lab manual. After you have completed the tutorial, you can complete the assessments for Lab 11.2, Lab 11.3, Lab 11.4, and so on.

Practice Tip

The assessments represent the different patients you will be processing through the lab procedures. Most labs present several assessments for processing; however, some labs have only one assessment.

3 When the NRx Security screen appears, log in to the NRx-based training software as the Primary User by typing STUDENT as the Login ID and PRACTICE as the Password. Press Tab or click Log In.

4 From the Rx Processing Tasks menu, click Search. Begin with Miguel Esparza's refill request from Figure 11.1. If no prescription number was presented, type in the patient's name (in Lastname, Firstname format), or if the prescription number was presented, type it into the Search field and click Find.

The prescription profile is color coded for quicker reference.

Black: Prescription is valid and has refills remaining;

Red: No refills remain, or the prescription has expired;

Purple: Prescription was placed into profile and has not been filled.

5 If you typed in the patient's name, follow Step 5a; if you typed in the prescription number, follow Step 5b.

5a

If you typed in the patient's name, the Patient Information profile will display. Click the Rx Profile icon on the top toolbar. When the Patient Profile listing the patient's prescriptions appears, double-click on the requested prescription. The Rx Summary screen will appear. Verify the patient name, medication name, and Last Filled date.

5b

If you typed in the prescription number, the Rx Summary screen will appear. Verify the patient name, medication name, and Last Filled date.

6 On the top toolbar, click the Print icon. From the drop-down menu, click Refill Request, and the Refill Request Options dialogue box will appear. Notice that the Print Call Physicians Form option is selected, and click OK. A preview of the Refill Authorization Request form will be displayed. Click Print this screen in the upper-right corner of the screen. A small window associated with your printer options will appear. Make the necessary selections for the printer you wish to use, and click as required to print the Refill Authorization Request form. Retrieve the printed form, and set it aside to be used in Part II of the lab.

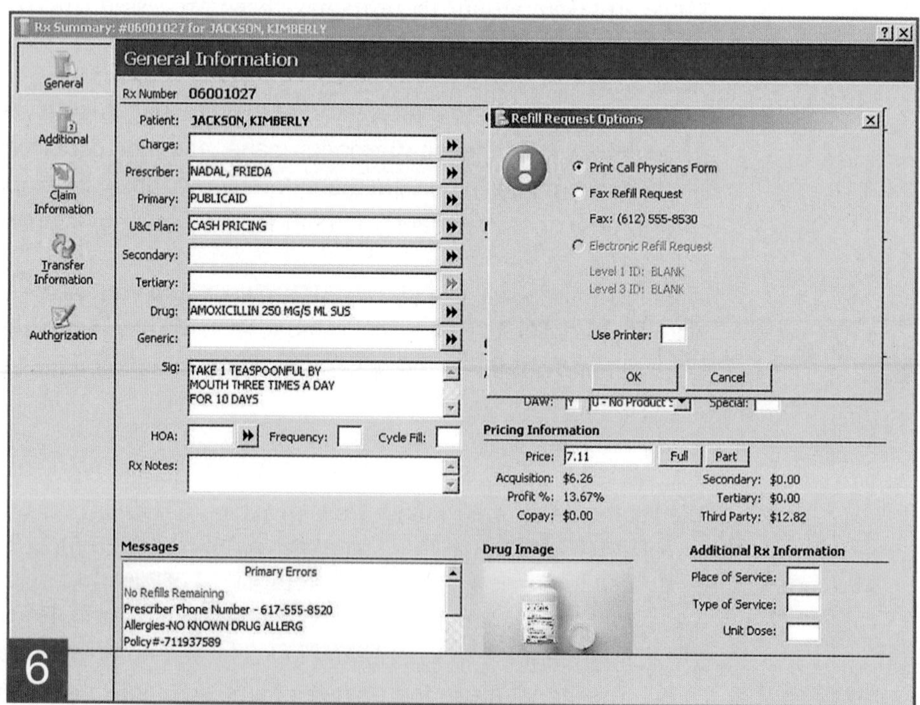

7 The tutorial will end. Click Close to close the tutorial and return to the Course Navigator.

© Paradigm Publishing, Inc.

8 After printing Mr. Esparza's Refill Authorization Request form, you may process the refill requests for the six remaining patients. Repeat Steps 2–7 with the remaining refill requests, proceeding in numerical order as presented in Figures 11.2–11.7 in your textbook and as Labs 11.2–11.7 on screen in the assessments listing. You will click the Submit button once you are satisfied that you have completed all the lab steps for each of the assessments. Clicking Submit will submit your assessment to your instructor and will bring you back to the Course Navigator, where you will be able to see your score. When you have processed all seven patients, proceed to Step 9.

9 Retrieve all seven printed Refill Authorization Request forms and stack them separately. You will use the Refill Authorization Request forms in the next step and should proceed now to Part II.

Part II: Phoning in the Refill Request

In this part of the procedure, you will seek authorization for the refills being requested. In practice, you may be required to fax the Refill Authorization Request form to the prescriber's office. However, refill requests are frequently communicated via telephone by following a specific procedure, as outlined in Steps 13–18.

To practice communicating refill requests, you will work with a partner, role-playing telephone conversations to simulate communication with a prescriber. Admittedly, because this is a practice scenario, there is no real telephone number to call and no actual prescriber to speak with. Nonetheless, you and your lab partner should do your best to role-play these pharmacy technician and prescriber conversations. The student pretending to be on the prescriber end of the phone line should sometimes pretend to be a prescriber or prescriber's office staff member and sometimes pretend to be a recorded voice on the office's refill message line.

Keep in mind that you and your partner should each write on your own stack of Refill Authorization Request forms when directed to do so. Although your two sets of forms should be identical, each student should write on her or his own forms to have documents to turn in to the instructor at the end of the lab.

10 Review the medication names on the seven Refill Authorization Request forms you have printed. If you are unsure how to correctly pronounce any of the names, ask your instructor or another student to model the pronunciations for you.

11 Select a partner, and keep at hand each student's stack of seven printed Refill Authorization Request forms. Keep one student's copy of *Pharmacy Labs for Technicians* open to these procedure steps, and open the other student's copy to the patient refill requests (Figures 11.1—11.7).

© Paradigm Publishing, Inc.

Practice Tip

You should switch roles partway through the procedure so that you each have a chance to role-play both sides of the conversation.

12 Decide who will play which role initially: one of you will play the role of the pharmacy technician calling for authorization, and the other will act as the prescriber or prescriber's office staff member and will either deny or approve the refill request. If you deny the request, you must offer justification for the denial; if you approve the request, you must state how many additional refills are permitted.

13 Telephone the prescriber's office for the first authorization request.

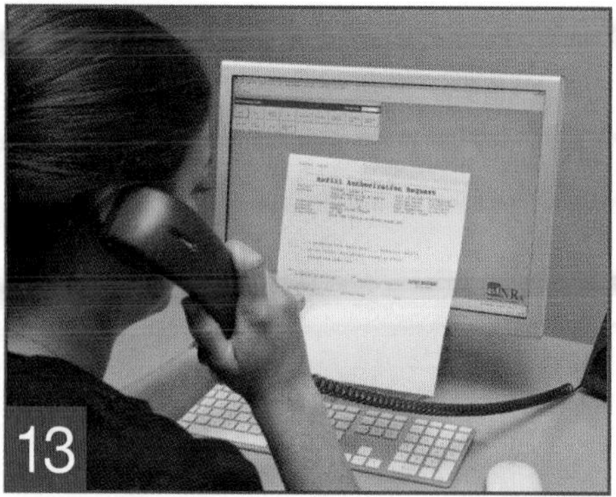

Pharmacy technician telephoning prescriber's office to request refill authorization

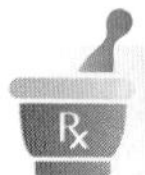

Work Wise

Some offices will have you speak to a person, and others will have pharmacy-specific refill message lines. In either case, remember to remain professional and courteous on the phone.

14 When the phone is answered, tell the person answering who you are, which pharmacy you are with, and that you have a refill authorization request. That person will either transfer you to the appropriate person or take the request immediately. If you get a recorded message, listen carefully to it before providing the information listed in Step 15.

15 Whether speaking to a person or on a message line, enunciate clearly and provide the following information, in this order:

Practice Tip

For one or two of the refill requests, the student in the prescriber role should simulate a recorded message line at the prescriber's office.

1. Patient's last name (Say it, and spell it out.)
2. Patient's first name (Say it, and spell it out.)
3. Date of birth (This is important, because you do not know how many John Smiths or Maria Garcias are seen at this office.)
4. Medication name (Say it, and spell it out.)
5. Strength
6. Quantity
7. Signa (either in signa form or as it appears on the sticky note or label)
8. Date written
9. Last date refilled or dispensed
10. Prescriber name (Say it, and spell it out.)
11. Your name, the name of the pharmacy you are with, and—most important—your call-back number
12. If you are on a message system, state the information again. If you are speaking to a person, repeat the information in the same order, or ask the person to repeat the information while you verify that it matches yours.

 © Paradigm Publishing, Inc.

16 If you are speaking to a person, you could receive authorization right away, or you might have to wait up to 48 hours. Ask for the person's name, and note that name, the date, and the time in a blank area on the Refill Authorization Request form. Similarly, when leaving a recorded message, expect a return phone call within 48 hours, and note on the form the date and time you left the message.

Practice Tip

Take special care when filling in the number of "additional" refills, because that number refers to fills authorized to take place after this one. For example, if the prescriber authorized only one refill, you must put a zero in the blank, because you are about to provide that one additional refill.

17 For the purposes of this lab, if authorization is not given right away or your request was left as a recorded message, all return phone calls should take place immediately during the role-play. Either during the initial call (if you receive authorization right away) or when the "prescriber" student calls back, the "pharmacy technician" student should record the prescriber's decision by checking off one of the three possible responses (Refills are Authorized, Refills are Denied, or Prescriber asks the patient to make contact) located at the bottom of the Refill Authorization Request form. If refills are authorized, be sure also to write the quantity of additional refills in the blank.

18 Follow Step 18a if the refill request was denied or Step 18b if the refill request was authorized.

18a If authorization was denied: Both students should write the reason for denial on the bottom of their own Refill Authorization Request form and set the forms aside for the moment. You will each have to submit these denied request forms to your instructor at the end of this lab. For now you may go on to process the next request, returning to Step 13. When you have received and recorded a response for all seven requests, you may proceed to Part III.

TAKE NOTE

At this point in pharmacy practice, the pharmacy technician would notify the patient—in person or over the telephone—of the denial and any special instructions given by the prescriber's office. If you wish to extend the role-play, you and your partner might play out such a conversation between the pharmacy technician and the patient.

18b If authorization was granted, you should temporarily put the approved Refill Authorization Request form aside and return to Step 13 to process the remaining requests. When you have received and recorded a response for all seven requests, you may proceed to Part III.

TAKE NOTE

At this point in pharmacy practice, the pharmacy technician would notify the patient—in person or over the telephone—of the approval and of when the refill will be ready. If you wish to extend the role-play, you and your partner might play out such a conversation between the pharmacy technician and the patient.

Part III: Further Discussion of the Refill Authorization Request Process—Roles, Skills, and Regulation

In this part of the lab, your class will meet as a whole and discuss three topics affecting the refill authorization request process: the evolving roles of pharmacy technicians and pharmacists in the process, the essential skills for professionally and successfully completing the process, and the variation in state-based regulation of the process.

Your instructor will facilitate the discussion and provide you with guidelines for participation. Keep those guidelines in mind as you work through the following steps as a class. The final step in this part instructs you in organizing your materials from Parts I and II and completing the lab.

19 Discuss the *evolving roles* of the pharmacist and the pharmacy technician in the process of obtaining refill authorization by considering the following questions or others posed by your instructor: The pharmacist and the pharmacy technician play central roles as members of the pharmacy team providing quality care to patients, but how do their roles differ for this process? What are the limitations of both roles for this process? What are the opportunities for growth in both roles in this process?

20 Discuss the *essential skills* for professionally and successfully obtaining refill authorization as a pharmacy technician by considering the following questions, or others posed by your instructor: What does it mean to "act professionally" when seeking refill authorization? What are the rules for telephone etiquette when communicating with the prescriber's office staff or with the office's refill message line? What other communication skills might you have or seek to obtain for professionally and successfully obtaining refill authorization?

 © Paradigm Publishing, Inc.

21 Discuss the *state-by-state variation in regulation* of the pharmacy technician's role in obtaining refill authorization by considering the following statements and questions or additional questions posed by your instructor: The role of the pharmacy technician can differ greatly from state to state. (For example, pharmacy technicians in Texas are allowed to obtain refill authorization via telephone and fax and to electronically generate a new prescription from an older record in the computer software, provided they update only the number of allowed refills. In Iowa, pharmacy technicians, at the discretion of the pharmacist, may receive new orders via telephone and other means. At the time this text was written, some states—including Colorado, Hawaii, and New York—do not regulate pharmacy technicians at all.) What regulations does your state's pharmacy act impose regarding this job activity? For example, does your state consider an over-the-phone authorization to be a new prescription, not a refill, even though the drug name, strength, and signa do not change?

22 **Conclusion:** Complete the tutorial and assessments 11.1–11.7. Collect the seven approved or denied Refill Authorization Request forms that you set aside in Step 18. Because you are not identified on the Refill Authorization Request forms, sign and date them. Turn in all printed items to your instructor. Then go to the Course Navigator, answer all questions in the Lab Review section, and submit your answers to your instructor.

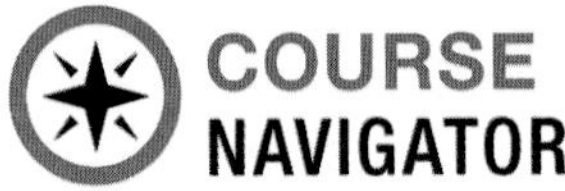

Access interactive chapter review exercises, practice activities, flash cards, and study games.

FIGURE 11.1
Refill Request Noted from Phone Call

Esparza, Miguel
09/12/1965
Humalog Insulin

FIGURE 11.2
Refill Request from Previous Fill Label

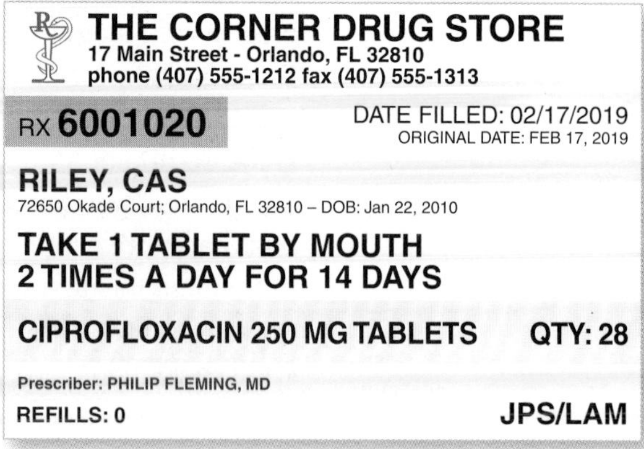
THE CORNER DRUG STORE
17 Main Street - Orlando, FL 32810
phone (407) 555-1212 fax (407) 555-1313

RX 6001020
DATE FILLED: 02/17/2019
ORIGINAL DATE: FEB 17, 2019

RILEY, CAS
72650 Okade Court; Orlando, FL 32810 – DOB: Jan 22, 2010

TAKE 1 TABLET BY MOUTH
2 TIMES A DAY FOR 14 DAYS

CIPROFLOXACIN 250 MG TABLETS QTY: 28

Prescriber: PHILIP FLEMING, MD
REFILLS: 0 JPS/LAM

FIGURE 11.3
Refill Request Noted from Phone Call

Jackson, Kimberly
06/23/2000
Amoxicillin
250mg/5mL

FIGURE 11.4
Refill Request Noted from Phone Call

Wilkins, Marquita
02/29/1996
Patanol

 © Paradigm Publishing, Inc.

FIGURE 11.5
Refill Request from Previous Fill Label

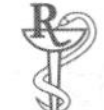

THE CORNER DRUG STORE
17 Main Street - Cedar Rapids, IA 52411
phone: (319) 555-1212 fax: (319) 555-1212

RX **6001019**

DATE FILLED: 02/20/2019
ORIGINAL DATE: FEB 20, 2019

KLEIN, JEFFREY
1157 North Plaza Avenue; Cedar Rapids, IA 52411 – DOB: Oct 18, 1991

TAKE 1 CAPSULE BY MOUTH 4 TIMES DAILY.

FLUOXETINE **QTY: 30**

Prescriber: ETHEL JACOBSON, MD
REFILLS: PRN **JPS/LAM**

FIGURE 11.6
Refill Request from Previous Fill Label

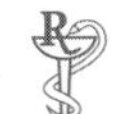

THE CORNER DRUG STORE
17 Main Street - Wasilla, AK 99654
phone: (907) 555-4444 fax: (907) 555-3333

RX **4776831**

DATE FILLED: 02/20/2019
ORIGINAL DATE: FEB 20, 2019

MALLOY, BRADLEY
20 Guarded Pass, Wasilla, AK 99654 – DOB: March 20, 1989

TAKE 1 TAKE BY MOUTH EVERY 4 TO 6 HOURS AS NEEDED FOR COUGH

PROMETHAZINE C CODEINE SYRUP **QTY: 180**

Prescriber: FRANK DAVIS, MD
REFILLS: PRN **JPS/LAM**

FIGURE 11.7
Refill Request Noted from Phone Call

Brenda Kreuger
02/27/1947
Xalatan

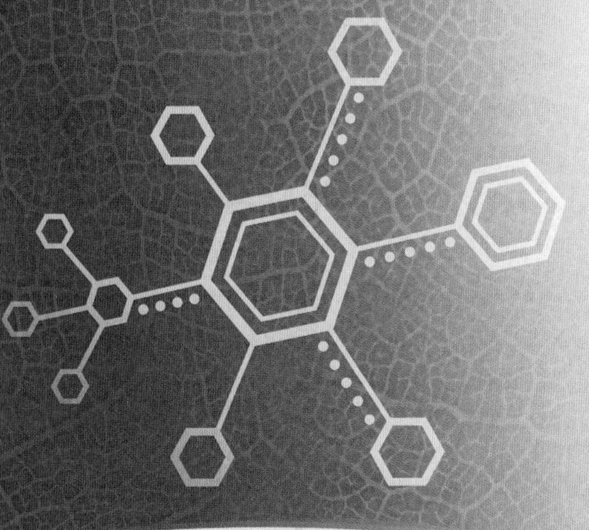

12

Processing Third-Party Claims

Learning Objectives

1 Accurately process patient prescriptions with third-party, or insurance, claims.

2 Understand how pharmacy management software processes third-party claims.

3 Understand why third-party claims are rejected.

4 Learn how to resolve common claim rejections using pharmacy management software.

Supplies

- NRx-based tutorial and assessments, available on the Course Navigator

Access additional chapter resources.

Submitting insurance claims will be a regular part of your work as a pharmacy technician. Because insurance companies act as a "third party" in the chain of events that moves payment from the first party (the patient) to the second party (the pharmacy), such processing is called "third-party adjudication" or "third-party processing." The word *adjudication* is related to *judging* and *judgment* and refers to someone in an outside position making a decision, or judgment, for those inside the situation.

In the case of **third-party adjudication**, the pharmacy submits an electronic claim to the third party, the insurance company. The insurance company then reviews the prescription claim and judges, based on the drug coverage plan the patient has already agreed to, whether and how much payment should be transmitted between those inside the situation (the patient and the pharmacy). Ultimately, the party (the insurance company), pays the pharmacy on behalf of the patient for part of the patient's prescription cost.

A third-party adjudication will take place on nearly all of the prescriptions in a community pharmacy and will be a significant part of your daily work. In an institutional pharmacy, however, pharmacy technicians do not often process third-party claims. Instead, you would only begin the process by entering orders into the computer system, and the institution's billing or medical records department would bill the patient's insurance company.

While processing claims, you may come across unfamiliar terms, including *adjudication*, *capture*, *BIN (bank identification number)*, *PCN (processor control number)*, *NDC (National Drug Code)*, *group code*, and *person code*. You may have encountered these terms in previous labs, but take some time now to review and learn them better as you practice processing third-party claims. **Capturing** (successfully submitting and obtaining payment on an insurance claim) is particularly relevant to this lab, for as you resolve common insurance rejections, you will need to update claims and capture a paid claim.

Once a claim is submitted, it will either be paid by the third party or be rejected. The most common rejections a pharmacy technician will encounter in community pharmacies are "NDC Not Covered," "Patient (PT) Not Covered/Invalid," and "Refill Too Soon." Most often, these rejections occur because patients are unfamiliar with particular coverage rules under their insurance plans. Many patients have the impression that the prescriber or pharmacy will track their insurance plan and readily know which products are covered. Although that would be ideal, it is not possible because of the wide variation in insurance plans. Therefore, additional communication must take place between the prescriber, the pharmacy, and the patient to resolve coverage questions. Most insurance issues may be resolved by a phone call to the insurance carrier or the prescriber's office. In fact, a good deal of your time as a pharmacy technician will be spent on the telephone, resolving third-party issues.

As a consequence of this communication and verification process, patients may understandably become frustrated. By the time patients reach the pharmacy to have their prescriptions filled, they have often been through quite a lot: they may have been sick for a few days prior to seeking medical attention, then they may have had to wait at the prescriber's office for a length of time, and now, perhaps in considerable pain or discomfort, they must wait at the pharmacy to receive their prescription. You can see how this situation could contribute to impatience and cause patient–pharmacy misunderstandings. Remember that patients are not directly angry with you, but are frustrated with the process itself. Because you are involved in the process, you can become a target of their frustration. Please do not take any misunderstandings personally, and try to remain calm and empathetic.

© Paradigm Publishing, Inc.

Procedure

Practice Tip

The assessments represent the different patients you will be processing through the lab procedures. Most labs present several assessments for processing; however, some labs have only one assessment.

At the end of this lab, you will find newly acquired insurance cards accompanying the associated prescriptions in Figures 12.1–12.6. You will use these figures through Parts I, II, and III of this lab to process a prescription claim for each patient. In Part I, you will enter the prescription claim data using Steps 1–14. Then either the prescription will process without incident or the software will notify you that the claim is rejected for one of three reasons: "NDC Not Covered," "Patient (PT) Not Covered/Invalid," or "Refill Too Soon." To resolve each rejection in Part II, you will be advised to go through Steps 15 and 16 under the section matching the rejection reason. In Part III, the final section of the lab, Steps 17–20 will guide you through printing labels and concluding the lab.

Admittedly, because this is a practice scenario, there is no patient present for you to speak with should the described situations arise or should you have questions about the prescription or insurance card. Nonetheless, when a procedure step asks you to communicate with a patient, imagine the patient is in front of you, and either whisper quietly to yourself as if having that conversation or silently imagine the patient's response. If your instructor permits it and time allows, you might also partner with another student to role-play these conversations between pharmacy technician and patient.

Part I: Processing the Prescription Claim

Practice Tip

Tip: Some pharmacy management software systems are case-sensitive, and in your pharmacy work you will need to be careful about using uppercase (capital) or lower case letters when typing in patient names and other data. However, for the purposes of these labs (Labs 8–14), you will not have to be concerned about case sensitivity.

1. Launch the Course Navigator learning management system. Click on Lab 12 in the left navigation pane, and then select NRx Tutorial and Assessments. When the menu for all available labs appears, click Tutorial 12.1.

2. The tutorial will launch in your browser, and you will be able to follow the steps online or in this lab manual. After you have completed the tutorial, you can complete the assessments, located under Assessments, for Lab 12.2, Lab 12.3, Lab 12.4, and so on.

3. When the NRx Security screen appears, log in to the NRx-based training software as the Primary User by typing STUDENT as the Login ID and PRACTICE as the Password. Click Log In.

4. On the Rx Processing Tasks menu, click Search.

5. When the Rx/Patient Search screen appears, type the patient's name in Lastname, Firstname format in the Search Criteria field (for the tutorial, you will use Figure 12.1 and enter "Donaldson, Vance"). Click Find or press Enter.

6 When the Patient Information screen appears, click Insurance Information at the bottom of the left menu bar. When the Patient Insurance Information screen appears, click the New icon on the top toolbar.

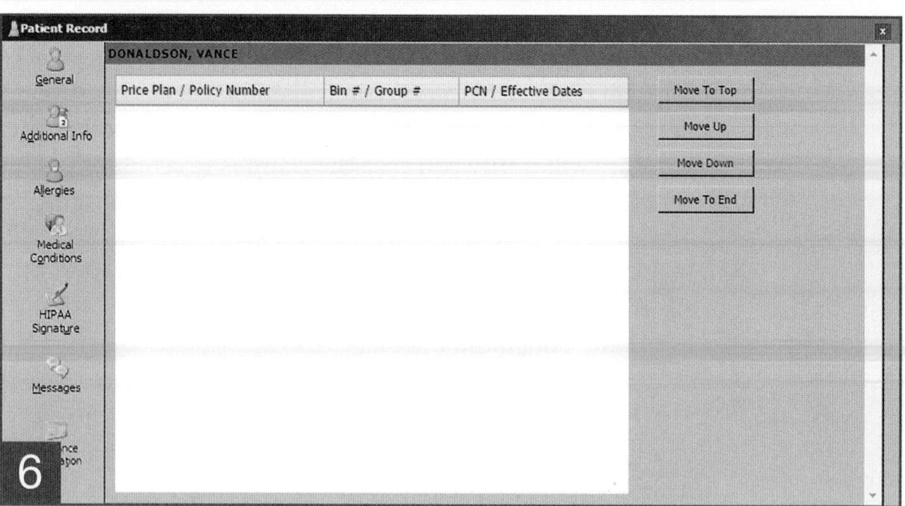

7 A blank Patient Insurance Record screen will appear. Click the double arrows to the right of the Payment Plan field.

If more than one plan shows the same name, match the BIN on the insurance card to the BIN on screen before selecting the plan name.

8 When the Price Plan Scan screen appears, enter the name of the third-party plan (located under the words "Insurance Card" on the patient's card) into the search field, and press Enter or click Find. Double-click the desired insurance plan or press the corresponding F-key.

9 The blank Patient Insurance Record screen will reappear. Enter the patient's insurance plan information from the insurance card into the appropriate fields. First, type in the Policy ID Number, and press Tab. Then, for the Group Number, you will have two options. If the insurance card indicates "None," move on to the Relationship field; if a Group Number is given, type it in, and then press Tab. If the card presents the Relationship category as "Not Specified," leave the field as is and click Save; if another Relationship category is given, click on the Relationship drop-down menu, and select the corresponding code number and name. Click Save.

If the same BIN comes up more than once, you can choose the correct PCN for the plan to help in adjudication.

 © Paradigm Publishing, Inc.

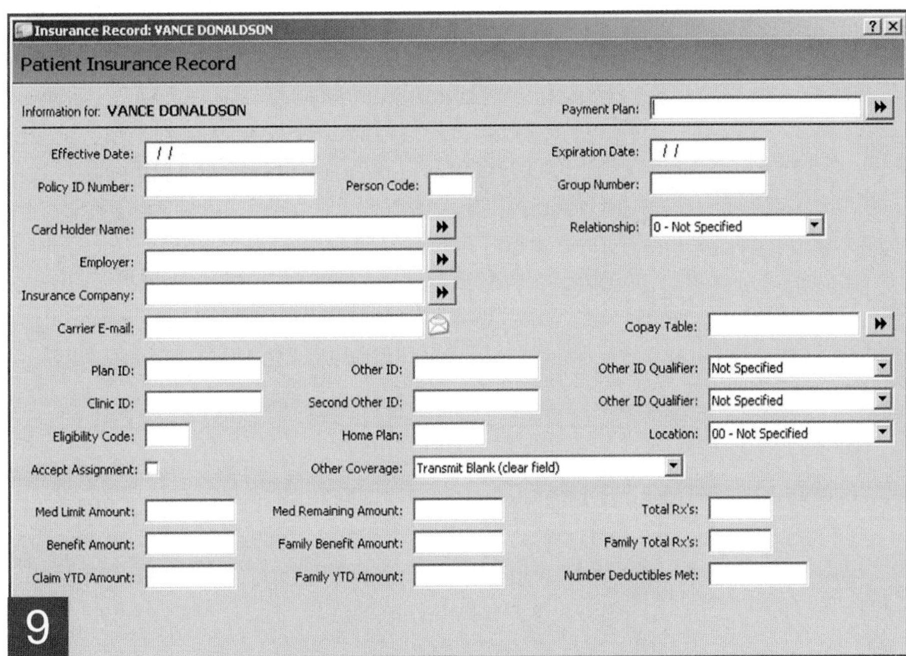

TAKE NOTE

Not all insurance carriers require the same information. All will require an ID number, but not all require a group number, person code, or relationship number. Note that you have relationship numbers on the insurance cards in this lab but not person codes. Keep in mind that person codes are slightly different from relationship numbers. Person codes tend to take the following form: 00-Unspecified; 01—Cardholder; 02—Spouse; 03, 04, 05, etc.—Children, sequentially numbered in birth order. Take extra care at your pharmacy job to ensure that you enter the proper item (person code or relationship number) according to the information listed on the patient's insurance card.

10 Press Esc to return to the Patient Payment Information screen. Click the Update Profile icon on the top toolbar. A Payment Change Detected dialogue box will appear displaying the message "The primary payment plan has changed for this patient. Do you wish to update the patient's prescription profile with the new payment plan?" Click Yes.

Tip: If you need help to process the prescription, review and follow the Procedure section of Lab 9.

11 Press Esc again to return to the Rx Processing Tasks menu, and process the prescription normally.

12 When you have processed the prescription through the step of clicking the Fill icon and clicking Fill in the Filling Options dialogue box, one of two things will happen. Either a Clinical Checking dialogue box or the prescription label preview screen will pop up (in which case you should proceed to print the label, referring again, if needed, to Lab 9, Steps 17—18), or the Rx Summary/General Information screen will remain on screen, unchanged. You should proceed to one of the two "If" sections below, according to whether you were able to print the label or not (because the prescription requires additional attention to resolve a claim issue).

If you were able to print the prescription label, it was successfully filled on a third-party plan. When you are sure the prescription label has printed and have picked it up from the printer, set it aside to turn in at the end of the lab. Click Next in the lower-right area of the label preview screen.

- When you return to the Course Navigator, you may process the next prescription by clicking on the assessments (Labs 12.2–12.6) in numerical order, referring to the corresponding Figure (Figures 12.2–12.6) for the associated patient data. Return to Step 4 to begin processing the next patient.

If the Rx Summary/General Information screen remains on screen, unchanged, and you were thus unable to proceed with printing the prescription label, a claim submission error has occurred. You should proceed to Step 13.

13 To view an explanation of the claim submission errors, press Esc, and return to the Rx Processing Tasks menu. Click the Electronic Claims Log button or press F4. Find the patient name on the log, and click it once to highlight it.

© Paradigm Publishing, Inc.

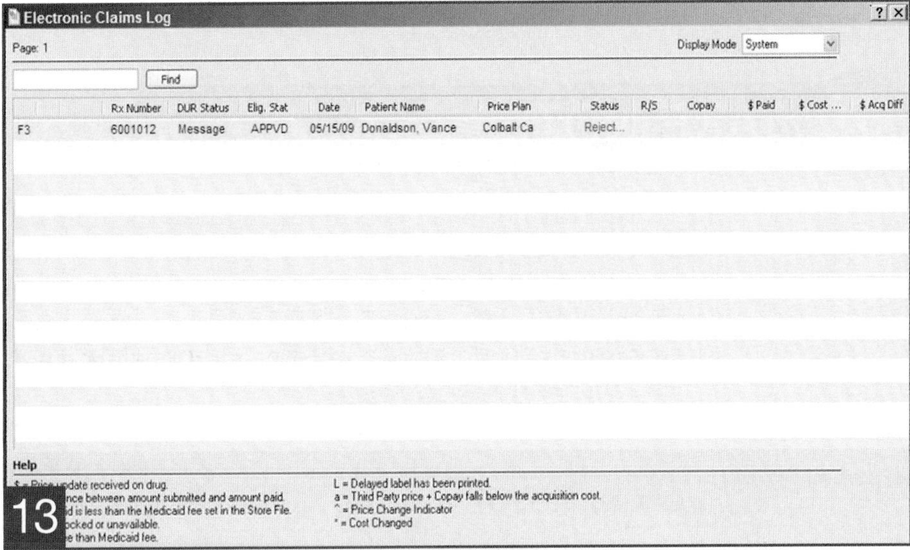

14 Click the Drug Utilization Review (DUR) button on the top toolbar and carefully review the information on the DUR screen. The data in the Conflict Description column determines which claim resolution section you should proceed to next, for Step 15 in Part II. Therefore, near the patient's prescription or insurance card, be sure to jot down all data appearing in the Conflict Description column, including the rejection reason (shown in red letters) and any additional messages regarding the rejection from the third-party provider. Press Esc.

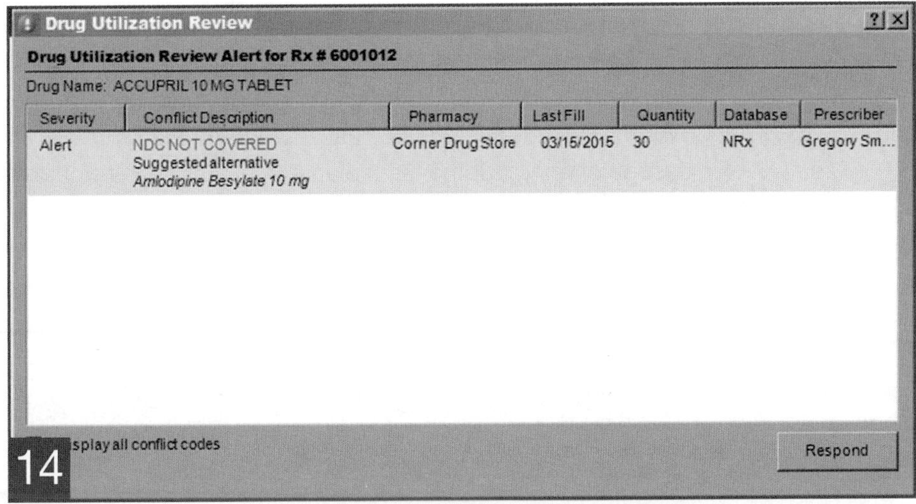

TAKE NOTE

Be sure to inform patients of the status of their prescriptions. In cases of rejection, patients may have helpful information to pass on to you, or they may become upset. It is important, however, to keep them fully informed so they are not waiting in the pharmacy unnecessarily. Be prepared to answer additional patient questions in such situations.

Part II: Resolving the Claim Rejection

In Part I, you either processed a patient's claim without issue or were told why a patient's claim was rejected. In Part II of the procedure, you will be shown how to correct a claim submission error based on rejection type. Move on to Step 15 within one of the three "If" sections below. Choose the section that corresponds to the claim rejection reason for the patient at hand. Take care to read the introductory paragraph for that section before proceeding. After you complete Steps 15 and 16 in the appropriate "If" section for a given patient, you will be clearly directed to Part III to perform Steps 17 and/or 18 to print labels, and, when you have completed all six assessments, to conclude the lab.

If "NDC Not Covered" causes the rejection, follow the instructions in this section: On the DUR Screen you viewed in Step 14, the "NDC Not Covered" conflict description may have been accompanied by a free-text message offering additional explanations, limitation reminders, or alternate drugs. In practice, if the message lists an alternate drug, you would ask the pharmacist to contact the prescriber's office to request a new prescription for the alternate. For the purposes of this lab, proceed as instructed in the following scenario (Steps 15[a] and 16[a]) to process this rejected patient claim.

TAKE NOTE

If the drug is not covered, you should alert the patient to the situation and inform him or her that, unless he or she wishes to pay the retail, or cash, price for the prescription, the pharmacist will need to contact the prescriber to request a new prescription for a medication that may be covered.

© Paradigm Publishing, Inc.

15a You received a message in Step 14 that Vance Donaldson's prescription was rejected because the NDC is not covered. The pharmacist then contacted the prescriber for clarification and received orders to change the drug to amlodipine besylate 10 mg with the same directions (i po QD), quantity (30), and refills (PRN). To take action on this patient's prescription, click the Correction icon on the top toolbar.

TAKE NOTE

In these "on hold" situations, patients will have to wait for the pharmacist to reach the prescriber. Thus, you should inform patients that resolution could take some time and that, while they are welcome to wait, going home is an option and the pharmacy will contact them when the prescription is ready. If patients become upset and begin to blame the pharmacy or the prescriber, explain that with so many insurance plans available, the prescriber or pharmacy cannot track each plan and drug formulary. Assure them that these situations are common, that you understand their frustration, and that they will be contacted as soon as the prescription is ready.

16a In the Rx Summary screen, update the drug name and strength by clicking on the denied drug in the Drug field. When that field turns blank, type in "amlodipine besylate 10 mg", and press Enter. Click Fill on the top toolbar. When the Filling Options dialogue box appears, click your cursor in the small Resubmit box so that a check mark appears, and then click Fill. The prescription should now process and fill without rejection. Skip over the next two "If" sections to Step 17 in Part III, where you will print the prescription label and be directed how to continue with or conclude the lab.

TAKE NOTE

If, in a case similar to Vance Donaldson's, it had been later in the day and the pharmacist phoned the prescriber's office only to find it closed, you would ask the patient to contact the physician's office the next day for a new prescription. You would place this prescription on hold in the patient's profile. The software would allow you to easily do so by clicking the Profile Only icon within the Correction process of the Electronic Claims Log. The prescription would then be on hold in the patient's profile, and a label would print with the prescription information but without the drug monograph.

If "Patient (PT) Not Covered/Invalid" causes the rejection, follow the instructions in this section: The DUR screen conflict description free-text message from the third party may have stated that the prescription was rejected because of data entry errors in the Patient Profile or Payment Info sections of the pharmacy software. It may also have been rejected because the patient has new insurance coverage or does not realize that the previous coverage has lapsed or been canceled. In such cases, you would review the patient's profile and payment information to ensure that the data on screen matches the data on the insurance card, updating as necessary. You might also have to contact the insurance company to verify coverage, either receiving verification or filling the prescription on a cash payment basis if the patient agrees. For the purposes of this lab, proceed as instructed in the following scenario (Steps 15^b and 16^b) to process this rejected patient claim.

15^b Kimberly Jackson's prescription was rejected because she is no longer covered by her old insurance plan. After you ask her if she has new insurance, she reveals that she does not currently have any insurance. You then ask if she agrees to cash payment for the prescription, and when she agrees, you click the Correction icon on the top toolbar.

16^b In the Rx Summary screen, you will need to update the Primary field from "PublicAid" to "Retail Pricing" to ensure that the prescription will not be billed to an insurance plan but will be paid at the moment at the retail, or cash, pricing level. To do so, click on the old insurance plan in the Primary field. When the field turns blank, type in "Retail Pricing", and press Enter or click the double arrows to the right of the Primary field. Click the Fill icon on the top toolbar. When then Filling Options dialogue box appears, click your cursor in the small Resubmit box so that a check mark appears, and then click Fill. The prescription should now process and fill without rejection. Skip over the next "If" section to Step 17 in Part III, where you will print the prescription label and be clearly directed how to continue with or conclude the lab.

If "Refill Too Soon" causes the rejection, follow the instructions in this section: The DUR screen conflict description free-text message from the third party may have indicated when the prescription was last filled, and that data can help you discuss the rejection with the patient. For example, either you or the pharmacist could ask the patient whether he or she remembers the prescription's last fill date and, if not, remind the patient of that date. You would then seek further information about why the refill request is being made early. For the purposes of this lab, proceed as instructed in the following scenario (Steps 15^c and 16^c) to process this rejected patient claim.

© Paradigm Publishing, Inc.

TAKE NOTE

When you engage patients in conversations about refilling too soon, some will recall that they still have a supply of the prescription. The situation can then be easily resolved by canceling the request or placing it on hold. However, some patients may become upset or angry, in which case it is always best practice to have a pharmacist or experienced technician intervene to calm the situation. When patients become argumentative and demand that a prescription be filled, the pharmacist may instruct you to change the primary price plan to Cash and fill the prescription.

15C Amala Gupta's prescription is for a controlled substance. It was last filled 16 days ago with a 20-day supply. Due to concerns in the pharmacy industry about potential abuse of controlled substances, it may not be prudent to fill the prescription early. In fact, the insurance company is not allowing an early refill, but is indicating the patient may refill in four days. You would remind the patient that she should have enough of the prescription remaining for four more days and ask her to return at that time to receive the fill when her insurance will cover the prescription. On the Electronic Claims Log screen, select the patient name, and click it once to highlight it.

16C Click the DUR button to return to the DUR screen describing the rejection details. Click the Reversal icon on the top toolbar. When the Reverse Claim dialogue box appears, notice that "Continue with reversal, only" is selected, and click Submit. The dialogue box Claim Reversal Results now advises you that this patient record is flagged for reversal. Click Ok. Because this fill has now been cancelled, a label will not be printed. Thus, as you move now into the final section of the lab (Part III), you should skip Step 17 (where a label would be printed) and proceed to Step 18, where you will be directed how to continue with or conclude the lab.

Part III: Printing Resolved Rejection Labels and Concluding the Lab

17 To print the prescription label, click Print this screen in the upper-right corner of the label preview screen. A small window associated with your local printer options will appear. Make the necessary selections for the local printer you wish to use, and click as required to print the screen. When you are certain that the prescription label has printed, set it aside to turn in at the end of the lab, and click Next in the lower-right area of the label preview screen.

© Paradigm Publishing, Inc.

18 When you return to the Course Navigator, you may process the next prescription by clicking on the next assessment (12.2–12.6), in numerical order, and referring to the corresponding Figure (12.2–12.6) for the associated patient data. Return to Step 4 to begin processing the next patient.

19 **Conclusion:** When you have processed all the patient claims in 12.1–12.6 and resolved any rejections by following the associated procedure steps, you may conclude the lab as follows. Click Submit to submit each assessment to your instructor. Turn in to your instructor all labels that you have set aside during this lab. Then go to the Course Navigator, answer all questions in the Lab Review section, and submit your answers to your instructor.

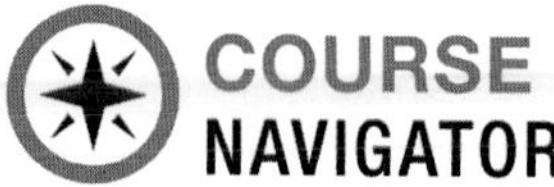

Access interactive chapter review exercises, practice activities, flash cards, and study games.

FIGURE 12.1
Patient Prescription and Insurance Card Data

Cobalt Care
Insurance card
VANCE DONALDSON
BIN: 00123
ID: ZVD996274638
GROUP: 11770
RELATIONSHIP: 01, CARDHOLDER
MEMBER SERVICES: 1-800-555-3232
CLAIMS/INQUIRIES: 1-800-555-6363

Rx
John Ashfield, MD
Greta Zlatoski, FCNP
Gregory Smythe, MD
44 Medical Pkwy.
Austin, TX 78704
(512) 555-1212 fax: (512) 555-1313

DOB May 15, 1987 DEA# ______
Pt. name Vance Donaldson Date 04/09/2019
Address 12 Maple Leaf Trail
Round Rock, TX 78664

Accupril
10 mg
30
i po QD

Refill PRN times (no refill unless indicated)
Gregory Smythe MD
______ License #

© Paradigm Publishing, Inc.

FIGURE 12.2
Patient Prescription and Insurance Card Data

FederalAide
Insurance card
MIGUEL ESPARZA
BIN: 999990
ID: 119875639
GROUP: B
RELATIONSHIP: 00, NOT SPECIFIED
MEMBER SERVICES: 1-800-555-3232
CLAIMS/INQUIRIES: 1-800-555-6363

Rx
Simona Brushfield, MD
2222 IH-35 South
Austin, TX 78703
(512) 555-1212 fax: (512) 555-1313

DOB Sep 12, 1965 DEA# ____
Pt. name Miguel Esparza Date 04/09/2019
Address 7583 E 11th St.
Austin, TX 78705

Humalog
100 Units/mL Vial
1 vial
12 units subQ qAM;
18 units subQ qPM pc

Refill PRN times (no refill unless indicated)
Simona Brushfield, MD MD
____ License #

FIGURE 12.3
Patient Prescription and Insurance Card Data

PublicAid
Insurance card
KIMBERLY JACKSON
BIN: 100009
ID: 711937589
GROUP: NONE
RELATIONSHIP: 02, SPOUSE
MEMBER SERVICES: 1-800-555-3232
CLAIMS/INQUIRIES: 1-800-555-6363

Rx
Frieda Nadal, MD
67 Savin Hill Ave
Boston, MA 02109
(617) 555-1212 fax: (617) 555-1313

DOB Jun 23, 2000 DEA# ____
Pt. name Kimberly Jackson Date 04/09/2019
Address 4590 Settling Glen Dr
Boston, MA 02109

Amoxicillin
250 mg/5 mL
150 mL
1 tsp po TID x 10D

Refill 0 times (no refill unless indicated)
Frieda Nadal MD
____ License #

FIGURE 12.4
Patient Prescription and Insurance Card Data

```
---------------------------------------------------------------------------
!!! -- START SECURED ELECTRONIC PRESCRIPTION TRANSMISSION -- !!!
---------------------------------------------------------------------------
FROM THE OFFICES OF PHIL JACKSON, MD; ETHEL JACOBSON, MD;
                    PETER JARKOWSKI, PA; EUGENE JOHNSON, DO

OFFICE ADDRESS:           67 EAST ELM
                          CEDAR RAPIDS, IA 52411
OFFICE TELEPHONE:         (319) 555-1212    TRANSMIT DATE: 04/09/2019
OFFICE FAX:               (319) 555-1313    WRITTEN DATE:  04/09/2019
---------------------------------------------------------------------------
TRANSMITTED TO            THE CORNER DRUG STORE
PHARMACY ADDRESS:         875 PARADIGM WAY
                          CEDAR RAPIDS, IA 52410
PHARMACY TELEPHONE:       (319) 555-1414
---------------------------------------------------------------------------
PATIENT NAME:             JEFFREY KLEIN     D.O.B.: OCT 18, 1991
PATIENT ADDRESS:          1157 NORTH PLAZA AVE
                          CEDAR RAPIDS, IA 52411
---------------------------------------------------------------------------
PRESCRIBED MEDICATION:    FLUOXETINE 20 MG
SIGNA:                    i PO QD
DISPENSE QUANTITY:        30
REFILL(S):                PRN
---------------------------------------------------------------------------
PHYSICIAN SIGNATURE:      [[ ELECTRONIC SIGNATURE ON FILE ]]
                          [[ FOR DR. ETHEL JACOBSON ]]

---------------------------------------------------------------------------
!!! -- END SECURED ELECTRONIC PRESCRIPTION TRANSMISSION -- !!!
---------------------------------------------------------------------------
```

ApolloHealth
Insurance card

JEFFREY KLEIN
BIN: 459872
ID: 882646507

GROUP: NONE
RELATIONSHIP: 02, SPOUSE

MEMBER SERVICES: 1-800-555-3232
CLAIMS/INQUIRIES: 1-800-555-6363

© Paradigm Publishing, Inc.

FIGURE 12.5
Patient Prescription and Insurance Card Data

PublicAid
Insurance card

AMALA GUPTA
BIN: 100009
ID: 778342987

GROUP: NONE
RELATIONSHIP: 01, CARDHOLDER

MEMBER SERVICES: 1-800-555-3232
CLAIMS/INQUIRIES: 1-800-555-6363

Rx
Sunjita Patel, MD
7612 N. HWY 27
Cedar Rapids, IA 52404
(319) 555-1212 fax: (319) 555-1313

DOB Aug 24, 1961 DEA# AP4756687
Pt. name Amala Gupta Date 04/09/2019
Address 5473 W 10th Street
Cedar Rapids, IA 52401

Lorazepam
0.5 mg
120 (one hundred twenty)
i po q4–6 h prn anxiety

Refill 5 times (no refill unless indicated)
Sunjita Patel, MD MD
License #

FIGURE 12.6
Patient Prescription and Insurance Card Data

Cobalt Care
Insurance card

KADE FROST
BIN: 10132
ID: ZVD526478695

GROUP: 22764
RELATIONSHIP: 02, SPOUSE

MEMBER SERVICES: 1-800-555-3232
CLAIMS/INQUIRIES: 1-800-555-6363

Rx
Robert Margerison, MD
Peter Blankenship, MD
Richard Burgraff, MD
Cassandra Poll, MD
7658 Apollo Str. Washington, DC 20001
(202) 555-2121 fax: (202) 555-2323

DOB Sept 03, 1994 DEA#
Pt. name Kade Frost Date 04/09/2019
Address 573 K Street NW
Washington, DC 20001

Truvada
30 (Thirty)
1 po qd

Refill 0 times (no refill unless indicated)
Robert Margerison MD
License #

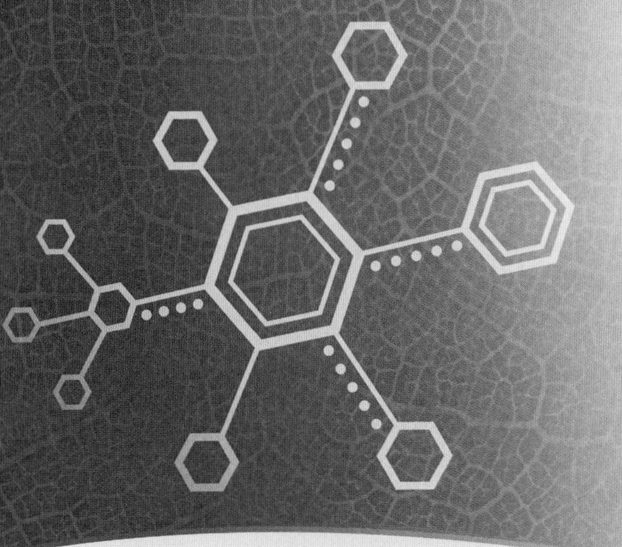

13

Verifying Cash Pricing

Learning Objectives

1 Understand the reasons for cash price payments in the community pharmacy.

2 Demonstrate proficiency in the use of computer software for prescription pricing.

Supplies

- NRx-based tutorial and assessments, available on the Course Navigator

Access additional chapter resources.

Previous prescription-preparation labs in this book have focused on patients who have a third-party, or insurance, plan. When a patient has insurance, the third party covers part of the prescription cost, and the patient often pays a set price, known as the **copay** amount, for the prescription. In copay situations, patients know that their cost will remain consistent. However, on some occasions, a pharmacy may not be able to accept a patient's insurance plan. As a pharmacy technician, you will then need to determine, or verify, how much the patient must pay for the prescription. This payment figure is known as the **cash price**.

Several factors can make cash price payment necessary. Sometimes a patient's insurance coverage is rejected because the patient is from another area of the country and the pharmacy is not contracted with the patient's insurance plan. At other times, the patient's insurance plan simply does not cover certain medications. When patients do not have a specific prescription benefit under the insurance coverage they carry, they must pay the cash price for the prescription. If applicable, they can then submit receipts to their insurance company for reimbursement under their medical benefits plan. In other cases, patients do not have any insurance coverage for prescriptions or have no health insurance at all, and cash price payment is their only option.

The cash price for prescriptions, like the price on most products sold in more than one outlet, can vary from pharmacy to pharmacy. Not all patients know this fact. Patients who must pay cash for their prescriptions and are aware of cash price variability will call many different pharmacies in their area to search for the best prescription price. Patients save money when using this smart shopping strategy, particularly when they do not have prescription coverage. Thus, in your pharmacy technician work, you will need to know how to look up cash prices for patients.

When you initiate such an inquiry within a computer software program, the screen will display several categories of information, often including the following:

- **Description** names the medication, whether brand or generic.
- **NDC number** is the National Drug Code.
- **Price plan** reveals the basis for the price, such as "cash pricing" (also known as "retail pricing").
- **Cost** displays what the pharmacy pays for the medication.
- **Markup** shows the amount of markup or the price increase to cover pharmacy operation costs.
- **Discount** notes any pricing discounts given to patients on this specific medication.
- **The % Profit-AWP** indicates the percentage of profit made from dispensing the medication compared with the average wholesale price, if available.
- **Acquisition cost** reveals how much it cost the pharmacy to purchase this amount of medication.
- **The % Profit-Margin** states the percentage of profit made above the cost of the medication.
- **Price** displays the price that should be quoted to the patient (notice that the size and prominence of the *Price* line make it easy for you to glance at the screen and quickly find this amount).

Procedure

In this lab, you will use the price quote feature of the NRx-based tutorial and assessments to verify cash pricing for the prescriptions listed on the worksheet at the end of the lab. As outlined above in the bulleted list, additional pieces of information will appear on screen for your reference.

1 Launch the Course Navigator learning management system. Click on Lab 13 in the left navigation pane, and then select Tutorials and Assessments. When the menu for all available labs appears, click the tutorial or assessment you wish to perform, beginning with Tutorial 13.1.

© Paradigm Publishing, Inc.

Usually several assessments are listed, representing the different patients you are processing through the computer software procedures. This lab is one of the few with only one assessment, Lab 13.2. Because all patient prescriptions are grouped together on one "Verifying Cash Pricing" worksheet at the end of this lab, no additional assessments are required.

2 The tutorial will launch in your browser, and you will be able to follow the steps online or in this lab manual. After you have completed the tutorial, you can complete the assessment for Lab 13.2.

3 When the NRx Security screen appears, log in to the NRx-based training software as the Primary User by typing STUDENT as the Login ID and PRACTICE as the Password. Click Log In.

4 On the Rx Processing Tasks menu, click Price Quote.

5 In the Drug field, enter the *first word* of the drug name (not the additional words or initials and not the numerals or units) as found on the lab worksheet at the end of the lab. Press Tab.

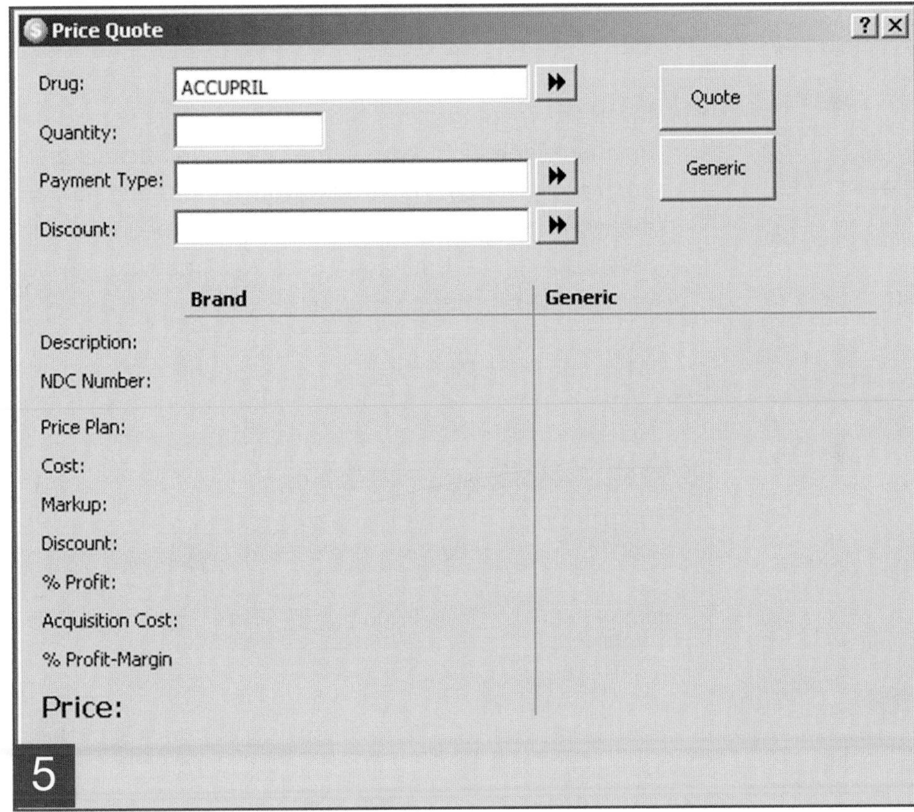

6 If the full drug name, strength, and form appear in the Drug field (because there is only one such drug to choose from and the software has populated the full details for you), you may proceed to Step 7. If the full drug description does not appear, the Drug Record Scan screen will appear instead (because the drug is manufactured in more than one strength or form, and you will have to choose). Carefully review your options. When you find the exact match to the drug listed on the worksheet, double-click it and proceed to Step 7.

TAKE NOTE

If multiple listings appear for the same drug description, be very careful to select the exact match by comparing the strength (for example, in milligrams, milliliters, and concentration) and the form (for example, as capsules, vials, and tablets). In some cases you will need to go a step further to eliminate a duplicate option. In those cases you must check that the number in the on-screen NDC column exactly matches the NDC number listed on the worksheet.

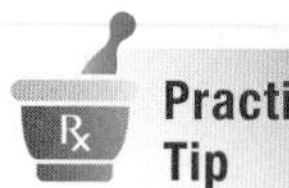

Practice Tip

As you proceed down the list of drugs on your worksheet, if the number you need to enter is already present in the Quantity field, simply press Tab.

7 When the Price Quote screen appears, make sure not to enter any data into the Discount field. If your cursor is not already there, click it in the Quantity field. Enter the quantity requested on the worksheet, and press Tab.

8 If you are entering the first drug, your cursor should now be in the Payment Type field. Type in the words "retail pricing," press Tab, and proceed to Step 9. However, if you are entering the remaining drugs on the worksheet, "retail pricing" will already be present in the Payment Type field, causing the Price Plan Scan to immediately appear. In those cases, you should proceed to Step 9.

9 When the Price Plan Scan appears, double-click Retail Pricing.

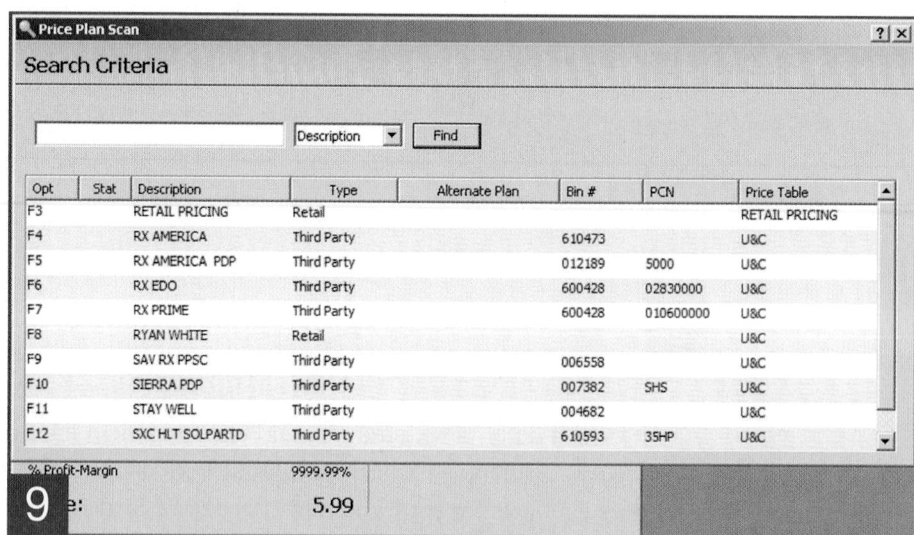

Price Plan Scan

Search Criteria

Description | Find

Opt	Stat	Description	Type	Alternate Plan	Bin #	PCN	Price Table
F3		RETAIL PRICING	Retail				RETAIL PRICING
F4		RX AMERICA	Third Party		610473		U&C
F5		RX AMERICA PDP	Third Party		012189	5000	U&C
F6		RX EDO	Third Party		600428	02830000	U&C
F7		RX PRIME	Third Party		600428	010600000	U&C
F8		RYAN WHITE	Retail				U&C
F9		SAV RX PPSC	Third Party		006558		U&C
F10		SIERRA PDP	Third Party		007382	SHS	U&C
F11		STAY WELL	Third Party		004682		U&C
F12		SXC HLT SOLPARTD	Third Party		610593	35HP	U&C

% Profit-Margin 9999.99%

9 e: 5.99

Practice Tip

Do not use the first price, the Cost, for the Acquisition Cost. You will find the Acquisition Cost farther down the list of data on the Price Quote screen. You will find the cash price in large, bold type at the very bottom, listed simply as "Price."

10 When the Price Quote screen returns, you will have the information you need to fill in the worksheet blanks. On the worksheet, record the requested data (the Acquisition Cost and the Cash Price) in the blanks on the right.

© Paradigm Publishing, Inc.

11 To determine the price for the next prescription listed on the worksheet, you may do one of the following:

11a If you need to change only the quantity and the drug name stays the same, click once on the existing quantity, which will disappear. Type in the new quantity. Press Tab two times. Repeat Steps 9 and 10.

11b If you need to change the drug name and quantity, click once on the existing drug name, which will disappear. Type in the next drug you wish to look up, and press Tab. Repeat Steps 6–10.

Be careful! Do not click the large red "X" found in the upper-right corner of the lab window. Doing so will close the entire lab, and your work will be lost.

12 When you have completed the worksheet for all 20 listed drugs and their quantity options, click the small black "X" in the upper-right corner of the Price Quote screen.

13 The Rx Processing Tasks menu will appear briefly. The tutorial will end. Click Close to close the tutorial and return to the Course Navigator.

14 **Conclusion:** Complete the tutorial and assessment 13.2. Sign, date, and tear out both pages of your completed worksheet, and turn it in to your instructor. Then go to the Course Navigator, answer all questions in the Lab Review section, and submit your answers to your instructor.

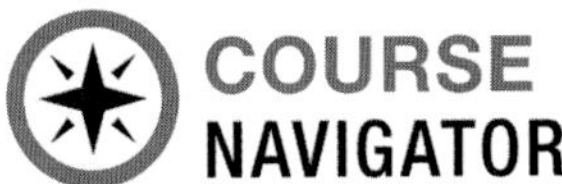

Access interactive chapter review exercises, practice activities, flash cards, and study games.

© Paradigm Publishing, Inc.

Name: ______________________ Date: ______________

Lab 13 Verifying Cash Pricing

Worksheet for Verifying Cash Pricing

Drug Description	NDC	QTY	Acquisition Cost ($)	Cash Price ($)
1. Accupril 10 mg tablets (from Tutorial 13.1)	00071-0530-23	30	________	________
2. Lorazepam 0.5 mg tablets	00378-0321-05	120	________	________
		60	________	________
3. Cephalexin 500 mg capsules	00093-3147-05	40	________	________
4. Alprazolam 2 mg tablets	00781-1089-05	120	________	________
5. Ciprofloxacin ER 500 mg tablets	00378-1743-89	28	________	________
		14	________	________
6. Humalog 100 units/mL vial	00002-7510-01	20	________	________
		10	________	________
7. Zolpidem tartrate 10 mg tablets	00054-0087-29	10	________	________
		5	________	________
8. Phenobarbital 64.8 mg tablets	00603-5167-32	90	________	________
9. Xalatan 125 mcg/2.5 mL	0013-8303-04	2.5	________	________
10. Amoxil 250 mg per 5 mL suspension	00029-6009-22	150	________	________
		75	________	________
11. Gentamicin 3 mg per mL drops	00168-0178-03	10	________	________

© Paradigm Publishing, Inc.

12.	Zyprexa 15 mg tablets	00002-4415-30	30	______	______
13.	Prednisone 2.5 mg tablets	00054-8740-25	32	______	______
			20	______	______
14.	Fluoxetine HCl 20 mg capsules	00406-0663-01	30	______	______
15.	Methylphenidate 20 mg tablets	00781-5754-01	60	______	______
			30	______	______
16.	Truvada 200 mg/300 mg tablets	61958-0701-07	30	______	______
			90	______	______
17.	Promethazine with codeine syrup	00472-1628-16	180	______	______
			473	______	______
18.	Azithromycin 250 mg tablets, Pack of 6	00093-7146-18	6	______	______
19.	Simvastatin 20 mg tablets	00093-7154-93	30	______	______
20.	Viagra 100 mg tablets	00069-4220-66	30	______	______
			10	______	______
			5	______	______

© Paradigm Publishing, Inc.

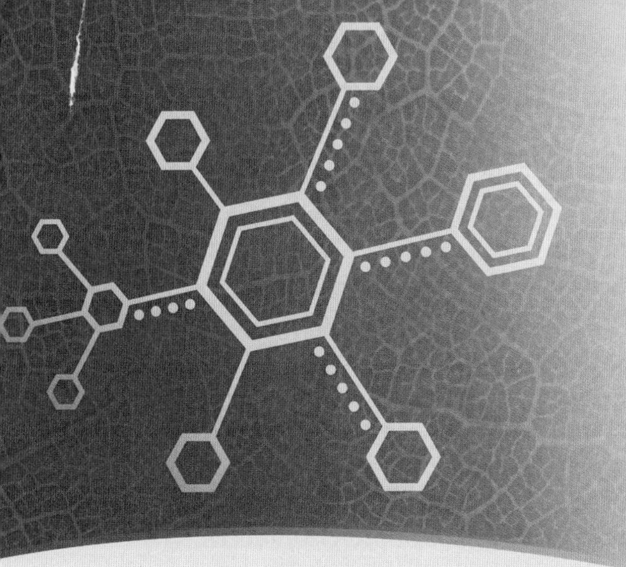

14

Producing an Audit Log

Learning Objectives

1 Demonstrate a basic understanding of using pharmacy management software for pharmacy audit log reporting.

2 Become more informed about the evolving roles of the pharmacist and the pharmacy technician in pharmacy administration.

Supplies

- NRx-based tutorials and assessments, available on the Course Navigator.

Access additional chapter resources.

Pharmacy technicians play a central role in assisting the pharmacist with prescription preparation in the community pharmacy setting. Such assistance improves when you are familiar with a variety of hard-copy and online resources and are confident about navigating within pharmacy software programs. When you take the initiative on a large number of daily responsibilities, both on the computer screen and at the counter, the pharmacist can focus on other duties, such as verifying prescriptions, counseling patients, administering immunizations, managing medication therapies, and overseeing the many components of pharmacy administration.

Medication Therapy Management is an area of increasing importance in pharmacy. This collaborative oversight of a patient's medications is covered more indepth in Lab 15.

The vast majority of these administrative duties requires the education and professional judgment of a licensed pharmacist. However, because the role of the pharmacist continues to shift toward patient **medication therapy management** tasks (the collaborative oversight of a patient's medications and their delivery), pharmacy technicians are increasingly assuming positions of greater administrative responsibility. Experienced pharmacy technicians, in particular, are moving up newly emerging and developing career ladders within independent and locally owned pharmacies and within hospital systems. Pharmacy technicians are also working as specialists, supervisors, and managers at all levels within the broader pharmaceutical industry. As the role of the pharmacist within direct patient care and medication therapy management continues to evolve, future pharmacy technicians will likely be asked to apply themselves to multiple pharmacy operations tasks.

One relatively new role that pharmacy technicians are taking on within pharmacy administration is report production. While several kinds of reports—including inventory management, pricing, accounts receivable, accounts payable, billing, third-party receipts, DEA prescribing, HIPAA compliance, controlled substance compliance, prescriber, and drug reports—can be run with pharmacy management software, the audit log is a frequently produced and reviewed report. The audit log provides (for a designated time period programmed by the user) a list of pharmacists who logged in to the computer system, the total number of prescriptions filled under each person's user ID, and a recap of every prescription filled. The log is often run at the end of the day (for just that one-day period), as a daily summary of prescription sales. The log breaks down those sales into four categories: first, a line-by-line list of prescriptions filled; second and third, newly filled prescriptions and refilled prescriptions broken down according to payment plan (cash price, Medicaid, or third party); and fourth, a cost analysis breakdown by payment plan. Details for each category include the following:

- **Line-by-line list of prescriptions filled:** This part of the log provides the prescription number, patient name, prescriber name, transaction number, drug name, quantity dispensed, dosage form unit (tablet, capsule, milliliter, etc.), original quantity prescribed, drug class, number of refills remaining, pharmacist logged in at the time, original date of prescription, date of last fill, price description, and price paid for each prescription.
- **Newly filled prescriptions by payment plan and refilled prescriptions by payment plan:** These parts of the log list the number of prescriptions filled for each payment plan, cost of each prescription, amount charged or billed for the total quantity of prescriptions, and **profit margin** (the difference between the pharmacy's prescription cost and amount charged to the patient or insurance provider) in dollars and also by percentage.
- **Cost analysis by payment plan:** This part of the log lists the number of prescriptions filled for each payment plan (cash price, Medicaid, and third party), total cost of prescriptions filled for each payment plan, total billed amount for all prescriptions, discounts applied to the price, amount of copays collected, applicable sales tax, profit margin (in dollars and by percentage) for the total prescriptions, average price, and average dollar profit margin for each payment plan.

Pharmacy management staff rely on the large amount of information provided by the audit log to estimate total profits, losses, overhead costs, and future sales and to schedule staff days and hours. You can contribute to pharmacy operations by using and understanding the audit log as part of your

© Paradigm Publishing, Inc.

pharmacy work. Building your awareness of the capabilities of the audit log and other pharmacy software reports increases your pharmacy management skills and adds value to your professional record, enhancing your ability to serve the pharmacy and its patients and, subsequently, to advance within the pharmacy profession.

Procedure

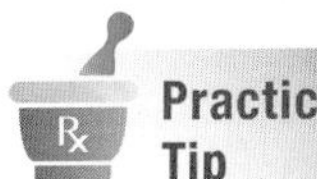

Practice Tip

Usually several assessments are listed, representing the different patients you are processing through the computer software procedures. This lab is one of the few with only one assessment, 14.2. Because all patient prescriptions are grouped together, printed on one audit log report, and examined further on the lab worksheet, no additional assessments are required.

In this lab, you will generate an audit log report and answer worksheet questions based upon on the report data.

1 Log in to the Course Navigator, and select Lab 14 from the left navigation pane. Then select Tutorials and Assessments.

2 Click the tutorial or assessment you wish to perform, beginning with tutorial 14.1.

3 When the NRx Security screen appears, log in to the NRx-based training software as the Primary User by typing STUDENT as the Login ID and PRACTICE as the Password. Click Log In.

4 Above the Rx Processing Tasks menu, click Reports on the topmost menu bar. On the menu that drops down, click Management, and on the next drop-down menu, click Daily Audit.

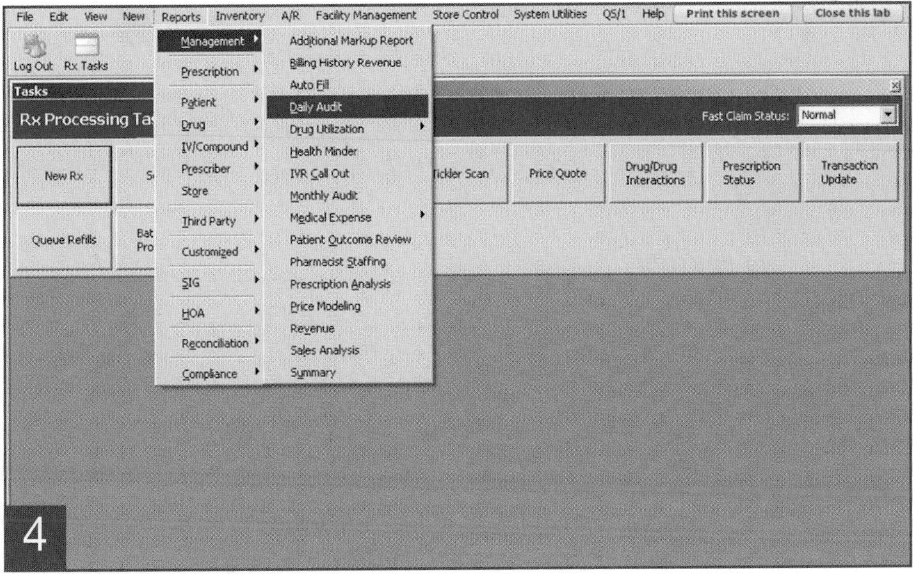

In your pharmacy work, you will probably be asked to produce an audit log report for a single, specific date and would enter that date in MM/DD/YY format. For example, if you wanted to process a report for December 21, 2019, you would enter the date as 12/21/19. At times you might also be asked to type in a range of dates or, as you do for this lab, to request a report for all available dates in the system.

5 The Select Options screen will appear. Click your cursor under the Value column, on the line corresponding to field [RX Transaction].Date Filled *Dflt. When a blank field opens up under your cursor, type in the word "All." Leave all other fields in their default, preset states, and click Next or press Enter.

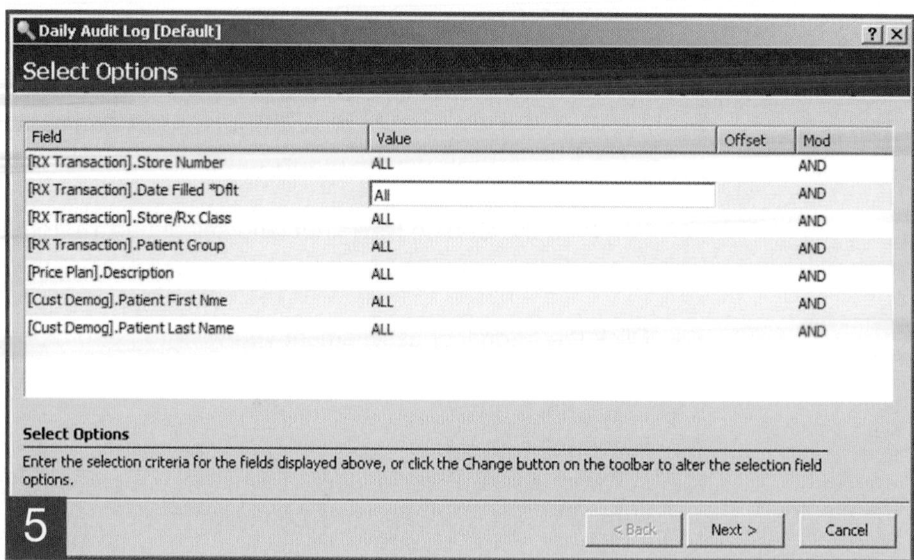

TAKE NOTE

The preset options are established for the purposes of this basic audit log lab. Because you are not yet trained to practice more detailed reports or more complex prescription processes, we are not discussing the advanced audit log report features in this lab. When you are at work in the field, you will be specifically trained to take advantage of additional pharmacy software capabilities to create the kinds of audit log reports (such as daily, monthly, drug-based, patient-outcome-based, and so on) that are useful to your individual pharmacy.

6 The Sort Options screen will appear. For the purposes of this lab, leave all values in their preset order, and click Next.

© Paradigm Publishing, Inc.

In pharmacy practice, you would be able to adjust these fields so that your audit log report is organized to meet your pharmacy's needs. For example, you could sort the data by store (if you are part of a larger chain of stores), by date filled, by prescription drug class (Schedules II, III, etc.), or by prescription number.

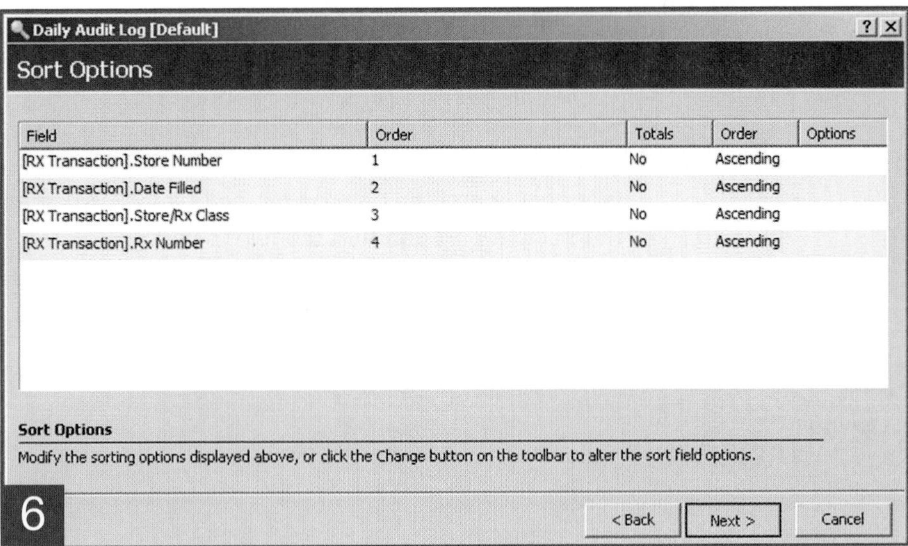

7 The Print Option Values screen will appear. Again, for the purposes of this lab, leave all values in their preset states, and click Finish.

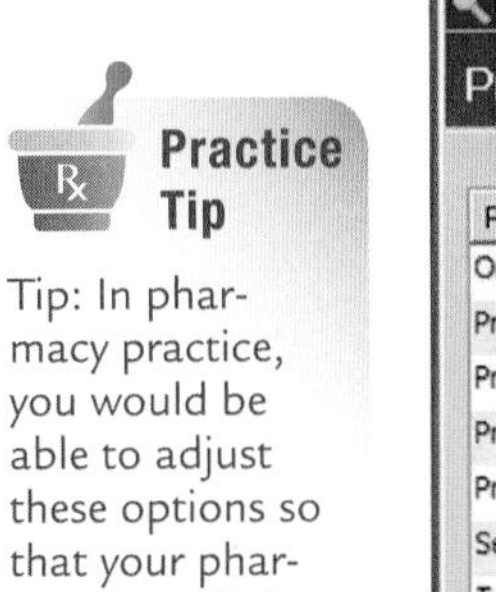

Tip: In pharmacy practice, you would be able to adjust these options so that your pharmacy's audit log report includes or excludes certain data, such as prescription signa, new prescriptions, or summary report totals.

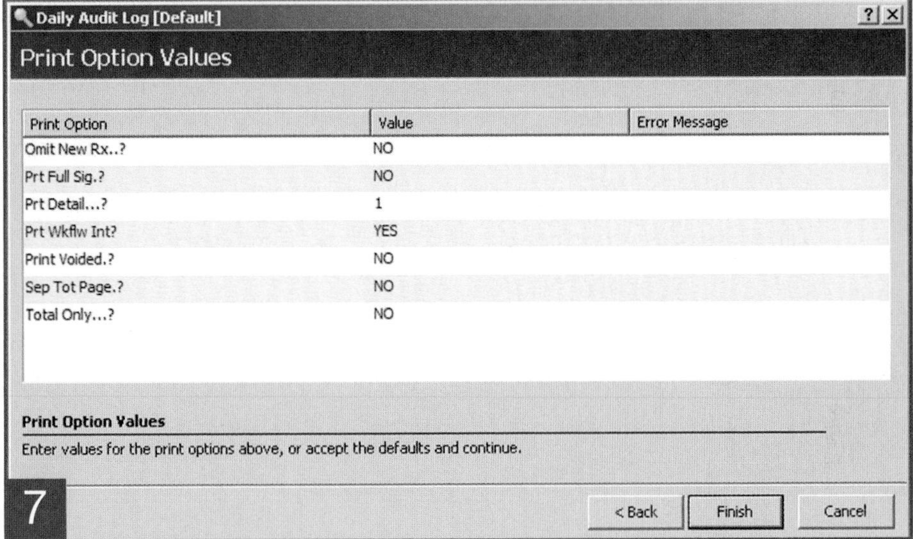

8 A preview of the audit log report for your pharmacy, The Corner Drug Store, will appear. Click Print this screen in the upper-right corner of the report screen.

9 A small window associated with your local printer options will appear. For this report to print properly, you will need to go into the Properties area of your printer options dialog box and select a *landscape* orientation for the layout. Click as necessary to make the remaining selections for your local printer to print the screen. When you are certain that the audit log report has printed, click Next at the bottom of the audit log report preview screen.

© Paradigm Publishing, Inc.

10 Repeat steps 1-9 to complete assessment 14.2.

11 **Conclusion:** Pick up the audit log report from the printer, and use it to answer the questions on the worksheet at the end of the lab. Write your name and the date on the completed worksheet and the printed audit log report and turn them in to your instructor. Then go to the Course Navigator, answer all questions in the Lab Review section, and submit your answers to your instructor.

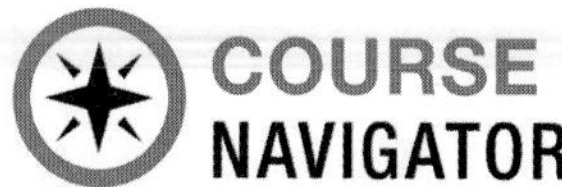

Access interactive chapter review exercises, practice activities, flash cards, and study games.

 © Paradigm Publishing, Inc.

Name: ______________________________ Date: ________________

Lab 14 Producing an Audit Log

Worksheet Based on Printed Audit Log Report

1. What prices did the following people pay for their prescriptions?

   a. Kimberly Jackson ____________

   b. Miguel Esparza ____________

   c. Marquita Wilkins ____________

   d. Lily Nguyen ____________

   e. Vance Donaldson ____________

   f. Jeffrey Klein (his C-II) ____________

   g. Amala Gupta ____________

   h. Cas Riley ____________

   i. Marco Domingo (for two prescriptions) ____________

   j. Brian Koch ____________

   k. Felicity Wruck (for two prescriptions) ____________

   l. Allison Sutter ____________

   m. Bradley Malloy (for two prescriptions) ____________

   n. Brenda Kreuger ____________

   o. Kade Frost ____________

2. What is the total amount collected by the pharmacy on the report? ____________
3. What is the total amount of copays collected on the report? ____________
4. What was the total average price for all prescriptions on the report? ____________
5. How many prescriptions did the pharmacist on duty fill? ____________
6. How many prescriptions were paid via third party? ____________
7. How many prescriptions were paid via cash pricing? ____________
8. What is the control schedule of Ms. Nguyen's Alprazolam? ____________

© Paradigm Publishing, Inc.

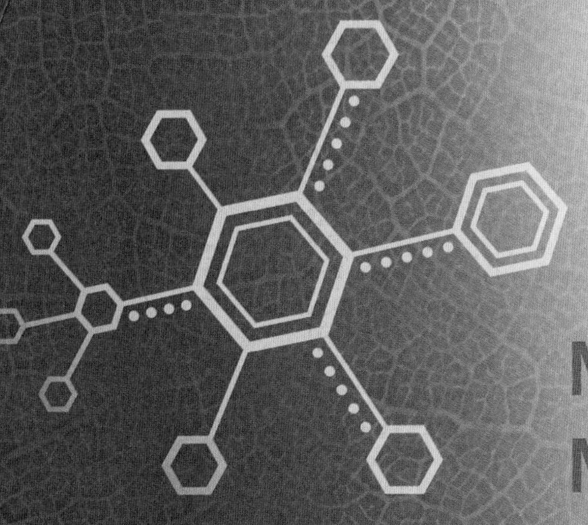

15

Medication Therapy Management

Learning Objectives

1. Identify the purpose of medication therapy management.
2. Describe the role of pharmacy personnel in medication therapy management.
3. Identify the responsibilities of the pharmacy technician in medication therapy management.
4. Review a patient profile and collect information for use in medication therapy management.

Supplies

- Medication therapy management forms

Access additional chapter resources.

Pharmacy practice continues to evolve, with pharmacists focusing more on the direct education and care of patients. Pharmacists' increased scope of practice includes administration of immunizations and improving the outcome of treatment through medication therapy management (MTM). **Medication therapy management** is a patient-focused, multistep process where a pharmacist may meet with a patient and his or her primary healthcare provider, such as a physician, nurse practitioner, or physician assistant, to recommend adjustments to the patient's medication therapy for better results. These adjustments may include the use of less expensive medications, the identification of potential medication interactions or adverse reactions, counseling on the best use of medications and durable medical equipment, counseling on complying with the medication regimen, and providing helpful information regarding disease-state management. Because this process is increasingly important to the long-term health of patients, a pharmacist may receive additional reimbursement from pharmacy benefit managers and other insurance companies for providing these specialized services.

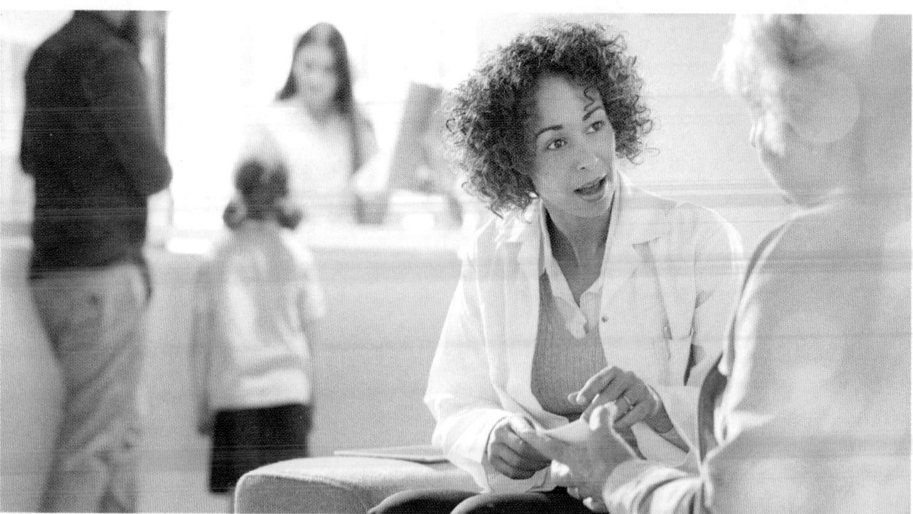

Patients meet with the pharmacist to discuss many different aspects of their medications, such as less expensive alternatives, possible medication interactions, and complying with the medication regimen.

MTM is a recognized practice by many states regulators and by federal law. The Medicare Modernization Act of 2003 identified three goals for MTM services: provide patient education and increase patients' understanding of their medications; improve medication compliance and adherence; and detect adverse reactions, including the misuse of medications. The practice of MTM requires professional judgment and special knowledge. Because of such knowledge, acquired during their education to earn the doctor of pharmacy degree and professional licensure, pharmacists are well equipped and qualified to work with other healthcare professionals in the provision of MTM services. Professional organizations such as the American Pharmacists Association (APhA), American Association of Colleges of Pharmacy (AACP), American College of Clinical Pharmacy (ACCP), and National Association of Chain Drug Stores (NACDS) endorse the model of pharmacist-led MTM. Many of these organizations also provide programs for pharmacists to earn specialty certification in the practice of MTM.

The MTM process is not as simple as the traditional method of filling a prescription and counseling a patient about his or her prescription. The MTM process is far more in-depth and requires significant communication and documentation, and its success can be measured by the improved health outcomes of patients.

Pharmacy technicians assist in the MTM process by facilitation of scheduling, patient coordination, data collection, research, chart construction, identification of health histories, documentation, and billing. These responsibilities do not always require the professional judgment of a pharmacist; however, they are often the barriers to the successful implementation of an MTM program due to limitations in time and the other required duties performed by pharmacists. As the front line in pharmacy care, pharmacy technicians are well-equipped to perform these vital tasks. By coordinating care, establishing appointments, and collecting data, pharmacy technicians facilitate the care of patients, which can lead to improved health outcomes.

© Paradigm Publishing, Inc.

The Information Collected in MTM

The information gathered in the process of building a patient chart can vary greatly depending on the scope of the pharmacy practice setting and the MTM appointment—an initial visit is much different than a follow-up or maintenance visit.

The most common points of data used in MTM include the following:

TABLE 15.1 Most Common Data Points Used in MTM

Data Point	Description	Example
Patient Name	Full name of the patient	Vance Michael Donaldson
Patient Address	Physical address	12 Maple Leaf Trail Round Rock, TX 78644
Date of Birth	Actual birth date	May 5, 1987
Gender	Identified patient gender	Male
Medical ID/ Record Number	Patient Unique Identifier (if applicable) from a medical chart, medication administration record, patient profile, or insurance card (not a Social Security number)	7751029
Height	Patient's height	6 ft/180 cm
Weight	Patient's weight	180 lbs/81.65 kg
Telephone Contact	Primary telephone number	(512) 555-1212
Medical History	Any historical information, such as diagnosis, medical conditions, allergies, and surgical procedures	Hypertension Allergy to penicillin No previous surgical procedures
Current Medication Regimen	A list of any prescription and OTC medications currently or recently taken by the patient, including name, strength, frequency of use, date started, date stopped, why stopped, and refill information	Accupril 10 mg Once daily Started May 5, 2016 Has not stopped 4 refills remain
Adherence Information	Information from the patient about whether he or she takes the medication as directed	"No, I sometimes forget to take my medication."
Additional Patient Information	Noticed side effects, general feeling, and quality of life	Patient indicates feeling of improved quality of life with no noticed adverse effect.
Primary Care Provider	Name and contact information for patient's primary care provider	Dr. Gregory Smythe (512) 555-1313
Lab Tests and Values	Relevant lab values to determine safety and effectiveness of drug therapy	International Normalized Ratio (INR) Prothrombin Time (PT), value of 2.2
Follow-Up Information	Any updates, instructions, and handouts for use by the patient for his or her follow-up appointment	Patient handouts, monograms, durable medical equipment, and other materials

Pharmacy technicians are perfectly poised to assist the pharmacist in providing MTM through the careful collection of data from patients. As pharmacy technicians are often the first and last people a patient will encounter while at a pharmacy, they have the opportunity to learn a lot about their patients. Thus, they play an important part in this complex, time-consuming, and critical process.

Procedure

In this lab, you will practice reviewing a patient profile and collecting relevant patient information for use by the pharmacist in an MTM session. You will become familiar with the most common data points used by a pharmacist in an interaction with a patient.

1. Using the information provided in Figures 15.1 and 15.2, complete two copies of the MTM form. Additional forms can be downloaded from the Course Navigator and printed out.

2. If a piece of information cannot be found or is unknown, clearly make a note on the form. Failing to do so could cause harm to the patient.

3. Complete one MTM form for the pharmacist and one for the patient. For documentation used by the pharmacist or other healthcare providers, the use of signa abbreviations is acceptable. For documentation used by a patient, use simple English. Remember to write clearly and legibly.

4. **Conclusion:** Turn in the completed worksheets to your instructor. Then go to the Course Navigator, answer all questions in the Lab Review section, and submit your answers to your instructor.

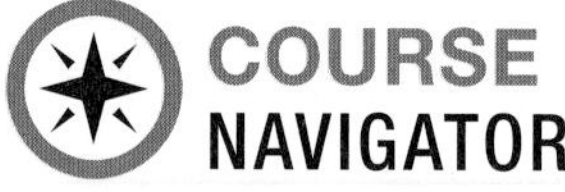

Access interactive chapter review exercises, practice activities, flash cards, and study games.

 © Paradigm Publishing, Inc.

FIGURE 15.1

++
++ MEDICATION HISTORY REPORT --- DATES: 04 APR 2018 TO 09 NOV 2019 ++
++

For: Donaldson, Vance (MALE)
Address: 12 MAPLE LEAF TRAIL
Round Rock, TX 78664
Birthdate: 05/15/1987
SSN: *** - ** - ****
RN: 8544218
Allergies: NKDA
Conditions: Hypertension

THE CORNER DRUG STORE
17 MAIN STREET
AUSTIN, TX 78704
PHARMACIST ON DUTY: JPS
Store Phone No.: (512) 555-1414
Provider No.: 4599992 DEA: FC1234563

DATE	RX # New/RF	DRUG/ITEM NAME NDC	QTY D/S	PRESCRIBER DEA #	PRICE	INS B/G
04/09/2019	6001012 RF	ACCUPRIL 10MG TAB 00071-0530-23	30 30D	G. SMYTHE FS1234563	20.00	Y B
03/09/2019	6001012 RF	ACCUPRIL 10MG TAB 00071-0530-23	30 30D	G. SMYTHE FS1234563	20.00	Y B
02/09/2019	6001012 RF	ACCUPRIL 10MG TAB 00071-0530-23	30 30D	G. SMYTHE FS1234563	20.00	Y B
02/09/2019	6005142 NEW	AZITHROMYCIN 250MG 00093-7146-18	6 5D	G. SMYTHE FS1234563	10.00	Y G
02/09/2019	2001143 NEW	VICODIN 5MG/300MG 00074-3041-53	20 5D	G. SMYTHE FS1234563	10.00	Y G
01/09/2019	6001012 RF	ACCUPRIL 10MG TAB 00071-0530-23	30 30D	G. SMYTHE FS1234563	20.00	Y B
12/09/2018	6001012 RF	ACCUPRIL 10MG TAB 00071-0530-23	30 30D	G. SMYTHE FS1234563	20.00	Y B
11/15/2018	6002076 NEW	AZITHROMYCIN 250MG 00093-7146-18	6 5D	G. SMYTHE FS1234563	10.00	Y G
11/09/2018	6001012 NEW	ACCUPRIL 10MG TAB 00071-0530-23	30 30D	G. SMYTHE FS1234563	20.00	Y B

++
++++++++++++++++++ END OF MEDICATION HISTORY REPORT ++++++++++++++++++
++

FIGURE 15.2

PHARMACY MEDICATION REPORT: SOUTHERN CALIFORNIA GENERAL HOSPITAL
1574 MEDICAL VISTA BLVD, IRVINE, CA 92617
TEL: 657-555-2000 PROV#: 55214875

PATIENT INFORMATION >>

Sutter, Allison M. MRN: 446378294 FEMALE DOB: 10/28/1975 HHGRTF
5672 Pas Robles Way Irvine, CA 92614 TEL: 657-555-8634
ALLERGIES: Penicillin PCP: Patterson, RHT: 160 cm WT:____
DX: APPENDICITIS ICD-10: K35.2
DATE of Admission: 04-15-2019 Discharge: 04-17-2019

PT admitted to ER for acute appendicitis	04-15-2019	0700	DR. Z. Janowski, Surgeon
XFER to surgical for immediate appendectomy	04-15-2019	0830	DR. Z. Janowski, Surgeon
XFER to PACU	04-15-2019	1350	DR. Z. Janowski, Surgeon
XFER to Med-Surg	04-15-2019	1615	DR. M. PHILLIPS, Hospitalist
PT DISCHARGE	04-17-2019	1730	DR. M. PHILLIPS, Hospitalist

PT MEDICATION DISCHARGE LIST

FLUOXETINE 20MG	Take 1 capsule by mouth daily	QTY: 30	Status: ACTIVE
LOVENOX 20MG	INJECT 20MG IM once a day > LAB VALUE > INR PT: 2.00	QTY: 10 04162019	Status: ACTIVE
CIPROFLOXACIN XR 500MG	Take 1 tablet by mouth once daily for 10 days	QTY: 10	Status: Active
TYLENOL w/CODEINE #3	Take 1-2 tablets by mouth every 4 to 6 hours as needed for pain. Not to exceed 4,000 mg of APAP in 24 hours.	QTY: 40	Status: Active
~~DIAZEPAM 5MG~~	~~Take 1 tablet by mouth~~ every 8 hours as needed	~~QTY: 10~~	~~Status:~~ discontinue

Patient to attend a follow-up appointment with Dr. Phillips on April 27, 2019 at 1pm and with Dr. Patterson on April 29, 2019 at 10:30am.

 © Paradigm Publishing, Inc.

Name: ______________________ Date: ______________

Lab 15 Medication Therapy Management

Worksheet

Patient Name: ______________________ DOB: __________ Gender: ______

Ht: _____ Wt: _____ Date of Session: ____________ Patient Record Number: ________

Allergies: ______________________ Diagnosis: ______________________

Address: ____

Telephone: ______________ PCP: ______________________________

Medical Conditions: ____

Surgical History: ____

Medication and Compliance Information: ______________________________

Lab Values: ____

Recommendations: ____

Follow-up: ____

Pharmacist Signature

Pharmacist Name/License No.

Date

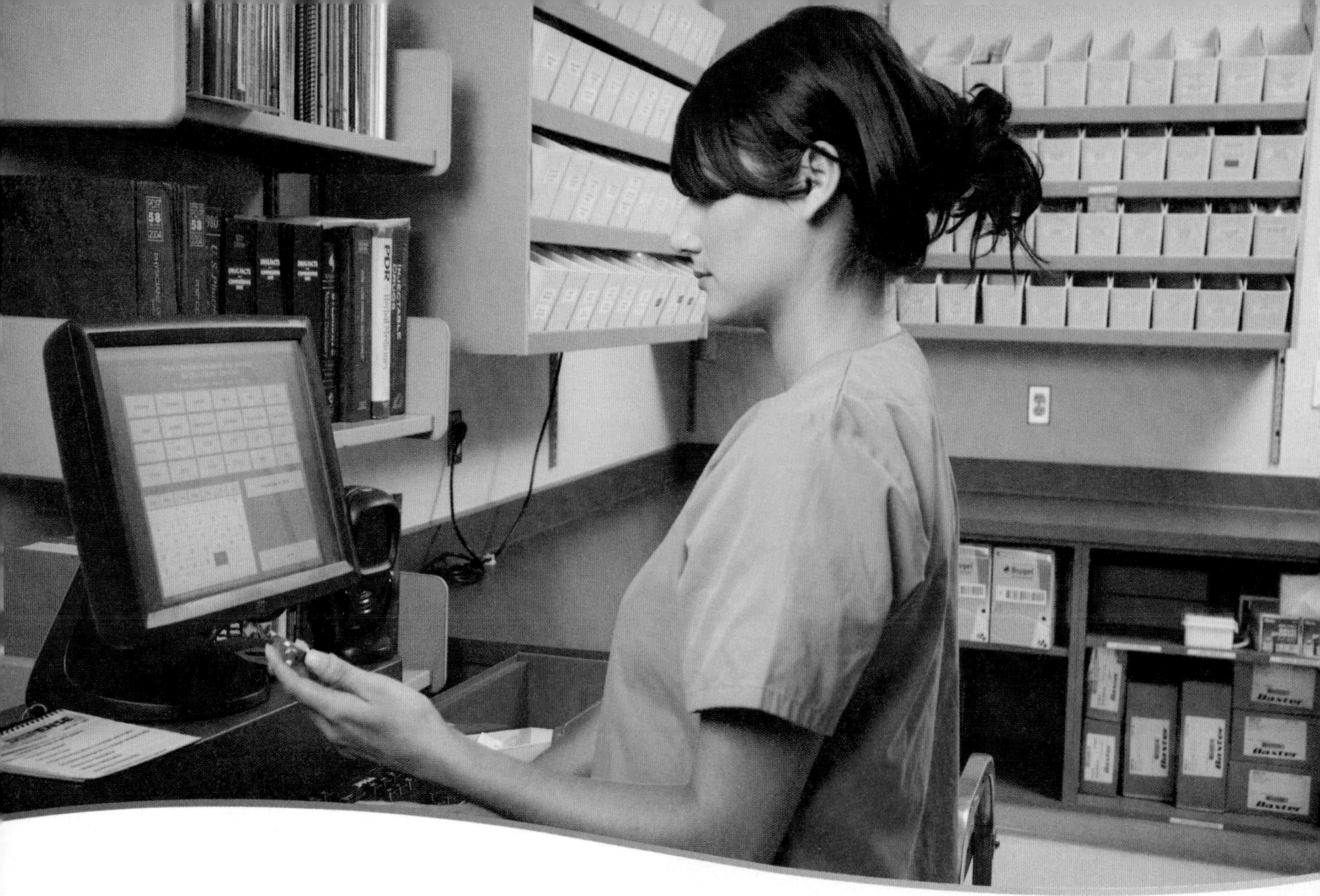

UNIT 3 Institutional Pharmacy Practice

A day in the life of a pharmacy technician...

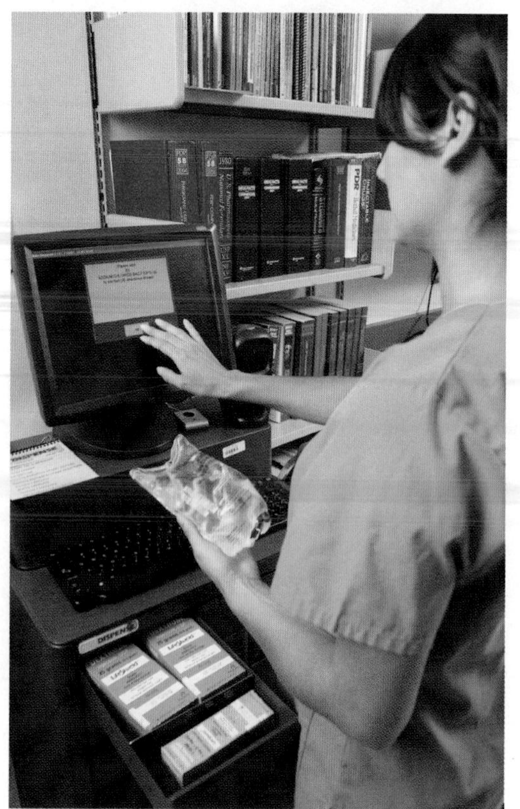

An ambulance pulls into the emergency room and doctors, nurses, and support staff throughout the hospital function as a team to care for the critically ill or injured patient. Multiple STAT medication orders arrive in the pharmacy for the newly admitted patient, along with a stack of urgent and routine orders for the hundreds of hospital patients who are undergoing treatment. The phone is ringing with doctors requesting drug information and nurses needing medication refills, or looking for a missing dose. Pharmacists are busy verifying medication orders sent through the computerized prescriber order entry (CPOE) system. Technicians are processing new orders, and the pneumatic tube system is dropping off more medication orders and refill requests. There is a backlog of crash carts to fill, floor stock is ready to be checked, and there is a unit clerk at the pharmacy window waiting to pick up medicine for a patient in the intensive care unit.

What is your role? How do pharmacy technicians function seamlessly in what amounts to controlled chaos?

Pharmacy technicians are vital members of the hospital team. All members of the team—physicians, nurses, pharmacists, pharmacy technicians, and a multitude of other support staff—must work together to care for patients who are recovering from injuries, diseases, or surgical treatments. Each team member must know the role he or she plays in effective patient treatment. The pharmacy technician must perform numerous tasks with speed and accuracy. Timely treatment, based on the accurate and precise delivery of pharmaceuticals, is essential to a patient's recovery.

This unit will guide you in the essential tasks of the hospital pharmacy technician, including 24-hour cart fill, floor stock checking, crash cart preparation, narcotic record keeping, automated dispensing machine filling, medication order processing, and medication reconciliation.

Performing these important tasks with speed, while maintaining 100% accuracy, will make you an indispensable member of the healthcare team.

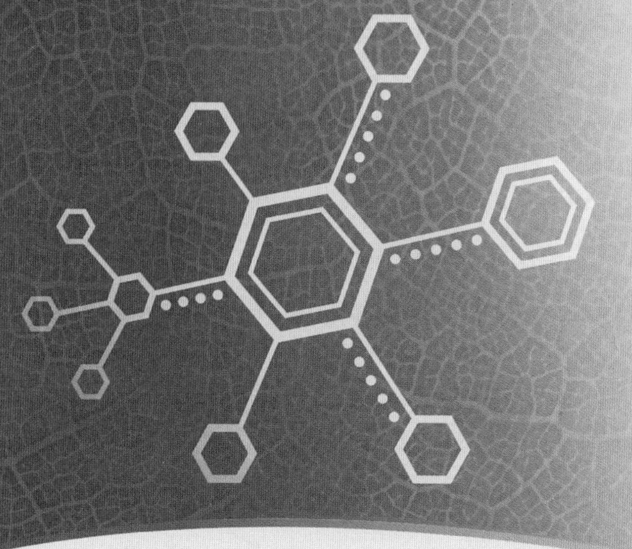

16

Filling a 24-Hour Medication Cart

Learning Objectives

1 Demonstrate proficiency in accurately performing a 24-hour cart fill.

2 Determine the location, label information, class, general use, signa, and abbreviations related to medications commonly used in a 24-hour cart fill.

3 Discuss the procedures for, and the importance of, each step in the 24-hour cart fill process.

Supplies

- Cart Fill Form
- Individual patient drawer, cassette, bin, or bag
- Access to a pharmacy lab stocked with common unit-dosed medications
- Access to standard pharmacy reference materials or the Internet

Access additional chapter resources.

The 24-hour cart fill is one of the most important basic functions that a pharmacy technician performs in institutional pharmacy practice. This process may be referred to as a *cart fill*, *medication pick*, *medication fill* or pick, or in similar terms as defined by the facility performing the procedure. Although cart fill specifics vary among institutions, the basic function is to quickly and accurately fill the required **unit-dosed** medications for one or more patients for a specified period of time. A **unit dose** is a medication packaged in a single-dose, one-time-use container. You might encounter slightly different terminology and procedures related to

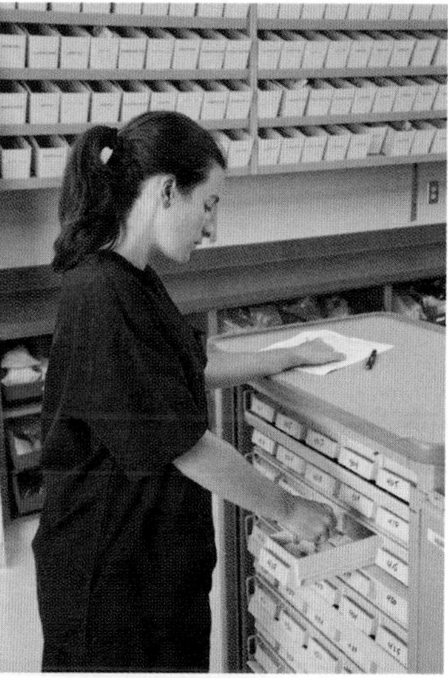

An important role of the pharmacy technician is to fill a medication cart.

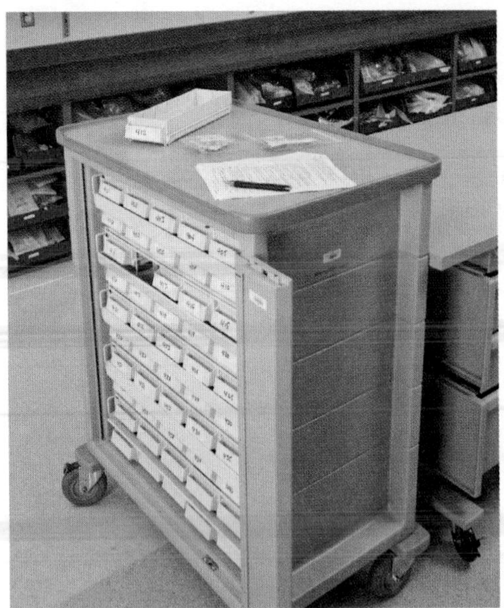

Medication cart

the process of filling a supply of medications for hospital patients.

For instance, some facilities might fill for a 24-hour supply, whereas others might fill for a 12-hour, 48-hour, 72-hour, or even 1-week supply. In addition, the container into which a facility places a patient's pick medications might be a drawer, tray, bin, cart, cassette, or resealable zipper bag. Some larger facilities even have automated robots instead of pharmacy technicians performing the cart fill.

Despite these differences, it is crucial that you always check the expiration date of every dose you put into the drawer. Rules regarding expiration dating vary from state to state, but they generally require that all medications used for cart fill have a minimum of one month of "good" dating left. If the dose's dating is not acceptable, then that dose may not be used in the cart fill.

Standard procedure requires filling the cart by referring to a Cart Fill Form or pick list. The form typically presents several categories of information:

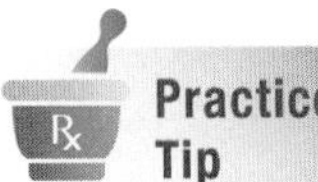

Practice Tip

In practice, you will often hear the terms "fast movers" to describe commonly prescribed medications, often kept in an area of the pharmacy that facilitates easy retrieval when filling the 24-hour medication cart, new prescriptions, or medication orders. The term "slow mover" refers to medications or pharmacy items that are not often prescribed. These are generally stored in an area of the pharmacy that is away from the busy, fast mover section.

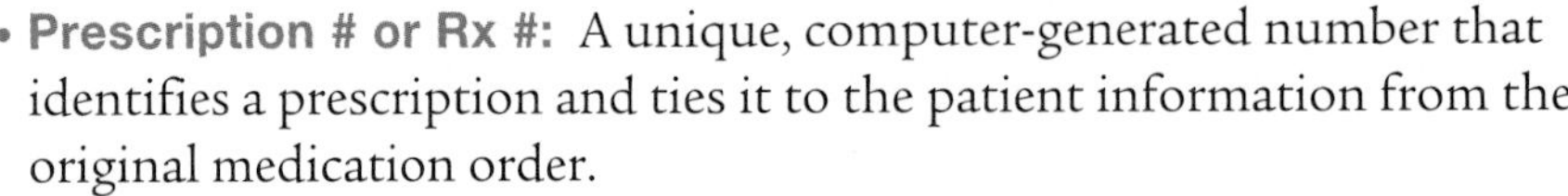

- **Prescription # or Rx #:** A unique, computer-generated number that identifies a prescription and ties it to the patient information from the original medication order.
- **Drug name:** Most hospitals arrange medications by generic name within various sections such as fast movers, slow movers, topicals, or injectables. Exceptions include combination drugs with more than one active ingredient, which are located under their brand names. However, such naming conventions may also vary between states and facilities.
- **Strength:** The strength of the individual tablet, capsule, ampule, or vial of the drug.
- **Directions:** The physician's directions for administration of the medication, including the route and the signa.
- **Number to dispense:** This number indicates the quantity of medication that you should place in the patient's drawer and is calculated based on the number of hours in the institution's fill period and the signa. Although in this lab you practice filling a medication cart based on a 24-hour fill period, the length of the fill period varies among institutions.

You will find an additional category on your Cart Fill Form, "Class or Primary Use," which is unique to this training lab. It has been added to help you learn the drug classifications and primary uses of many common medications.

© Paradigm Publishing, Inc.

Procedure

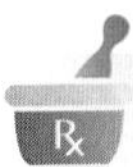

Practice Tip

In practice, you will fill 24-hour supplies of medications for multiple patients. Be sure to verify the patient's name and room number; or make use of barcode technology to ensure that you place the patient's medications into the correct drawer.

For this lab, you will perform a 24-hour cart fill for one patient. You will find one version of a Cart Fill Form (version 16.1) at the end of this lab. Do not begin filling out that form until your instructor offers guidance. While you *may* be assigned to fill out that particular form, your instructor may instead give you a different form (numbered 16.2 or higher). He or she will probably have several different Cart Fill Forms to hand out, differing slightly in the quantities and items being requested. This form variety will prevent students from all having to be in the same part of the room at the same time. Your lab work can flow more smoothly and be completed within the allotted class time if you work on different forms. Thus, please do not begin performing the steps below until your instructor informs you which Cart Fill Form to use.

1 Be sure to put your name and today's date on the Cart Fill Form.

2 Using the directions and signa, calculate how many doses you will need to fill a 24-hour supply of medications for the assigned patient. Write your answers for each medication in the "Number to Dispense" column on your Cart Fill Form.

3 Using pharmacy reference materials or the Internet, look up the class or primary use of each drug, and record the information on your Cart Fill Form in the "Class or Primary Use" column. Write a few words describing the class or primary use of each drug (e.g., antihypertensive, analgesic, used to lower blood sugar, or used to treat upper respiratory infections).

TAKE NOTE

When performing an actual cart fill, you will not be required to look up or record the class or primary use of the medication. For the purposes of this lab, looking up the drug information will help you to familiarize yourself with various drugs and their uses.

4 To help you locate the medication in the pharmacy, look up the brand/generic name of any drug on the Cart Fill Form that is unfamiliar to you.

5 Obtain the drugs you require from the appropriate pharmacy area. Be sure that each drug and its dose match exactly what is on the Cart Fill Form.

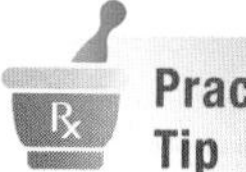

Practice Tip

Watch out for abbreviations such as EC, ER, SR, or CR. Drug names followed by these abbreviations are different from drugs of the same name without them

6 Place the appropriate amount of each drug into the patient's drawer (see the "Number to Dispense" column).

7 **Conclusion:** Fold up the completed Cart Fill Form, and place it in the drawer with the medications for your instructor to check. Then go to the Course Navigator, answer all questions in the Lab Review section, and submit your answers to your instructor.

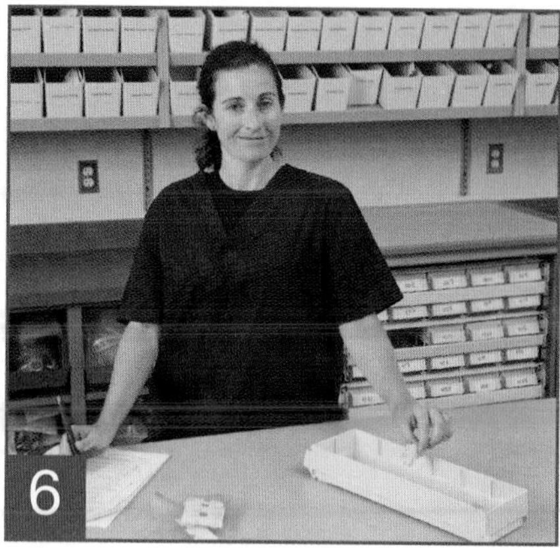

Pharmacy technician filling a medication cart drawer

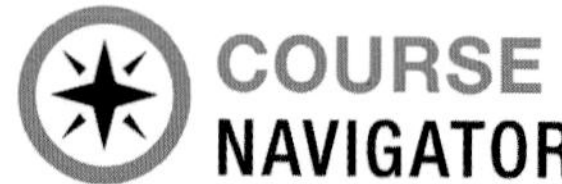

COURSE NAVIGATOR

Access interactive chapter review exercises, practice activities, flash cards, and study games.

© Paradigm Publishing, Inc.

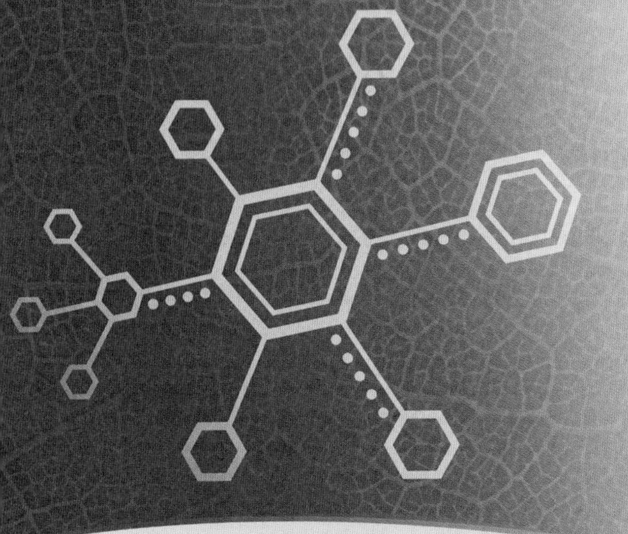

17 Filling and Checking Floor Stock

Learning Objectives

1 Demonstrate skill and accuracy in filling and checking floor stock.

2 Determine and discuss the rationale and procedures for filling and checking floor stock.

3 Identify the key terms and abbreviations used when filling floor stock.

Supplies

- Floor Stock Request Form (FSRF)
- Access to a pharmacy lab stocked with floor stock items
- Access to a brand/generic handbook, pharmacy resource materials, or the Internet

Access additional chapter resources.

Most hospitals keep a small supply of certain medications on each floor or unit. This supply is commonly referred to as **floor stock** or **unit stock**. The number and types of medications kept in floor stock vary between facilities and even between floors or units of the same hospital. Floor stock medications generally include those items that need to be administered immediately, such as nonnarcotic analgesics, antiemetics, antipyretics, and certain intravenous (IV) solutions.

Some institutions store floor stock items in an automated drug storage and dispensing system (ADSDS) that is located on each floor or unit. The ADSDS is specially designed for security and tracking of refilled and dispensed items. While there are many similarities between filling regular floor stock and filling an ADSDS, the procedure is somewhat different than what you will follow for this lab. For the purposes of this lab, you will follow procedures for filling the type of floor stock that is typically stored in a secure area of the nursing unit, but not in an ADSDS. You will learn more about filling an ADSDS in Lab 21.

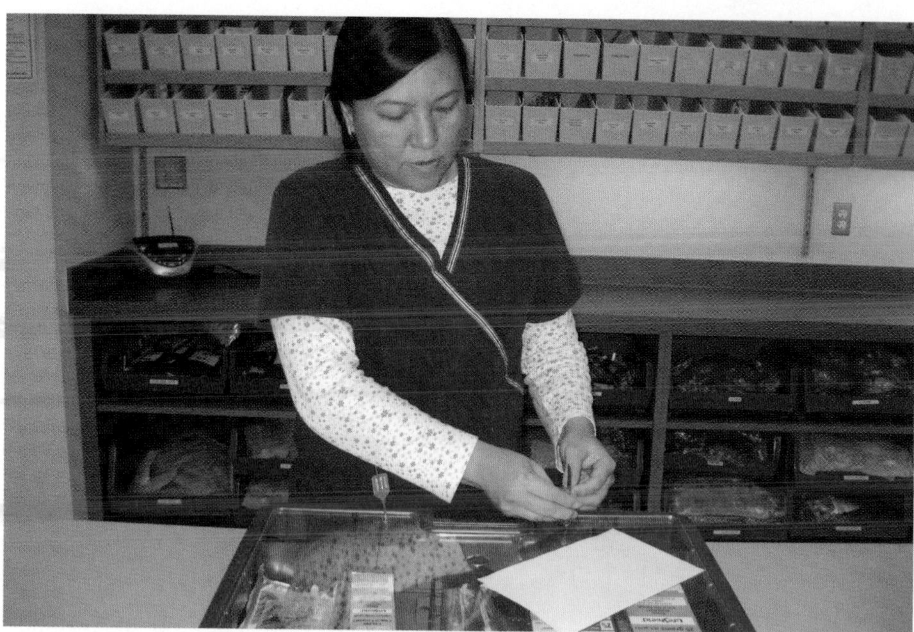

Pharmacy technician checking floor stock

When a pharmacy is very busy, the time it takes from the moment the physician writes an order until the pharmacy fills it and returns it to the nurse for administration—often referred to as the "turnaround time" of a pharmacy medication—can be quite long. The need to administer "STAT," "now," and initial doses quickly is the primary reason for having floor stock. Your timely and accurate filling and checking of floor stock items on the Floor Stock Request Form (FSRF) ensures that these medications are available to the nursing staff for immediate administration to patients.

Your role as a pharmacy technician requires familiarity with key terms used for filling and checking floor stock. Key terms include the following:

- **Unit:** The floor or nursing unit that placed the floor stock request. The unit may be identified by name, letter, abbreviation, or number (e.g., obstetrics, ICU, or fourth floor).
- **Par level:** The total amount of a particular medication that the requesting unit keeps on hand when fully stocked.
- **Fill #:** A number requested by designated nursing unit personnel to indicate the amount of each drug to be filled by the pharmacy in order to bring it up to par level. (The par level minus the actual amount on hand equals the fill #.)
- **Filled by:** The initials of the pharmacy staff member filling the FSRF.
- **Checked by:** The initials of the pharmacy staff member checking the FSRF.
- **The double check:** This procedure takes place when pharmacy technicians do both floor stock procedures (filling and checking) rather than having a pharmacist, nurse, or other hospital staff member check a technician's fill work. The double check is allowed in many, but not all, states.

 © Paradigm Publishing, Inc.

You should be aware that standard floor stock generally does not include the following:

- **Critical care medications:** Critical care items are commonly kept in a crash cart that is brought to the bedside for emergency administration to patients experiencing respiratory or cardiac arrest.
- **Medications requiring pharmacy compounding:** Some medications, such as creams, ointments, special oral solutions, and IV solutions with additives, require compounding in the pharmacy. The pharmacy sends such medications, whether prepared under nonsterile conditions or via strict aseptic technique, to the nursing unit as needed, based on physician's orders.
- **Narcotics:** These medications are kept in a separate, high-security area. Access to narcotics is restricted to authorized personnel, and special record keeping is required for their administration.

Procedure

This lab contains three procedure sections. You will learn the procedures for filling and checking a standard FSRF by practicing these two procedures separately as Part I: Filling Floor Stock and Part II: Checking Floor Stock. You will use the same FSRF for both parts. After you complete both of those procedures, you will turn in the single FSRF to your instructor, as described in the final part, Part III: Completing This Lab.

Part I: Filling Floor Stock

You will now fill a standard floor stock request using an FSRF. Note that one FSRF is included at the end of this lab. However, you may or may not be assigned to fill that particular form. Your instructor will probably choose to hand out several different FSRFs.

Therefore, it is important that you do not begin filling an FSRF until your instructor advises you which form to use. The forms differ slightly in the quantities and items being requested so that students will fill and check different requests, enabling the lab work to flow smoothly and be completed within the allotted class time. Once you have your designated FSRF in hand, you will begin with the first medication and proceed line by line, filling one medication at a time.

1. Because this lab will ask you to check the expiration date of each floor stock dose to make sure it is acceptable, you must first determine your state's expiration date requirements. Your instructor will have verified these state regulations, so you should ask about them now.

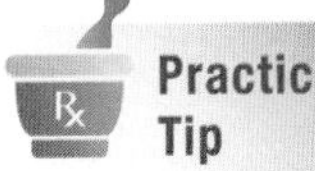

Practice Tip

Once a medication is returned to the unit and added to that unit's floor stock, the total amount of that medication will generally equal the par level. However, there are rare occasions when, based on temporarily increased usage, the nursing unit will request that a medication be refilled above the standard par level.

2 Look up the brand and generic names of any medications on the FSRF that you are unfamiliar with. Note that you will fill *only* the medications and amounts written in the "Fill #" column. When the "Fill #" column is left blank, you will not fill that medication.

3 Find the first item to be filled. Make sure that what you are pulling from the pharmacy stock matches exactly what is ordered on the FSRF. The name, strength, form, and number of items must all exactly match the FSRF.

4 Pull out the correct number of that item (i.e., the number in the "Fill #" column) and place it on an uncluttered section of counter or tabletop.

5 Check the expiration date of each dose to make sure it is acceptable.

6 Moving down the FSRF, continue to pull the correct number of each requested item (i.e., those with a quantity listed in the "Fill #" column).

7 Once you have pulled all of the items with a quantity in the "Fill #" column, arrange them so that the order of the items on the counter matches that on the FSRF. Organizing in this way makes the checking process more efficient.

8 Write your name and today's date in the blanks at the top of the Lab 17 worksheet, the FSRF. Near the bottom of the FSRF, write your name in the "Filled by" blank and the date in the "Today's date" blank.

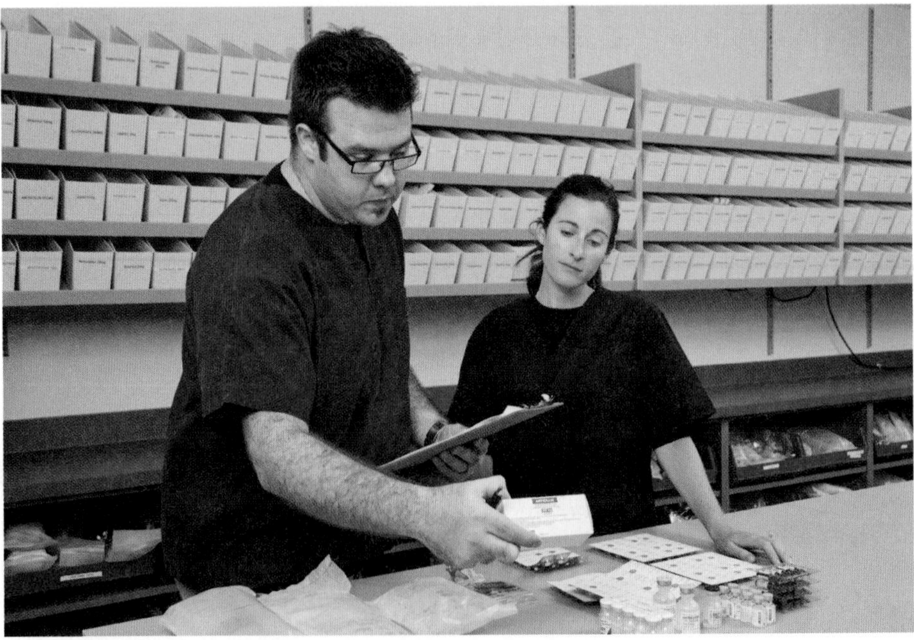

Pharmacy technician performing a double check

 © Paradigm Publishing, Inc.

Part II: Checking Floor Stock

While properly filling floor stock medications is crucial, it is also imperative that your checking process be thorough and accurate. Because many states allow technicians to perform the double check (described in the key terms section of this lab) on standard floor stock items, you will now pair up with another student in the lab to do the double check.

Remember the importance of being thorough and accurate. When you receive the other student's completed FSRF, you will again begin with the first medication and proceed line by line, carefully checking one medication at a time.

As the "checker," you must check that the drug name, strength, form, expiration date, and quantity match what is on the FSRF. Before you begin, have a pen or pencil ready to mark on the FSRF any errors you find while checking. When you are done checking the fill, you will be asked to point out the errors to the student who filled the FSRF, to count up the errors, and to write down the total number of errors on the FSRF.

9 Find another student to perform a floor stock check on your work, and have that student begin the check, starting with Step 10.

10 On the completed FSRF, check the first item requested in the "Fill #" column. Verify that the name of the medication filled matches exactly what is ordered on the FSRF. If you find an error, circle the medication name.

11 Verify that the strength of the drug matches what is on the FSRF, and circle any strength errors you find.

12 Verify that the formulation (form) of the drug matches what is on the FSRF, and circle any form errors you find.

13 Verify that the technician filled the quantity that the nursing unit requested, and circle any quantity errors you find.

14 Check the expiration date of each dose to make sure it is acceptable, and note any dating problems near the medication line you are currently checking.

15 Repeat Steps 10–14 with the next medication on the FSRF, continuing until you have checked all items and noted any errors found.

16 Add up the total number of errors you have circled or noted on the FSRF. Write this number at the bottom of the FSRF in the "Number of errors caught by checker (and corrected by filler)" blank, and write your name in the "Checked by" blank.

© Paradigm Publishing, Inc.

Part III: Completing This Lab

17 Get together with the student who filled the stock for the FSRF you have just checked, and reexchange your FSRFs. Point out any errors you found to that student. He or she should now correct those errors. After your own FSRF has been returned to you and your errors have been pointed out, you should correct any errors you made in your filling procedure.

18 **Conclusion:** Ask your instructor for a final check. The instructor will check what you have *filled* on your FSRF and will also verify what you have *checked* by looking at the other student's FSRF. Then go to the Course Navigator, answer all questions in the Lab Review section, and submit your answers to your instructor.

Access interactive chapter review exercises, practice activities, flash cards, and study games.

© Paradigm Publishing, Inc.

Name: ______________________ Date: ______________

Lab 17 Filling and Checking Floor Stock

Floor Stock Request Form

Unit Obstetrics

Fill #	Medication Being Requested (name, strength, form)	Par Level
8	Acetaminophen 325 mg tablets	10
5	Acetaminophen 500 mg caplets	10
	Amoxicillin 250 mg capsules	6
	Amoxicillin 500 mg capsules	6
3	Azithromycin 250 mg tablets	5
	Ciprofloxacin 500 mg tablets	2
	Dexamethasone 8 mg/2 mL for injection (vial)	4
2	Diphenhydramine 25 mg capsules	8
2	Dextrose 5% in water 1,000 mL (IV bag)	6
1	Dextrose 5% in 0.45 sodium chloride 1,000 mL (IV bag)	4
	Dulcolax 5 mg tablets	6
3	Furosemide 20 mg tablets	5
1	Furosemide 40 mg tablets	5
8	Ibuprofen 200 mg caplets	10
	Ibuprofen 600 mg caplets	10
	Maalox 30 mL oral liquid (unit-dose cups)	2
	Mylanta 30 mL oral liquid (unit-dose cups)	2
	Metoclopramide 10 mg tablets	4
	Promethazine 50 mg/2 mL for injection (ampule)	2
1	Sodium chloride 0.45% 1,000 mL (IV bag)	4
6	Sodium choride 0.9% 30 mL vial (bacteriostatic)	10
5	Sodium chloride 0.9% 1,000 mL (IV bag)	8
	Tobramycin 40 mg/1 mL for injection (multidose vial)	1
	Tucks Pads topical (jar)	1

Filled by ______________________ Today's date ______________

Number of errors caught by checker (and corrected by filler) ______________

Checked by ______________________

Instructor final check ______________ Number of errors missed by checker ________

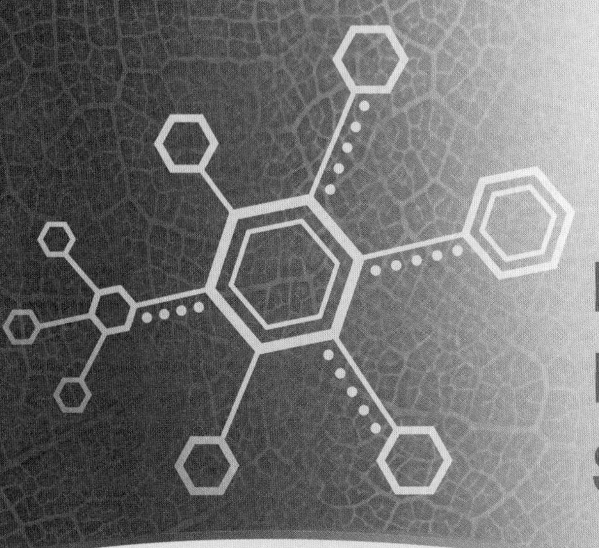

18 Filling and Recording Controlled Substance Floor Stock

Learning Objectives

1. Demonstrate proficiency in the counting and preparation of controlled substance floor stock based on a Controlled Substance Floor Stock Refill Form.
2. Demonstrate accuracy in record keeping related to the filling of controlled substance floor stock.
3. Discuss the procedures and rationale for filling controlled substance floor stock and related record-keeping procedures.

Supplies

- Access to a narcotic cabinet, vault, or room stocked with common C-II through C-V narcotics for floor stock use
- Access to a brand/generic handbook
- Access to a sample C-II perpetual log book
- Access to a sample C-III through C-V perpetual log book
- Controlled Substance Floor Stock Refill Form
- Counting tray and spatula
- Calculator
- Black pen
- Red pen

Access additional chapter resources.

In an institutional setting, all controlled substances are kept in a secure, double-locked location in the pharmacy, where access to the medications are restricted only to authorized pharmacy personnel. These controlled substances are dispensed in a manner similar to standard floor stock; however, unlike regular floor stock, there are a number of special record keeping and security procedures that must be followed.

The area where controlled substances are stored in the pharmacy is called the **narcotic cabinet**. While many of the medications kept in the narcotic cabinet are classified as narcotics, there are other types of drugs that may also be stored in the cabinet, including anti-anxiety medications, stimulants, and steroids. Any medication that is identified as a controlled substance by the 1970 Controlled Substances Act is secured in the pharmacy narcotic cabinet. In larger institutions, a full-time pharmacy technician is often responsible for the operation of the

FIGURE 18.1 Drug Enforcement Administration Form

See Reverse of PURCHASER'S Copy for Instructions

No order form may be issued for Schedule I and II substances unless a completed form has been received (21 CFR 1305.04).

OMB Approval No. 1117-0010

TO (Name of Supplier) | STREET ADDRESS

CITY AND STATE | DATE | **TO BE FILLED IN BY SUPPLIER**

SUPPLIER'S DEA REGISTRATION NO.

LINE No.	**TO BE FILLED IN BY PURCHASER**					
	No. of Packages	Size of Package	Name of Item	National Drug Code	Packages Shipped	Date Shipped
1						
2						
3						
4						
5						
6						
7						
8						
9						
10						

SAMPLE

◀ LAST LINE COMPLETED (MUST BE 10 OR UNDER) | SIGNATURE OF PURCHASER OR ATTORNEY OR AGENT

Date Issued	DEA Registration No.	Name and Address of Registrant
10302014	AA4720581	Get Well Pharmacy 1000 Healthline Road Wellness, TX 70000
Schedule: 2, 2N, 3, 3N, 4, 5		
Registered as a: TRAINING ONLY	No. Of this order Form: 002235985	

DEA FORM-222 (Oct. 1992) | **U.S. OFFICIAL ORDER FORMS - SCHEDULES I & II** DRUG ENFORCEMENT ADMINISTRATION SUPPLIER'S Copy 1 | **75841302**

narcotic cabinet. Smaller institutions might require the pharmacy technician to work with controlled substances only on an as-needed basis or in special situations, such as when compounding or delivering controlled substances to the nursing unit. The technician responsible for handling controlled substances will likely receive specialized, on-the-job training.

Many institutional pharmacies require pharmacy technicians to carry out all aspects of pharmaceutical controlled substance-related duties. These duties include ordering, pulling, counting, record keeping, filling, delivering, providing quality assurance, and placing the controlled substance floor stock in a secure area on the unit. To order controlled substance floor stock from wholesalers and other suppliers, a Drug Enforcement Administration (DEA) Form 222 is used. An example of such a form is shown in Figure 18.1.

Many facilities have an automated system that utilizes barcode technology to track and record additions and withdrawals of controlled substances from the narcotic cabinet. In these facilities, the perpetual inventory—a record of every item that is entered into or removed from the narcotic cabinet—is an electronic record that is tied to a pharmacy software system that would automatically alert the narcotic technician or pharmacist of any discrepancy in the perpetual inventory record. However, some facilities manually record all withdrawals and additions in perpetual log books. The technician is often responsible for the record keeping (recording all controlled substance withdrawals and additions) of perpetual log books.

 © Paradigm Publishing, Inc.

FIGURE 18.2 Perpetual Inventory Record

Perpetual Inventory Record

____
Drug name, strength, and dosage form

____________________ ____________________
NDC Manufacturer

Date	Invoice #	Department/Floor/Unit #	Qty +/–	Balance	Initials	Verified by

The **perpetual log book** is an official, legal record of all activity relating to medications stored in the narcotic cabinet. The perpetual log book contains pages entitled Perpetual Inventory Record forms (Figure 18.2) or Controlled Substance Record forms. Because there is generally one perpetual log book for C-II narcotics and a different perpetual log book for C-III through C-V narcotics, you should make sure you are using the correct book for each entry. Some aspects of controlled substance record-keeping may vary between facilities and states, such as the color of pen that is to be used and the unit identification information that is recorded on the perpetual log. However, the step-by-step procedures taken in controlled substance record keeping will generally be similar to what you will perform in this lab. Due to the importance of keeping an accurate controlled substance record, you must become familiar with and practice these standard controlled substance perpetual log book procedures:

- Make all entries or additions into the perpetual log in black pen.
- Record withdrawals and negative balances in red pen. Note that only the number should be in red, not the entire line entry.
- Note errors by drawing a single line through the entire line entry. The initials of the person making the correction should be written next to the strikethrough and circled.
- Errors in the narcotic records must remain traceable and legible Therefore, never erase or scribble out errors, and note that it is *never acceptable* to use white-out or similar products.

© Paradigm Publishing, Inc.

- Always record information in the perpetual log on the next available line. There should never be an open or empty line in the perpetual log.
- Never write information on the bottom of a perpetual log sheet below the preprinted spaces. Rather, once you have filled the last available line on the page, you *must* start a new sheet.
- To start a new sheet, transfer the drug name, strength, dosage form, manufacturer, and National Drug Code (NDC) number from the drug bottle onto the appropriate space at the top of the new sheet. Transfer the balance or actual count number into the first available balance space on this new sheet.

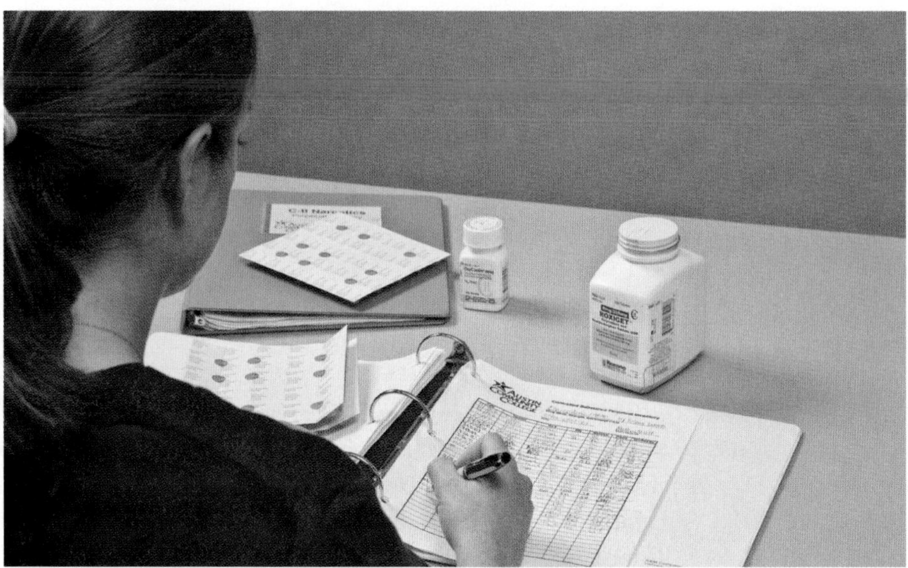

Pharmacy technician entering information into the perpetual log

In order to provide the utmost security, be sure that controlled substances, the keys to the narcotic cabinet, and all controlled substance records are kept under your supervision while working in this area. These items should never be left unattended or unsecured. All controlled substance records must be kept on hand in the pharmacy for a minimum of two years. The board of pharmacy for your state, the DEA, and other regulatory agencies may ask to review controlled substance records, including the perpetual log books, so immediate access to these records is essential. It should be noted that significant deficits on a perpetual log must be investigated and resolved. This investigation is first performed by pharmacy personnel, which may include the narcotic technician, the pharmacist on duty, and the pharmacist-in-charge. If it is determined that there has been a significant loss of a controlled substance, it must be reported to the DEA on Form 106. What constitutes a significant loss is dependent upon the schedule of the controlled substance and the amount of medication that is being reported as missing or stolen. Consult the DEA website or your state board of pharmacy for further guidance on responding in cases of significant loss of controlled substances.

 © Paradigm Publishing, Inc.

Procedure

In this lab, you will fill a Controlled Substance Floor Stock Refill (CSFSR) Form and record the dispensed controlled substances in the appropriate perpetual log books.

1. Read through the CSFSR Form completely. If necessary, look up the brand or generic medication names with which you are unfamiliar.

2. Open the appropriate (either C-II or C-III through C-V) perpetual log book, and find the first medication listed on the CSFSR Form. Verify that the NDC number, drug name, strength, and form that are listed on the perpetual log match exactly what is ordered on the refill form.

3. Using a black pen, record today's date in the "Date" column on the first available line of the perpetual log for this medication. Under the "Department/Floor/Unit #" field, write the words "actual count." Record your initials under the "Initials" field. Leave the "Invoice #," "Qty +/–," and "Balance" fields blank for now.

4. Open the narcotic cabinet and locate the first item ordered on the CSFSR Form. Pull out the bin or tray containing that medication. Verify that the NDC number, drug name, strength, and form match exactly what is ordered and that all of the medications to be dispensed have acceptable expiration dates. Expiration dating requirements may vary between states and facilities, so consult your instructor to determine acceptable expiration dates for items used in this lab.

5. Count all tablets or capsules in the medication bin. Be sure to count everything in the bin, including unopened bottles, partial bottles, and unit-dose medications. If necessary, use a counting tray and/or calculator.

6. Using a black pen, record the total number counted from this bin in the perpetual log book in the "Balance" field. Record your initials in the appropriate place on the same line.

7. Pull the requested number, as specified for the first drug on your CSFSR Form, out of the bin. The medication must be in unit-dose form. Consult your instructor if you do not have enough unit-dosed medication to fill the entire order.

8. On the next available line for this medication (i.e., the line directly below the actual count), record today's date; the department, floor, or unit name and/or number as it appears on your CSFSR Form; and your initials in the appropriate fields.

TAKE NOTE

Be aware that in some facilities, the recording of both entries and withdrawals are made in black pen. Refer to your facility policy and procedure manual for specific procedures for narcotic record keeping.

9 Using a red pen, record the amount that you pulled from the bin in the "Qty +/–" field. This number should match the number ordered by the department, floor, or unit.

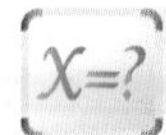

Math Morsels

Your formula is "Actual Count or Balance Minus Amount Dispensed (or Qty +/–) Equals Amount Remaining in Bin."

10 From the "Balance" (the actual count found in the first entry line), subtract the number to be dispensed (the number recorded under the "Qty +/-" field of the second entry line). This new count should be recorded, in black, under the "Balance" field of the second entry line and should be equal to the amount left in the bin.

11 Remember that when you are working with a perpetual log, the actual count must match the remaining balance that was written by the previous person recording entries for that medication. If you see a narcotic discrepancy during your work, report it immediately to your instructor. A narcotic discrepancy is a disagreement between the actual count of a narcotic and the amount listed in the perpetual log or narcotic record.

12 Move from the perpetual log to the CSFSR Form. Fill in the "Starting Balance," "# Dispensed," and "Remaining Balance" information that you determined for the first medication listed on the CSFSR Form.

13 Place to the side, temporarily, the amount that was just filled for the first medication ordered.

14 Fill the other medications on the CSFSR Form, following the same procedures listed above.

15 **Conclusion:** Once all of the medications on the CSFSR Form have been filled and recorded in the perpetual log book(s) and you have filled in the necessary information on the CSFSR Form, write your name and today's date on the form and ask for an instructor to check your work. Then go to the Course Navigator, answer all questions in the Lab Review section, and submit your answers to your instructor.

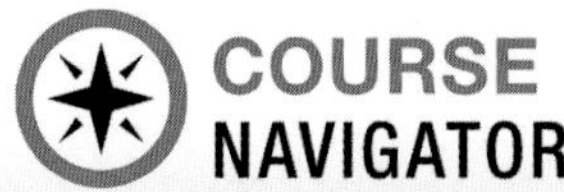

Access interactive chapter review exercises, practice activities, flash cards, and study games.

© Paradigm Publishing, Inc.

Name: ______________________________ Date: ________________

Lab 18 Filling and Recording Controlled Substance Floor Stock

Controlled Substance Floor Stock Refill Form (18.1)

Department/Floor/Unit Name or Number ______Obstetrics______

Floor Stock Controlled Substances Ordered by This Unit:

Tylenol #3 tablets X 50

Starting Balance _______ # Dispensed _______ Remaining Balance _______

Vicodin 5 mg/325 mg tablets X 25

Starting Balance__________ # Dispensed _______ Remaining Balance_______

Morphine 10 mg prefilled syringes X 20

Starting Balance__________ # Dispensed _______ Remaining Balance_______

Instructor's initials ________________________ **Assignment grade** ______________

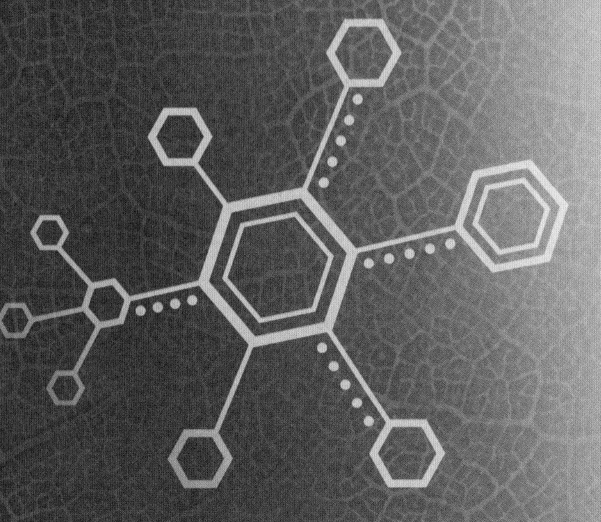

19

Preparing Oral Syringes

Learning Objectives

1 Demonstrate competence in the preparation of oral syringes.

2 Demonstrate accuracy in basic math calculations related to the preparation of oral syringes.

3 Discuss the procedures and rationale for preparing oral syringes.

Supplies

- Ibuprofen oral suspension × 1 pint
- 10 mL oral syringe × 1
- 5 mL oral syringe × 1
- 3 mL oral syringe × 1
- Oral syringe caps × 3
- Rubber oral syringe bottle adaptor
- Paper and pencil for calculations
- Nitrile, vinyl, or similar gloves, if desired
- Calculator

Access additional chapter resources.

Many **enteral** medications are available in an oral solid form that delivers medication through a patient's gastrointestinal tract. In some cases, the patient is unable or unwilling to swallow a capsule or tablet, and the physician may instead request the oral liquid form of the medication. Some oral liquid medications are available prepackaged in unit-dose cups. However, many oral liquid medications are supplied to hospital pharmacies in the original bulk bottle. In order to deliver the proper dosage to multiple patients in the most sanitary and cost-effective manner, the pharmacy technician will prepare individual doses in oral syringes by withdrawing the doses from the bulk bottle. This preparation process requires a special bottle adaptor that fits into the mouth of the bottle to facilitate easy withdrawal of the medication. A schematic illustration of oral syringe preparation is shown in Figure 19.1.

FIGURE 19.1
Schematic Illustration of Oral Syringe Preparation

The syringe tip is seated inside the opening of a rubber bottle adaptor, which is seated inside the mouth of a bulk bottle of oral liquid.

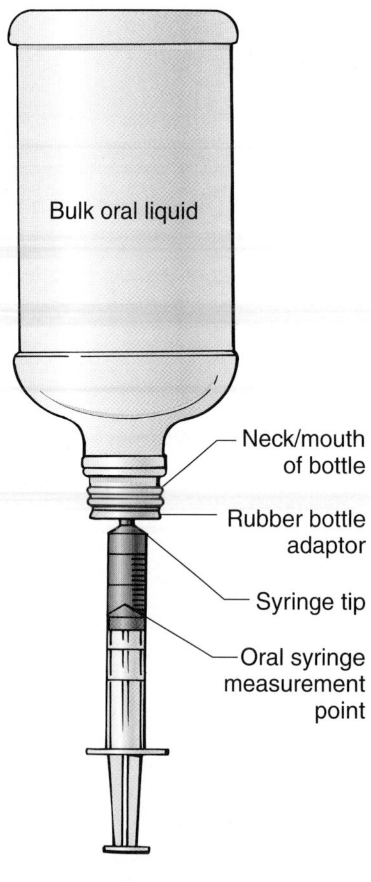

Preparing oral syringes requires that you first perform precise calculations to determine the amount of liquid to draw into each syringe. You will use a basic formula called "ratio and proportion" to calculate how much liquid is needed for each individual dose. The calculation is based on the concentration of the liquid medication in the bulk bottle and the dose you desire to prepare, and it requires some familiarity with pharmaceutical math. An explanation of these basic calculations is provided on page 211.

Most oral syringes are administered by squirting their contents directly into the patient's mouth. Some oral syringes are administered by nurses, who introduce a syringe's contents through a patient's nasogastric tube (NG tube or NGT). As illustrated in Figure 19.2, an NG tube is inserted into the patient's nose, continues past the throat, and ends in the stomach. Using an oral syringe with an NG tube eliminates the need to swallow, which may be difficult for some patients, and delivers medications and food directly to the patient's stomach. Remember that oral syringes are for one-time use only; they must be disposed of in the trash after the dose has been administered to the patient.

FIGURE 19.2
Enteral Feeding Tube Sites

Insertion sites for NG, G, and J tubes. Gastric tubes (G tube), and jejunostomy tubes (J tube) may also be used to administer medications via oral syringe.

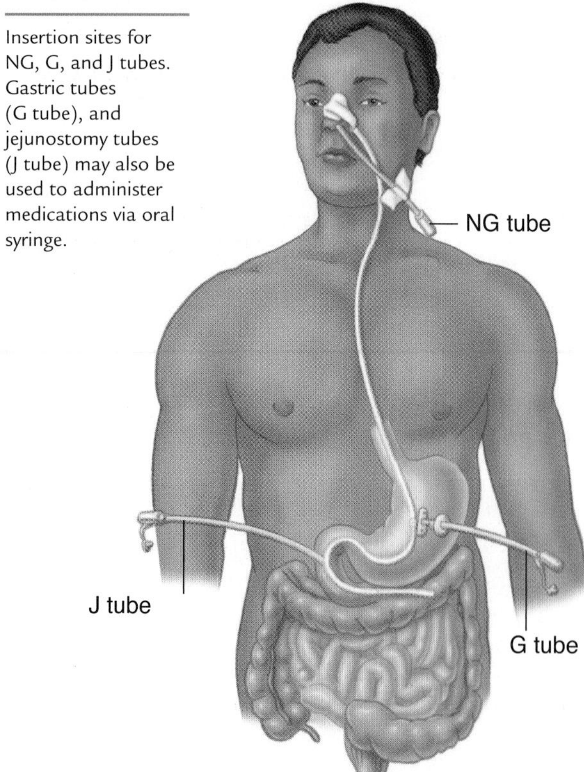

© Paradigm Publishing, Inc.

General Explanation of the Dose Calculation Process:

To determine the amount of liquid to draw into each syringe, you will use a basic "ratio and proportion" formula. Your calculation will provide you with an answer to the question, "How much liquid will I need to withdraw from the bulk bottle for an individual dose?"

First, look on the oral medication bottle label, and find the concentration as provided in milligrams per milliliter. Write down the number in fraction form:

$$\left.\frac{\text{Number of milligrams}}{\text{Number of milliliters}}\right\} \text{as stated on the medication label}$$

TIP: *To be accurate and clear when using ratios and proportions, always write down the abbreviations for the units (e.g., mg, mL, etc.) you are working with when you write down the numbers.*

Next to this concentration ratio, place an equals sign, and then write down the number of milligrams in the desired dose over *x* milliliters (the amount you are solving for):

$$\frac{\text{Number of milligrams (from medication label)}}{\text{Number of milliliters (from medication label)}} = \frac{\text{Number of milligrams in desired dose}}{x \text{ milliliters}}$$

You have created an equation communicating that one ratio is equivalent to another ratio. You can now cross multiply (work in a diagonal direction) and then divide to calculate the missing *x* value in your equation and answer your dosage question:

- Multiply the Number of milligrams in desired dose by the Number of milliliters (from medication label).
- Take the result, and divide it by the Number of milligrams (from medication label).
- Your answer is the missing value, *x* milliliters, the amount that you need to withdraw.

Specific Dose Calculation for This Lab:

In the following Procedure section, you will prepare three doses of ibuprofen. Below is the calculation process for one of those doses. Use this model to complete your calculations for the remaining two doses when you reach Step 4 of the Procedure section.

For the ibuprofen 200 mg dose, your initial question is, "How many milliliters do I need to withdraw from the bulk bottle for the desired dose of ibuprofen 200 mg?"

Your bulk ibuprofen medication bottle label indicates a concentration of 100 mg/5 mL. Thus, your two equivalent ratios result in this formula:

$$\frac{100 \text{ mg}}{5 \text{ mL}} = \frac{200 \text{ mg (in this desired dose)}}{x \text{ millilters (to be drawn up)}}$$

- First you cross multiply: 200 mg × 5 mL = 1,000 mg/mL
- And then you divide: 1,000 mg/mL ÷ 100 mg = 10 mL
- This final number, 10 mL, is your missing value for *x* and the answer to your question, "How many milliliters do I need to withdraw from the bulk bottle for the desired dose of ibuprofen 200 mg?"

Procedure

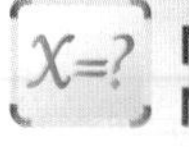

Math Morsels

Read the explanation, and use the formula provided on the previous page to perform your dose calculations. Your instructor will guide you in practicing the calculations, and you should ask for additional instruction as needed.

In this lab, you will calculate three individual doses of oral liquid medication and prepare the doses using oral syringes and a bottle adaptor. The doses you will draw up are ibuprofen 200 mg, ibuprofen 100 mg, and ibuprofen 50 mg.

1 Wash your hands thoroughly.

2 Gather the listed supplies. To prevent accidental stains on your clothing, you may wish to wear medical scrubs or a lab coat when performing this lab. Your instructor may also direct you to wear gloves while performing this lab. If so, gather those supply items.

3 Verify that the ibuprofen bulk bottle label indicates a concentration of 100 mg/5 mL.

TAKE NOTE

Certain medications require you to take special precautions to protect yourself when preparing oral syringes. In those situations, you would likely be required to wear gloves and goggles for eye protection. Read the manufacturer label and/or your facility policy and procedure manual to determine if the drug you are working with requires special protection.

4 On a separate sheet of paper, neatly perform your calculations to answer this question for each of the three desired ibuprofen doses: "How many milliliters will I need to withdraw from the bulk bottle to prepare this dose?" You will show your instructor your calculations sheet at the end of the lab.

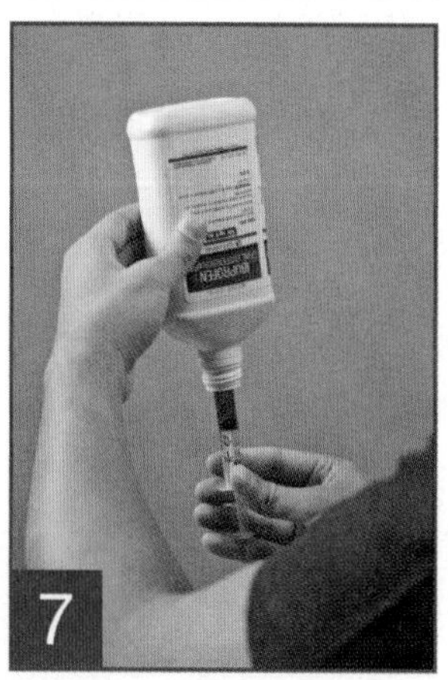

7

5 Remove the cap from the pint bottle of ibuprofen. Attach the bottle adaptor with a gentle twisting motion. The bottle adaptor should be firmly seated in the bottle top so that only the top one or two rings of the adaptor are visible. Do not push on the adaptor with too much force, or it will fall directly into the liquid and render the bottle's contents unusable.

6 Select an appropriate syringe for the dose you are preparing, choosing the size closest to the desired dose while ensuring that the entire dose fits. Also select an appropriate syringe cap, noting that they are available in different sizes and that the cap should fit tightly and securely on the syringe tip.

© Paradigm Publishing, Inc.

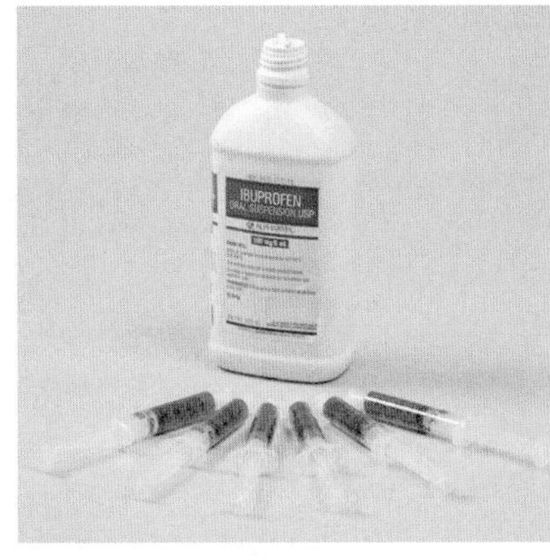

Capped oral syringes

7 Insert the tip of the first oral syringe into the hole on top of the bottle adaptor. Invert the bottle and syringe so that the syringe is now below the bottle.

Practice Tip

If, upon inverting the bottle, you notice the medication leaking, then the syringe was not firmly seated in the bottle adaptor. To correct this problem, turn the bottle and syringe upright, and gently push and twist the syringe downward to attach it more firmly to the bottle adaptor.

8 Pull down on the plunger so fluid starts to flow into the syringe. Once the syringe is about one-third full, push up forcefully on the plunger to expel all air bubbles and fluid back into the bottle.

9 Pull down on the plunger again so fluid starts to flow into the syringe, and then quickly push up on the plunger to expel the air bubbles and fluid. Repeat this process several times in quick succession. This technique is called **crushing**. Crushing forces all of the air bubbles out of the syringe and allows only fluid to fill the syringe when you later draw up the full, prescribed volume.

10 Once the air bubbles have been removed by using the crushing method, pull down on the plunger until you have the desired volume of fluid in the syringe. Take the measurement where the shoulder of the black stopper at the end of the syringe plunger meets the proper graduation on the syringe barrel.

11 Invert the bottle and syringe again so that the bottle is right-side-up and the syringe is upside-down. Holding only the syringe barrel, remove the syringe in a twisting, pulling motion to break the suction that has been created. Once the suction is released, the syringe should easily detach from the bottle adaptor.

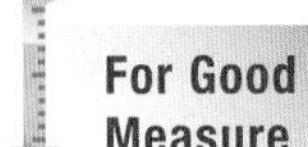

For Good Measure

Removing the bubbles when the syringe is only one-third full is important. You would find the crushing process very difficult if the syringe were more full or if you had drawn up the final, proper volume.

12 Place the properly fitting syringe cap firmly onto the syringe tip, and set the syringe aside. Repeat the complete procedure for both remaining doses, and place all three capped syringes on the work surface next to the ibuprofen bottle.

13 **Conclusion:** Write your name and today's date on the sheet where you performed the math calculations. Ask your instructor to check all three filled syringes, the medication bottle, and your calculations. Then go to the Course Navigator, answer all questions in the Lab Review section, and submit your answers to your instructor.

Access interactive chapter review exercises, practice activities, flash cards, and study games.

© Paradigm Publishing, Inc.

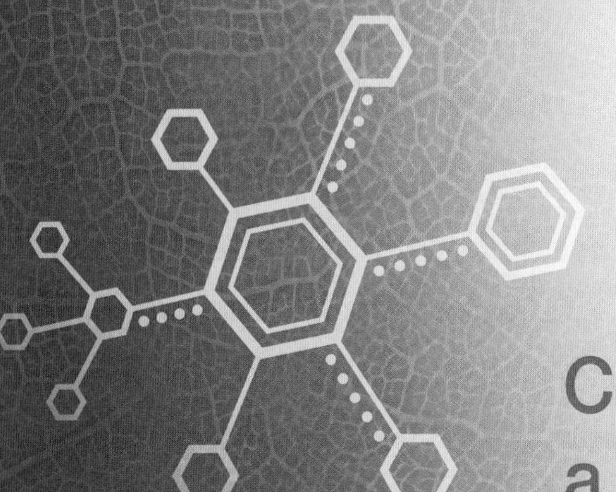

20

Charging and Refilling a Crash Cart

Learning Objectives

1 Identify and discuss the rationale for the preparation and use of a crash cart.

2 Demonstrate proficiency in initiating patient charges for crash cart medications.

3 Demonstrate skill and accuracy in filling a crash cart.

Supplies

- Access to a pharmacy lab stocked with standard emergency medications
- Access to a crash cart, tray, or tackle box
- Crash Cart Charge Form
- Crash Cart Refill Form
- Access to a brand/generic handbook

Access additional chapter resources.

In a hospital it is vital to have a crash cart on hand for treating respiratory or cardiac arrest and other potentially fatal emergency conditions. Be aware that this cart may also be referred to as a "crash tray," "code cart," or "tackle box," or by other names individual facilities may have developed. Many large facilities keep a crash cart on each floor or nursing unit, often in a specified location.

The arrangement and contents of crash carts vary widely among institutions. For example, due to the differences in body size and physiology, there are significant differences in the types and strengths of medications found in crash carts that are used to treat adult patients and those used to treat pediatric patients. As a general rule, adult crash carts are stocked with emergency medications such as epinephrine, atropine, and nitroprusside. The cart may also contain standard IV base solutions, IV tubing, and a limited supply of syringes, needles, and other medications or supply items. Most of the items in the crash cart will be for **parenteral** use, most frequently administered intravenously, because a patient who is

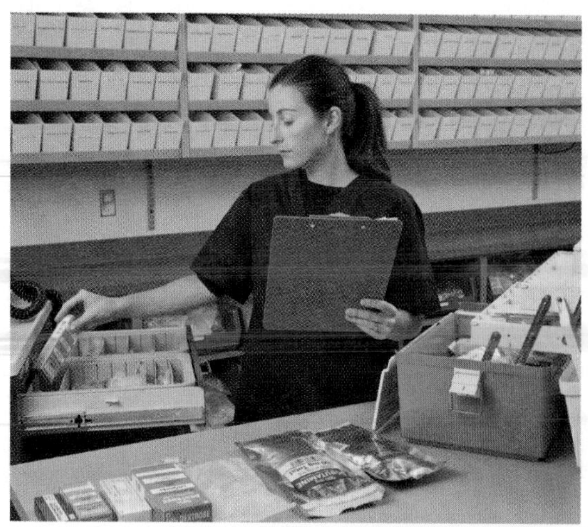

Pharmacy technician checking and refilling a crash cart

experiencing respiratory or cardiac arrest is generally unable to take oral medications. Parenteral is any route of administration other than sublingual, enteral, or topical, such as intravenous or intramuscular. Because crash carts need to be immediately accessed, facilities often use tamper-evident plastic locks, which can be easily opened in emergency situations.

When a hospital patient goes into cardiac or respiratory arrest, a **code** is called by hospital staff and is usually announced on an overhead paging system. A code is a life-threatening situation when a patient is in cardiac or respiratory arrest. The code may also be referred to as a "code blue," "code zero," "crash," "zero," or by another term preferred by the facility. A designated code team—a group of doctors and nurses trained in emergency medical care—commonly responds and assumes treatment of the patient. At that time, the charge nurse (or other designated person) unlocks the crash cart, and the code team removes medications and supplies from the crash cart to treat the patient. Except in the case of such code use, the crash cart must be kept locked at all times. At the time of a code, the tamper-evident lock will be broken open so that items in the crash cart can be accessed by the code team.

Once the code has ended, the crash cart is returned to the pharmacy to be refilled and to determine which items should be charged to the patient. Some larger institutions employ barcode and/or radio-frequency identification (RFID) technology, which allows pharmacy technicians to scan items in returned crash carts to quickly determine which items need to be refilled, replace items that are outdated, and bill the patient. However, most institutional pharmacies still manually refill and charge crash carts; therefore, accurate and timely initiation of patient charges and crash cart refilling are crucial tasks often performed by the pharmacy technician.

As a technician, you must inventory the used crash cart and charge the patient for any items that were used during the code by recording the information on a Crash Cart Charge (CCC) Form. You must also refill medications that were used to treat the patient and check expiration dates on all cart medications, replacing anything that does not have—in most states—a minimum of six months of acceptable dating. Since crash cart expiration dating policies may vary between states and facilities, in practice, you will need to determine your state's requirements and/or your facility's policies regarding acceptable expiration dating for crash cart items, and be sure that only those items that meet acceptable expiration dating requirements are refilled in the crash cart.

For the purposes of this lab, a minimum of six months is considered acceptable. The number of each item that is to be refilled and recorded on a Crash Cart Refill (CCR) Form will be determined by subtracting the number on hand in the cart from the par level (the number to be kept in the cart when it is full). The technician puts the resulting quantity (the refill number) into the cart.

 © Paradigm Publishing, Inc.

Procedure

This lab requires you to practice two related procedures: initiating patient charges and refilling the crash cart. During the first procedure, you will use the CCC Form to charge the patient for medications and supply items used during the code. During the second part of the procedure, you will use the CCR Form to check medication expiration dates and refill the crash cart in preparation for its return to the nursing unit to be used in a future code.

Part I: Charging the Patient

First, you will use a CCC Form to charge the patient for items used during the code. Your instructor will tell you, based on supplies available in your lab, whether to use the CCC Form provided at the end of this lab or to wait for a different form to be handed out to you.

1. If necessary, look up the brand/generic names of any CCC Form medications with which you are unfamiliar.

2. Verify crash cart expiration dating with your instructor before beginning the lab. Six months is generally acceptable, but this may vary somewhat from state to state, and between different facilities.

3. Open the top drawer of the crash cart (or the first section of the tray). Find the first item listed on the CCC Form. Note that the drawer may be divided into multiple sections, and the first section should match the first item listed on the CCC Form.

4. Count the number of the first item in the crash cart. This quantity should exactly match the item's par level as listed on the CCC Form. If it does not, the difference reflects the quantity of that item used to treat the patient and now to be replaced. Write the refill number on the corresponding line on the CCC Form.

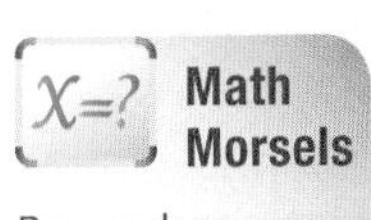

Remember that Par Level – Number on Hand = Number to be Refilled.

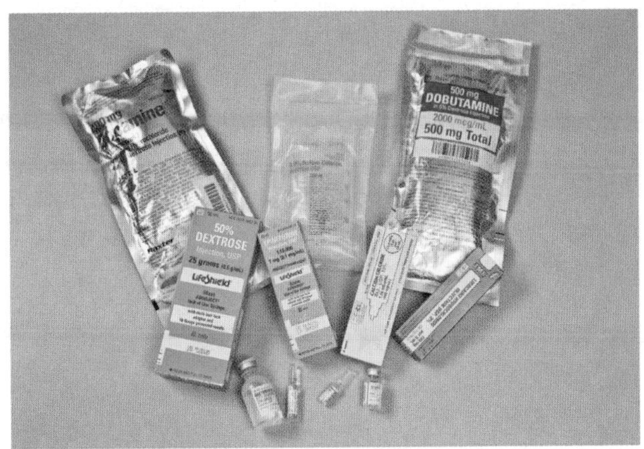

Common emergency medications stocked in crash carts

In an institutional setting, the Crash Cart Charge Form would now be used to enter patient charges into the facility's computerized billing system. For the purposes of this lab, however, the computer-based, data entry portion of the charging process will be skipped.

5 Continue down the CCC Form, recording the refill number for each item listed. Once you have completed the CCC Form, write your name and today's date on the assignment. Temporarily set the CCC Form aside to await your instructor's check.

Part II: Refilling the Crash Cart

You will now use a CCR Form to check expiration dates and refill the crash cart. Your instructor will tell you, based on supplies available in your lab, whether to use the CCR Form provided at the end of this lab or to wait for a different form to be handed out to you.

6 Locate the item in the crash cart or tray that corresponds to the first item listed on the CCR Form. Find the expiration date for each dose of medication (which may be an ampule, vial, syringe, IV bag, or other supply) for this first item. Each refilled item must have a minimum of six months remaining prior to its expiration date. If the item does not comply (i.e., it expires less than six months from today's date), remove it from the crash cart or tray.

For example, if you are refilling four adenosine 6 mg vials and each one has a different expiration date, you will write down only the earliest expiration date.

7 If necessary, refill this item to match the par level, replacing any missing (i.e., used) doses or any doses you removed due to unacceptable expiration dating. Be sure that the replacement doses have at least six months of acceptable expiration dating. Place these items into the appropriate section of the crash cart, tray, or tackle box.

8 Write down the earliest expiration date—the one expiring first—for this item.

9 Repeat the entire procedure (checking expiration dates, removing and refilling as needed, and recording the earliest expiration date) for each item listed on the CCR Form until the entire cart has been refilled (brought up to par level) with items that have acceptable dating.

10 **Conclusion:** Write your name and today's date on the CCR Form. Retrieve the CCC Form that you set aside, and then ask for an instructor check. The instructor will check both crash cart forms—the CCC Form, to verify that you have properly charged the patient, and the CCR Form, to verify that you have refilled each item properly and recorded the correct expiration dates. Then go to the Course Navigator, answer all questions in the Lab Review section, and submit your answers to your instructor.

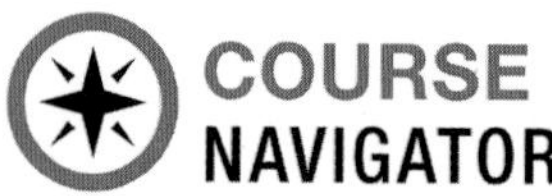

Access interactive chapter review exercises, practice activities, flash cards, and study games.

© Paradigm Publishing, Inc.

Name: ______________________ Date: ______________

Lab 20 Charging and Refilling a Crash Cart

Crash Cart Charge Form

Medication/Supply Item	Par Level	Number to Charge Patient
Vented IV tubing	2	
Bacteriostatic normal saline 30 mL vial	4	
Dextrose 50% 25 gram syringe	1	
Sodium bicarbonate 8.4% 50 mL syringe	2	
Heparin 5,000 units/mL syringe	4	
Naloxone 0.4 mg/mL syringe	2	
Lidocaine 2% prefilled syringe	2	
Dexamethasone 4 mg/mL vial	1	
Atropine 0.1 mg/mL 10 mL syringe	3	
Furosemide 100 mg/10 mL vial	2	
Acyclovir 500 mg vial	1	
Adenosine 3 mg/mL vial	1	
Calcium chloride 10% prefilled syringe	2	
Potassium chloride 2 mEq/mL 20 mL vial	2	
Theophylline 400 mg in 500 mL IV bag	2	
Dopamine 1,600 mcg in 250 mL IV bag	1	
Sodium chloride 0.9% 1,000 mL IV bag	4	
Dextrose 5% in water 1,000 mL IV bag	4	
Diphenhydramine 50 mg vial	2	
Epinephrine 1:10,000 syringe	4	
Solu-Medrol 125 mg vial	2	
Lopressor 10 mg vial	2	
Cardizem 20 mg vial	4	

© Paradigm Publishing, Inc.

Name: ______________________ Date: ______________

Lab 20 Charging and Refilling a Crash Cart

Crash Cart Refill Form

Medication/Supply Item	Par Level	Expiration Date
Vented IV tubing	2	
Bacteriostatic normal saline 30 mL vial	4	
Dextrose 50% 25 gram syringe	1	
Sodium bicarbonate 8.4% 50 mL syringe	2	
Heparin 5,000 units/mL syringe	4	
Naloxone 0.4 mg/mL syringe	2	
Lidocaine 2% prefilled syringe	2	
Dexamethasone 4 mg/mL vial	1	
Atropine 0.1 mg/mL 10 mL syringe	3	
Furosemide 100 mg/10 mL vial	2	
Acyclovir 500 mg vial	1	
Adenosine 3 mg/mL vial	1	
Calcium chloride 10% prefilled syringe	2	
Potassium chloride 2 mEq/mL 20 mL vial	2	
Theophylline 400 mg in 500 mL IV bag	2	
Dopamine 1,600 mcg in 250 mL IV bag	1	
Sodium chloride 0.9% 1,000 mL IV bag	4	
Dextrose 5% in water 1,000 mL IV bag	4	
Diphenhydramine 50 mg vial	2	
Epinephrine 1:10,000 syringe	4	
Solu-Medrol 125 mg vial	2	
Lopressor 10 mg vial	2	
Cardizem 20 mg vial	4	

© Paradigm Publishing, Inc.

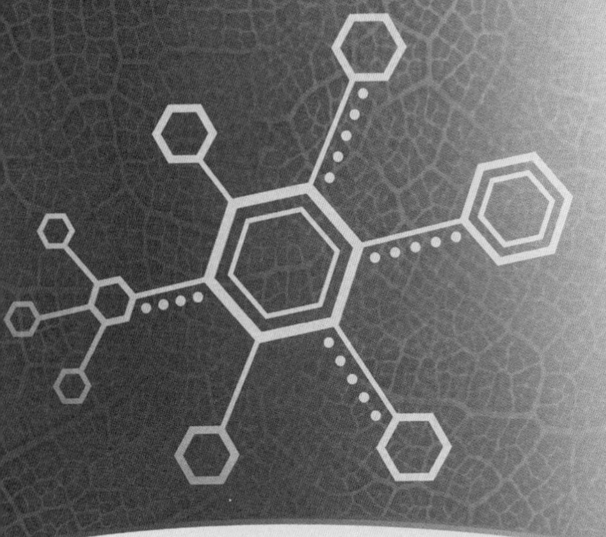

21 Filling an Automated Drug Storage and Dispensing System

Learning Objectives

1. Demonstrate skill and accuracy in the process of filling an automated drug storage and dispensing system.
2. Determine and discuss the rationale and procedures for using an automated drug storage and dispensing system for pharmacy products.

Supplies

- An Automated Drug Storage and Dispensing System Refill Request Form
- Access to a pharmacy lab stocked with items commonly found in an automated drug storage and dispensing system cabinet or tower
- Access to an automated drug storage and dispensing system cabinet or tower and its networked computer
- Access to a brand/generic handbook

Access additional chapter resources.

Many large hospitals use an **automated drug storage and dispensing system (ADSDS)** to assist with storing, dispensing, tracking, and charging some pharmaceuticals. The ADSDS generally consists of a cabinet or tower with an attached laptop computer that is networked to the pharmacy department. Each floor or unit of the hospital commonly has such a system.

Several different types or brands of ADSDSs are used in the institutional pharmacy setting. Some of the more common systems include Pyxis, Accudose, SureMed, MedDispense, and Omnicell. Although the systems have some procedural differences, they are all very similar in how they store, dispense, and track pharmaceuticals.

Hospitals invest in an ADSDS for speed, accuracy, cost savings, and security. In particular, the system provides nursing staff with immediate access to many medications and supply items, allowing the staff to avoid waiting for the pharmacy to fill the order. Because the system automatically

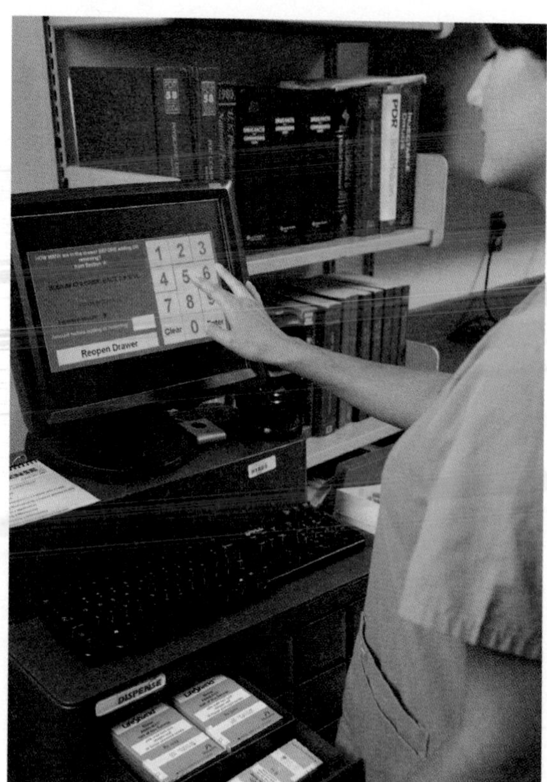
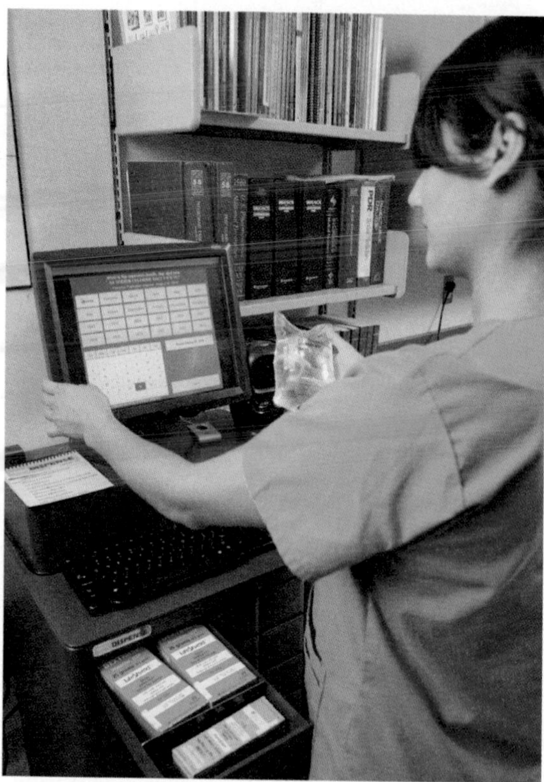

Pharmacy technician logging medications into the ADSDS (left) and placing drugs into specific drawers (right)

prints out an accurate list for cabinet refills and patient charging, the chance for human error is reduced, and labor costs are saved. Most importantly, the system offers a secure environment for pharmaceutical storage, because each item is tracked along its path from the pharmacy, to the nurse, and to the patient. Being careful to check and double-check medication counts is important to avoid creating a **count discrepancy**, a disagreement between the actual count of a medication in the ADSDS and the amount displayed on the verification screen. Doing so can help prevent you from being suspected of the serious offense of **drug diversion** (stealing or otherwise illegally taking or using drugs from the facility).

Your primary role in working with an ADSDS is to refill the system inventory according to the ADSDS Refill Request Form. The ADSDS on each nursing unit automatically generates this form. Each cabinet on each hospital unit or floor produces a separate refill form. Your job is to fill all the items on every refill form. In some institutions, you may also be responsible for delivering the medications to the unit and placing them into the individual ADSDS cabinets. In other settings, the nurse or unit assistant delivers and places the medications into the individual ADSDS units.

© Paradigm Publishing, Inc.

Procedure

In this lab, you will refill medications for an ADSDS. You will also properly enter the refilled items into the ADSDS's computer system and insert the medications into the ADSDS cabinet. Your instructor may have you complete multiple repetitions of this lab to help you build speed and accuracy. It is vital that you pay close attention to accuracy with regard to the drug name, strength, number to refill, expiration date, computer entry, and proper placement within the ADSDS.

1 Verify acceptable expiration date requirements with your instructor before beginning this lab.

2 Look up the brand/generic names of any medications listed on the ADSDS Refill Request Form with which you are unfamiliar.

3 Find the first item to be filled. Make sure that what you are pulling from the pharmacy stock matches *exactly* what is ordered on the ADSDS Refill Request Form. The drug name, strength, dosage form, and amount ordered must all match those on the ADSDS Refill Request Form.

4 Pull out the correct amount of that item, and place it on an uncluttered section of counter or table top.

5 Check the expiration date of each dose to be sure it is acceptable. Set aside expired doses or those with unacceptable dating, and point them out to your instructor. Do not include these doses in your count for refilling the ADSDS.

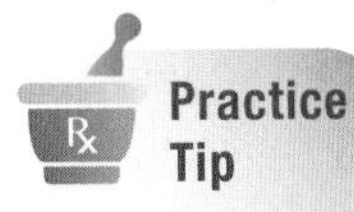

Your work with an ADSDS may require you to process ADSDS Refill Request Forms for multiple nursing units. In such cases, be sure to keep the items from each ADSDS Refill Request Form separate and clearly labeled so that you supply the correct items into each nursing unit's ADSDS.

6 Continue down the refill sheet, pulling the correct amount of each requested item.

7 Once you have pulled all of the items on the ADSDS Refill Request Form, arrange them in such a way that what is on the counter matches (from left to right) what is ordered on the ADSDS Refill Request Form (from top to bottom). This extra organizational step makes the checking process more efficient.

8 Write your name and today's date on the ADSDS Refill Request Form, and ask for an instructor check.

9 Once your instructor has completed the check, take the ADSDS Refill Request Form and the medications to the ADSDS.

Practice Tip

Medications may be stored in the ADSDS by brand or generic name. Procedures may vary from state to state or among institutions.

Practice Tip

To avoid creating a count discrepancy, be sure to double-check the count in the drawer before verifying or denying the count in the computer.

Practice Tip

Again, to avoid creating a count discrepancy, be sure to double-check the count that you are adding before entering the number into the computer.

10 Enter your login and password, which have been provided by your instructor, into the computer. Enter the first medication name into the computer. The cabinet will automatically open the drawer (sometimes referred to as a *cell*) containing this medication.

11 Once the drawer opens, the computer will ask for verification of the medication count. Count the units (the exact number of pills, vials, bags, suppositories, etc.) in the drawer.

12 If the count in the drawer matches the computer's count, answer "yes" or enter the matching quantity. If the count in the drawer does not match the computer's count, answer "no" or enter the correct quantity into the computer. The computer will generate a discrepancy, or error, report, which will require later resolution by the nursing unit director and pharmacy quality assurance technician.

13 The computer will display the question, "How many do you wish to add?" Enter the exact number of units (pills, vials, bags, suppositories, etc.) of the medication you are placing into the designated drawer.

14 The computer will ask you to verify the new count and close the drawer. Carefully follow the steps listed on the computer.

15 Repeat this process for each medication on the ADSDS Refill Request Form.

16 Once you have placed all medications into the cabinet, log out of the computer. Logging out will cause the computer on the ADSDS to generate a receipt or printout. The receipt will list the actual count of everything in each drawer that you opened, track items added to the drawer, and highlight any discrepancies. Verify that the receipt contains your login name and the correct date.

17 **Conclusion:** Give the receipt and the completed ADSDS Refill Request Form to your instructor. Then go to the Course Navigator, answer all questions in the Lab Review section, and submit your answers to your instructor.

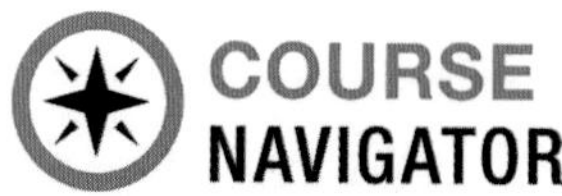

Access interactive chapter review exercises, practice activities, flash cards, and study games.

© Paradigm Publishing, Inc.

Name: ______________________ Date: ______________

Lab 21 Filling an ADSDS

Automated Drug Storage and Dispensing System Refill Request Form

Medication Name and Strength	Number to Refill	Instructor Check
Acetaminophen 325 mg tablets	10	______
Acetaminophen 500 mg caplets	8	______
Ampicillin 125 mg vials	6	______
Ampicillin 250 mg vials	3	______
Ampicillin 500 mg vials	11	______
Ampicillin 1,000 mg vials	2	______
Bacteriostatic NS 30 mL vials	9	______
Cimetidine 150 mg tablets	1	______
Diphenhydramine 25 mg tablets	10	______
Heparin lock flush 100 units/5 mL	6	______
Furosemide 20 mg tablets	4	______
Metoclopramide 5 mg/mL vial	3	______
MOM 30 mL unit-dose cup	2	______
Promethazine 25 mg/1 mL ampule	4	______
D_5W 100 mL IVPB	2	______
NS 50 mL IVPB	5	______
D_5W 1,000 mL IV	2	______

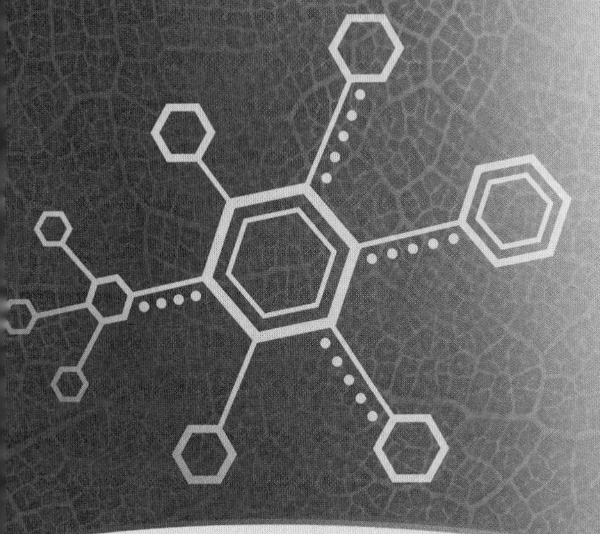

22 Medication Reconciliation

Learning Objectives

1 Describe the purpose of the medication reconciliation process.

2 Describe the role of the pharmacy technician in the medication reconciliation process.

3 Reconcile a patient-provided list of medications to a new or existing medical record.

Supplies

- Drug reference book(s) or Internet sites

Access additional chapter resources.

Practice Tip

To learn more, about The Joint Commission, visit http://PharmLabs3e.ParadigmCollege.net/Joint_Commission.

Practice Tip

To learn more about the Institute for Safe Medication Practices, visit http://PharmLabs3e.ParadigmCollege.net/ISMP.

Web

As medical science progresses, the management and treatment of disease states grow increasingly simple and increasingly complex. This may seem to be a paradox; however, with steadily increasing numbers of options for effectively treating diseases, the need for the healthcare team to maintain an accurate list of medications in the treatment of a hospital patient is very important. To ensure that a patient's medication history is accurately maintained and updated throughout the continuum of care, The Joint Commission strongly emphasizes the need to carefully document medication therapy throughout the treatment process within a hospital, from admission through discharge.

The weakest point for this communication, as identified by The Joint Commission and the Institute for Safe Medication Practices (ISMP), is when a patient is moved (transferred) from one care unit to another. During the transfer process, communication concerning the patient's treatment can break down because of the number of people involved, the lack of standardized procedures for moving a patient, the potential for shift change, and other factors. When combined, these contributing factors can potentially lead to a medication error.

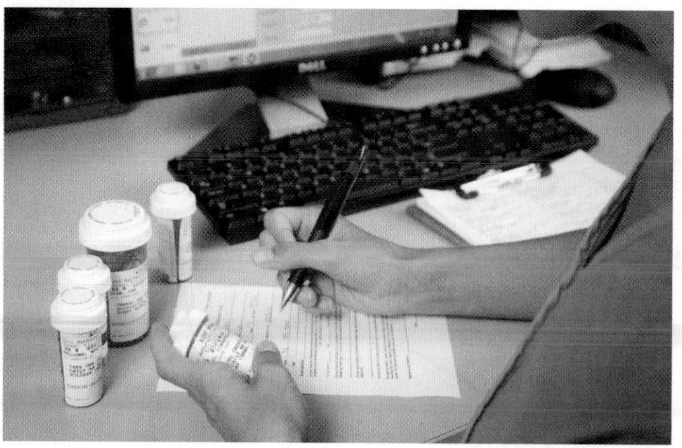

A pharmacy technician reviewing a patient's prescription bottles

As a means to prevent further lapses in communication, The Joint Commission includes the medication reconciliation process in its National Patient Safety Goals (NPSG), which are a part of the hospital accreditation process. Goal 03.06.01 of the NPSG states that "there is evidence that medication discrepancies can affect patient outcomes. Medication reconciliation is intended to identify and resolve discrepancies—it is a process of comparing the medications a patient is taking (and should be taking) with newly ordered medications. The comparison addresses duplications, omissions, and interactions, and the need to continue current medications." The ISMP also strongly promotes medication reconciliation as a means of eliminating medication errors.

One of the fastest growing areas of responsibility of institutional pharmacy technicians lies in the medication reconciliation process, in which they have a significant role. As a pharmacy technician, you may be asked to interview a patient and reconcile a list of medications at any point in the continuum of care. The most common points include admission and discharge, though pharmacy technicians may also help in the reconciliation process when patients present themselves to the emergency room or any other unit in the hospital. These units include intensive care, intermediate care, labor and delivery, outpatient surgery, and medical-surgical.

Medication reconciliation may occur in many ways. Often a patient will bring his or her prescription bottles from home, and the medication reconciliation technician must review each of the prescription bottles to determine if the prescriptions are still valid and are currently being taken by the patient. Sometimes the technician will contact the prescriber or the pharmacy where the prescription was filled in order to get the most current medication information for the patient. However, the first step is an initial interview with the patient, designated caregiver, or designated agent, followed by review of a patient-provided list. The list is then transcribed to a document or a computer system for inclusion in the medical record. It serves as a reference to aid the physician or other healthcare providers in establishing medication therapy while the patient is treated at the hospital.

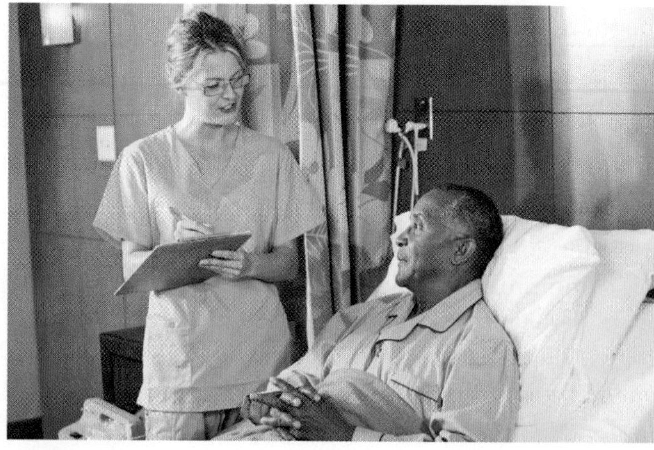

A pharmacy technician interviewing a patient about his medications

 © Paradigm Publishing, Inc.

Patients or their agents may not be able to provide accurate medication history because of injury, language barriers, being too young to communicate effectively, or disability. In the event that the patient cannot or will not communicate with the staff, does not know the details of his or her medication history, or is otherwise incapacitated, it may be necessary to call the patient's local pharmacy (if identified), next of kin, pharmacy benefits provider, or insurance company to obtain the list of medications. This process of obtaining information from third parties occurs more often than not, and while it is a potentially cumbersome process, it's important for you to work diligently to obtain the list and provide the highest level of care to each patient as you develop his or her medication history. The goal is to compile the best possible medication history during the reconciliation process. According to the NPSG Elements of Performance for the medication reconciliation process, "the types of information clinicians use to reconcile medications include (among others) medication name, dose, frequency, route, and purpose. Organizations should identify the information that needs to be collected to reconcile current and newly ordered medications and to safely prescribe medications in the future."

The other, equally important goal is to respect the dignity and privacy of the patient. You may be working in an area where many other people, including patients, family members, healthcare providers, staff, and others, will be present. You will be speaking about health information protected under the Health Information Portability and Accountability Act (HIPAA), and it is crucial that you make a diligent effort to protect this information, even if it means asking other people in the room to leave while you speak to the patient. Regardless of the others' reactions, your duty is to protect the patient.

To properly obtain a patient's medication history through a direct interview of the patient or the patient's representative (family member, other healthcare provider, or insurance company), there are several steps to follow:

1. Identify yourself by full name, role, department, and the purpose for your visit.
2. Verify the identity of the patient to ensure that you have the right patient and the right set of patient records. Each time you speak to a patient, even if you have spoken to him or her before, it is a best practice to verify the patient's name, date of birth, and patient ID number. This may be accomplished by speaking to the patient, looking at the patient's identification bracelet, and cross-referencing this information with the patient's chart information.
3. If other people are present in the room, ask the patient if he or she prefers that other people leave the room while you discuss his or her medication history, which is personal and protected information.
4. Ask the patient to verify his or her height, weight, and allergies to ensure appropriate medication dosing. There are many medications used in a hospital that must be accurately dosed using this information.

5. Ask the patient to name each prescription medication he or she takes, one medication at a time, and to provide the following information for each:
    a. Name
    b. Strength
    c. Route of administration
    d. Frequency of dosage
    e. Purpose
    f. Date/time of the most recent dose
6. Ask the patient to name each over-the-counter (OTC) medication he or she takes, one medication at a time, and to provide the following information for each:
    a. Name
    b. Strength
    c. Route of administration
    d. Frequency of dosage
    e. Purpose
    f. Date/time of the most recent dose
7. Ask the patient to name each herbal supplement or vitamin he or she takes, one supplement or vitamin at a time, and to provide the following information for each:
    a. Name
    b. Strength
    c. Route of administration
    d. Frequency of dosage
    e. Purpose
    f. Date/time of the most recent dose
8. Once the list is completed, it may be necessary to transcribe it into a computer system or a fresh document, depending on the facility's policies and procedures.

TAKE NOTE

While it may not seem important to obtain a list of OTC medications and herbal supplements, these items can interact or interfere with prescription medications used in the hospital. Another critical fact is that not every patient fully understands the use or intent of a medication. As an example, a pharmacy technician asked if the patient was on medication. The patient stated that he was not. When asked about any vitamins or supplements, the patient indicated he was taking a supplement and handed the technician a bottle of isoniazid, a legend drug used to treat tuberculosis. Because of this potential for confusion, it is important for the medication history to be as accurate and complete as possible.

© Paradigm Publishing, Inc.

Once completed, the list should be added to the patient's chart for review by the healthcare team as a point of reference for treatment and development of medication orders.

In many cases, a patient may be able to provide you with his or her own list of medications and supplements. This will aid in the process, but it is still necessary to interview the patient or patient representative for information on the last dose taken. If this information is not known, it is important to note this on the completed document.

Once the medication reconciliation process is finished, you may be asked to interview more patients and complete their medication histories or to return to the pharmacy to assist in order preparation. The medication reconciliation process is crucial to medication safety and should be executed with the most attentive care.

Procedure

Practice Tip

Many times, patient medication lists will contain spelling or other errors. You also have to read carefully to avoid misunderstanding a patient's handwriting.

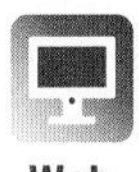

Web

1. Using the information provided in the following patient medication lists (Figures 22.1, 22.2, 22.3 , and 22.4), complete a Paradigm Hospital Medication Reconciliation Document (provided at the end of this lab).

2. If a piece of information is not known, make a note indicating as such—never guess, and never assume. This could cause serious and potentially fatal harm to the patient.

3. The use of signa abbreviations is accepted in many cases; however, there are many abbreviations that are prohibited in a hospital setting. When preparing the medication reconciliation document, be mindful to avoid these restricted abbreviations: http://PharmLabs3e.ParadigmCollege.net/Do_Not_Use.

4. When you have finished the list, be sure to fill in the Created by Name/Credential, Dept, and Date lines with the appropriate information.

5. **Conclusion:** Submit the completed forms to your instructor for review and grading. Then go to the Course Navigator, answer all questions in the Lab Review section, and submit your answers to your instructor.

TAKE NOTE

Medication reconciliation is a critical step in the continuum of care. Many medications sound alike and have similar dosing. When preparing a patient's medication history, a critical eye for detail is vital for the well-being and safety of the patient.

FIGURE 22.1
A Handwritten Form

Molly Summers is sitting in the ER in acute care after having an incident at a supermarket. She has been in pleasant spirits since she arrived. She stated that she took her medication through last night, but did not take anything today, April 17, 2019, other than one nitroglycerin tablet at the supermarket this morning around 7 a.m. She stated that she is allergic to shellfish and penicillin. In her interview, she stated that she is 5 feet, 8 inches tall and weighs approximately 250 pounds. She presents the following handwritten form with worn edges and multiple creases from having been folded and kept in her wallet for an extended period of time.

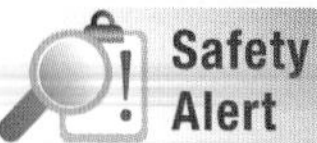

While patients may have a list of their medications, they sometimes contain misspellings or other errors. The pharmacy technician should make sure to verify the correct medication, spelling, and dosage when performing medication reconciliation.

Prescription Medications

Medication Name	Dose/How often?
Nitrogliserin	0.4 mg under the tongue for chest pain
Asperin	81mg in the morning
Alprazalam	1mg every 6 hours or as needed for my ~~anx~~ nerves
Glocotrol	5mg 2x/day
Xalatan Eye Drops	1 in left eye when I go to bed
Humulin 70/30	50 units in the morning
Lantis	22 units at bed time

 © Paradigm Publishing, Inc.

FIGURE 22.2
A Handwritten List of Medications and Supplements

A family member, Gloria, provides the pharmacy technician a handwritten list of George Miller's medications and supplements. In an interview, Gloria states that George was relatively compliant with his medications. George collapsed around 2 p.m., when they were at the movies. George had taken his medications at 8 a.m. and through noon today, Saturday, April 13, 2019. He takes his evening medications around 7 p.m. and his nighttime medications around 10 p.m. George has no allergies. He was born on September 8, 1965; is 6 feet, 2 inches tall; and weighs 200 pounds.

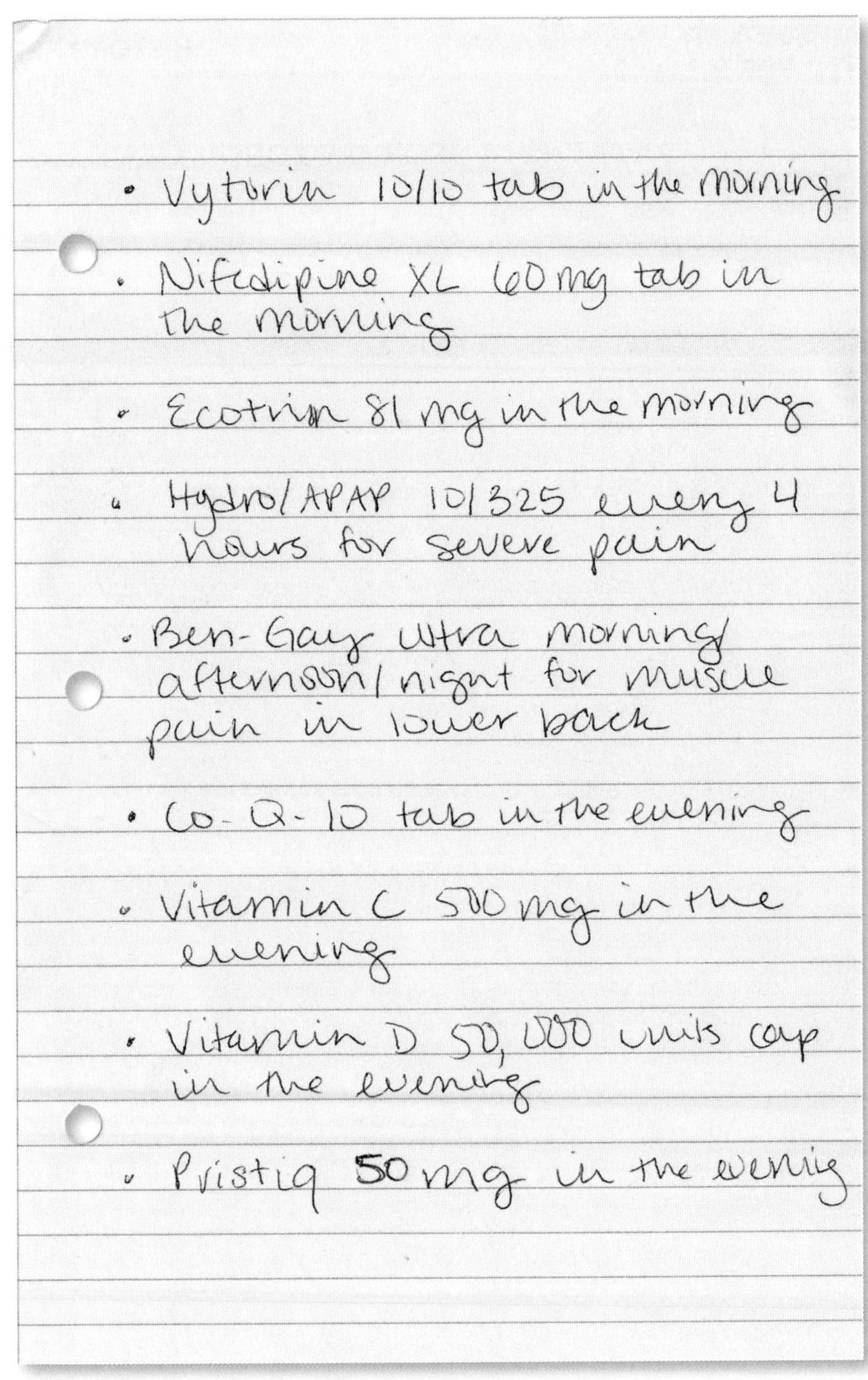

- Vytorin 10/10 tab in the morning
- Nifedipine XL 60 mg tab in the morning
- Ecotrin 81 mg in the morning
- Hydro/APAP 10/325 every 4 hours for severe pain
- Ben-Gay Ultra morning/afternoon/night for muscle pain in lower back
- Co-Q-10 tab in the evening
- Vitamin C 500 mg in the evening
- Vitamin D 50,000 units cap in the evening
- Pristiq 50 mg in the evening

FIGURE 22.3
A Typed Document from a Local Pharmacy

The patient arrived unconscious but had an old prescription bottle in her purse. The pharmacy faxed a typed document to the hospital emergency room at the request of a pharmacy technician.

The Corner Drug Store
875 Paradigm Way – Austin, Texas 78704
(512) 555-1212 – telephone

PATIENT PRESCRIPTION HISTORY REPORT

PATIENT INFORMATION

FELICIA JOHANSEN
1457 North Lamar Blvd
Austin, Texas 78738
(512) 555-1212

DOB: 04/27/1955
Height: 5ft 7in Weight: 115lbs
ALLERGIES: PCN, Codeine

Insurance
Apollo Health (115609)
ID: GT334918; Grp: RX12
PC: 00

Prescription	QTY	Directions	Prescriber	Date Written	Last Filled
PLAVIX 10MG TABLETS	30	TAKE 1 TABLET BY MOUTH DAILY	CARDOZA, FRANCISCO MD	01/12/19	02/13/19
LISINOPRIL 10MG TABLETS	30	TAKE 1 TABLET BY MOUTH DAILY	CARDOZA, FRANCISCO MD	01/12/19	02/13/19
SYNTHROID 0.05MG TABLETS	30	TAKE 1 TABLET BY MOUTH EACH MORNING BEFORE BREAKFAST	CARDOZA, FRANCISCO MD	01/12/19	02/13/19
LIPITOR 10MG TABLETS	30	TAKE 1 TABLET MY MOUTH AT BEDTIME	CARDOZA, FRANCISCO MD	01/12/19	02/13/19
PROTONIX 40MG TABLETS	30	TAKE 1 TABLET BY MOUTH EACH MORNING FOR GERD.	CARDOZA, FRANCISCO MD	01/12/19	02/13/19
ROZEREM 8MG TABLETS	10	TAKE 1 TABLET BY MOUTH AT BEDTIME AS NEEDED FOR SLEEP	CARDOZA, FRANCISCO MD	10/08/18	12/10/18

 © Paradigm Publishing, Inc.

FIGURE 22.4
Prescription Labels

A patient admitted to the hospital brought his current prescription medication bottles with him.

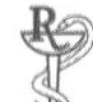

THE CORNER DRUG STORE
17 Main Street - Orlando, FL 32810
phone (407) 555-1212 fax (407) 555-1313

RX **6598774**

DATE FILLED: 03/04/2019
ORIGINAL DATE: 10/01/2018

STRICKLAND, MARK
896 Burnet Road, Austin, TX 78757 – DOB: November 24, 1993

TAKE 1 TABLET BY MOUTH EVERY DAY FOR PrEP.

TRUVADA 200MG/300MG TABLETS **QTY: 30**

Prescriber: MARCO GRANETO, MD
REFILLS: 1 **JPS/LAM**

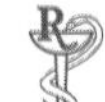

THE CORNER DRUG STORE
17 Main Street - Orlando, FL 32810
phone (407) 555-1212 fax (407) 555-1313

RX **6598775**

DATE FILLED: 03/04/2019
ORIGINAL DATE: 10/01/2018

STRICKLAND, MARK
896 Burnet Road, Austin, TX 78757 – DOB: November 24, 1993

TAKE 1 TABLET BY MOUTH DAILY.

LOSARTAN/HCTZ 100MG/12.5MG GENERIC FOR HYZAAR 100MG/12.5MG TABLETS **QTY: 30**

Prescriber: MARCO GRANETO, MD
REFILLS: 7 **JPS/LAM**

Name: ______________________ Date: ____________

Lab 22 Medication Reconciliation

PARADIGM HOSPITAL MEDICATION RECONCILIATION DOCUMENT

PATIENT INFORMATION	LIST OF ALLERGIES	Height (inches)
NAME ____________ D.O.B. ____________ GENDER: ☐ MALE ☐ FEMALE	____ Initial here for NO KNOWN ALLERGIES	____________ Weight (kg) ____________

Medication Name	Dose	Route	Frequency	Special Instructions	Last Dose	Status
Alprazolam	0.5mg	PO	Q 4 hours	PRN Anxiety	02/22/19 1645	EXAMPLE
						☐ ACTIVE D/C ☐
						☐ ACTIVE D/C ☐
						☐ ACTIVE D/C ☐
						☐ ACTIVE D/C ☐
						☐ ACTIVE D/C ☐
						☐ ACTIVE D/C ☐
						☐ ACTIVE D/C ☐
						☐ ACTIVE D/C ☐
						☐ ACTIVE D/C ☐
						☐ ACTIVE D/C ☐

Please provide the name, relationship, and phone number for the source of information contained on this document if other than patient:

Created by Name/Credential: ____________________ Dept: ________ Date: ________

Reviewed by Name/Credential: ____________________ Dept: ________ Date: ________

Ordered by physician: ____________________ **Date:** ________

Name: ________________________ Date: ______________

Lab 22 Medication Reconciliation

PARADIGM HOSPITAL MEDICATION RECONCILIATION DOCUMENT

PATIENT INFORMATION	LIST OF ALLERGIES	Height (inches)
NAME ______________ D.O.B. ______________ GENDER: ☐ MALE ☐ FEMALE	____ Initial here for NO KNOWN ALLERGIES	____________ Weight (kg) ____________

Medication Name	Dose	Route	Frequency	Special Instructions	Last Dose	Status
						☐ ACTIVE ☐ D/C
						☐ ACTIVE ☐ D/C
						☐ ACTIVE ☐ D/C
						☐ ACTIVE ☐ D/C
						☐ ACTIVE ☐ D/C
						☐ ACTIVE ☐ D/C
						☐ ACTIVE ☐ D/C
						☐ ACTIVE ☐ D/C
						☐ ACTIVE ☐ D/C
						☐ ACTIVE ☐ D/C
						☐ ACTIVE ☐ D/C

Please provide the name, relationship, and phone number for the source of information contained on this document if other than patient:

Created by Name/Credential: ______________________ Dept: ________ Date: ________

Reviewed by Name/Credential: ______________________ Dept: ________ Date: ________

Ordered by physician: ______________________ **Date:** ________

© Paradigm Publishing, Inc.

Name: ______________________ Date: ______________

Lab 22 Medication Reconciliation

PARADIGM HOSPITAL MEDICATION RECONCILIATION DOCUMENT

PATIENT INFORMATION	LIST OF ALLERGIES	Height (inches)
NAME ______________ D.O.B. ______________ GENDER: ☐ MALE ☐ FEMALE	____ Initial here for NO KNOWN ALLERGIES	______________ Weight (kg) ______________

Medication Name	Dose	Route	Frequency	Special Instructions	Last Dose	Status
						☐ ACTIVE ☐ D/C
						☐ ACTIVE ☐ D/C
						☐ ACTIVE ☐ D/C
						☐ ACTIVE ☐ D/C
						☐ ACTIVE ☐ D/C
						☐ ACTIVE ☐ D/C
						☐ ACTIVE ☐ D/C
						☐ ACTIVE ☐ D/C
						☐ ACTIVE ☐ D/C
						☐ ACTIVE ☐ D/C
						☐ ACTIVE ☐ D/C

Please provide the name, relationship, and phone number for the source of information contained on this document if other than patient:

Created by Name/Credential: ______________________ Dept: ________ Date: ________

Reviewed by Name/Credential: ______________________ Dept: ________ Date: ________

Ordered by physician: ______________________ **Date:** ________

Name: ______________________________ Date: ________________

Lab 22 Medication Reconciliation

PARADIGM HOSPITAL MEDICATION RECONCILIATION DOCUMENT

PATIENT INFORMATION	LIST OF ALLERGIES	Height (inches)
NAME ____________________ D.O.B. ____________________ GENDER: ☐ MALE ☐ FEMALE	____ Initial here for NO KNOWN ALLERGIES	____________ Weight (kg) ____________

Medication Name	Dose	Route	Frequency	Special Instructions	Last Dose	Status
						☐ ACTIVE ☐ D/C
						☐ ACTIVE ☐ D/C
						☐ ACTIVE ☐ D/C
						☐ ACTIVE ☐ D/C
						☐ ACTIVE ☐ D/C
						☐ ACTIVE ☐ D/C
						☐ ACTIVE ☐ D/C
						☐ ACTIVE ☐ D/C
						☐ ACTIVE ☐ D/C
						☐ ACTIVE ☐ D/C
						☐ ACTIVE ☐ D/C

Please provide the name, relationship, and phone number for the source of information contained on this document if other than patient:

Created by Name/Credential: ______________________ Dept: ________ Date: ________

Reviewed by Name/Credential: ______________________ Dept: ________ Date: ________

Ordered by physician: ______________________ **Date:** ________

© Paradigm Publishing, Inc.

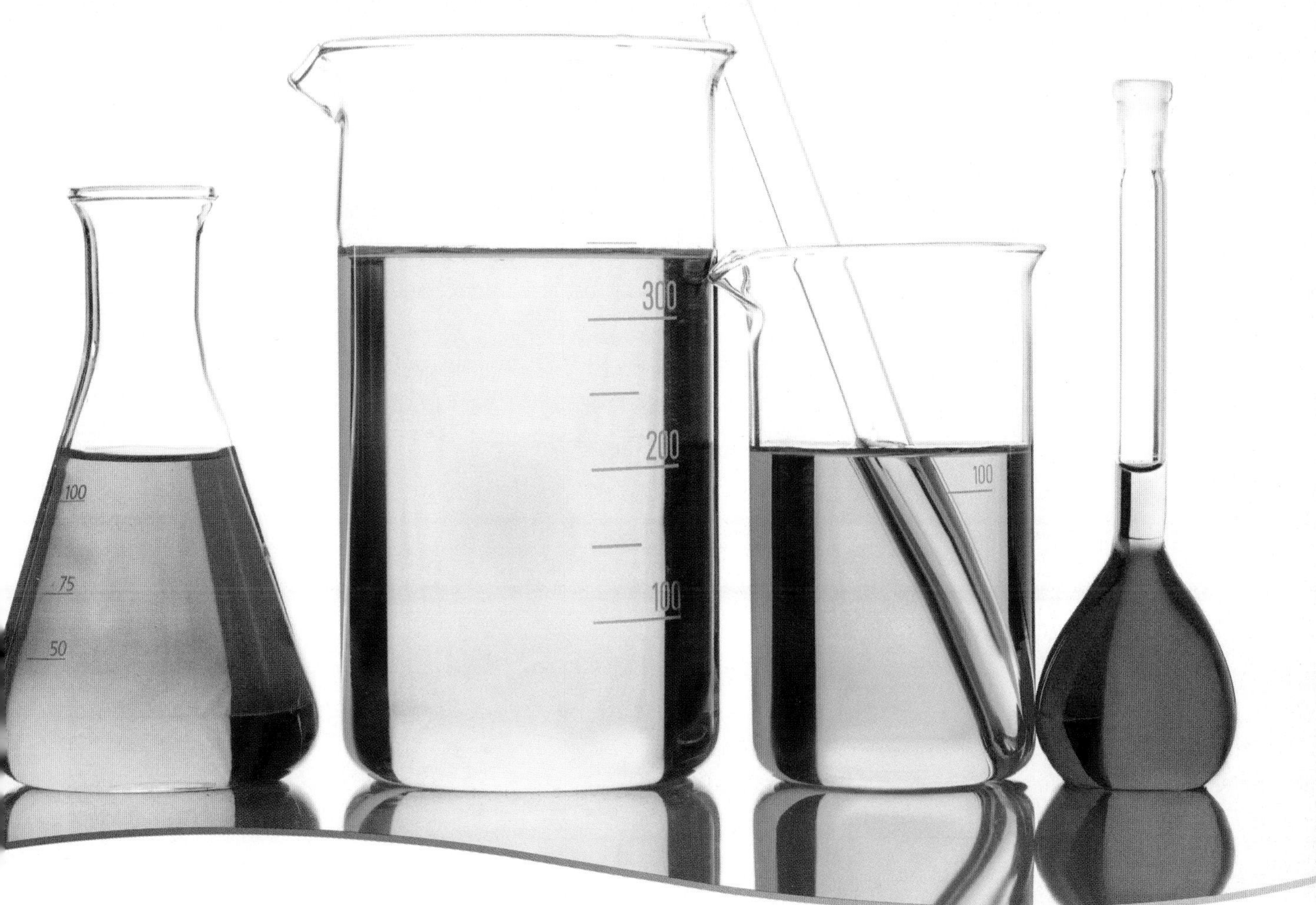

UNIT 4 Nonsterile Extemporaneous Compounding

A day in the life of a pharmacy technician...

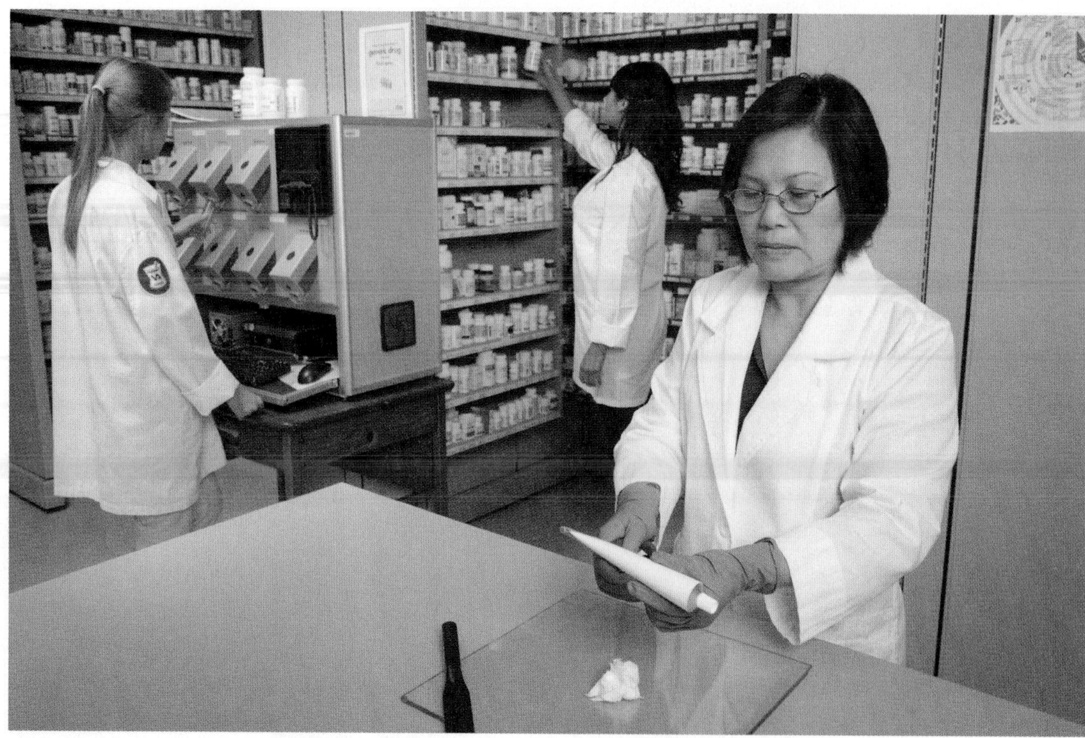

Grasshoppers Solution, Costanzi's Solution, testosterone cream, medicinal lollipops, pain capsules—preparing compounded prescriptions such as these is all in a day's work for the pharmacy technician in the extemporaneous compounding environment.

Pharmacy technicians with special training in extemporaneous compounding prepare medications for patients who require a drug or dosage form that is not commercially available. Some patients require medications that are free of allergenic inactive ingredients such as dyes or preservatives; other patients require unique combinations or dosages of medication. Certain medications that may only be available as a tablet or capsule might be ground into a powder and administered topically based on the patient's individual needs.

Pharmacy technicians who prepare extemporaneously compounded pharmaceuticals must have strict attention to detail and prepare the medication according to a specific recipe.

This unit will guide you through the essential tasks related to extemporaneous compounding, including the use of a mortar and pestle, digital scale, weighing boat, and various graduated cylinders. You will learn how to prepare solutions, ointments, and creams according to pharmacy recipes. These tasks are the foundational aspects of extemporaneous compounding.

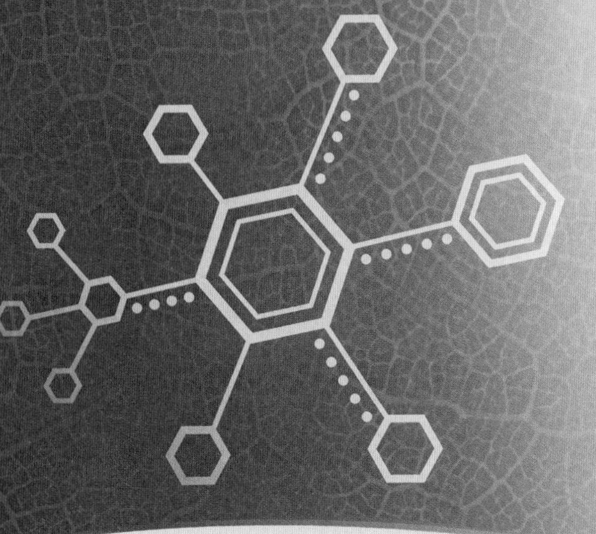

23

Reconstituting Powders

Learning Objectives

1 Demonstrate skill in measuring diluent and reconstituting powder medications for oral use.

2 Demonstrate competence in calculations related to reconstituting powder medications for oral use.

3 Discuss the rationale for and procedures related to reconstituting powder medication for oral use.

4 Practice common pharmacy calculations related to the preparation of oral liquid medications.

5 Become familiar with the compounding log as a means of recording the measurements, ingredients, and procedures used in compounding nonsterile products.

Supplies

- Augmentin 125 mg/5 mL (100 mL bottle)
- Reconstitube® (or similar, 100 mL or larger device attached to a water supply)
- Auxiliary labels
- Medication labels
- Calculator

Access additional chapter resources.

Introduction to Extemporaneous Compounding for Labs 23–28

Prior to the mass production of prepared pharmaceutical products in the 1940s and 1950s, pharmacies prepared individualized medications per prescription orders from prescribers. This individualized preparation was termed **compounding** and included compressing tablets, creating suspensions, and filling capsules with a requested strength or amount of medication. Pharmacy technicians are still called upon to perform many types of extemporaneous, or nonsterile, compounding procedures, including preparing oral solutions, suppositories, capsules, troches, lozenges, creams, ointments, gels, and pastes. Today, compounding is required under several circumstances, including as a response to patients' unique needs, manufacturer-based difficulties, and physician-initiated requests. This type of compounding is often referred to as **extemporaneous compounding**. Additionally, extemporaneous compounding is sometimes referred to as *nonsterile compounding*.

In November 2013, the US Pharmacopeial Convention (USP) (a scientific nonprofit organization that sets standards for the identity, strength, quality, and purity of medicines, food ingredients, and dietary supplements) released significant revisions to Chapter <795> Pharmaceutical Compounding–Nonsterile Preparations. This chapter provides the minimum enforceable regulations on the preparation of nonsterile pharmaceutical products. Many states adopt these federal guidelines as a direct or indirect part of their state's pharmacy act (rules and regulations of pharmacy practice adopted as law in each state). As a pharmacy technician, you will be required to understand these guidelines in the daily execution of your job duties.

With patient safety being the primary focus of these regulations, pharmacy technicians must be aware of and responsible for how products are prepared and how the final product is dispensed to the patient. The environment, the equipment used, and all ingredients in the process must be properly maintained and cleaned. This helps prevent cross-contamination and ensures the safety of pharmacy personnel and patients alike.

The revisions to USP Chapter <795> became officially enforceable in January 2014. The importance of these regulations is summarized by the final bullet point in the *Training* section of the revised chapter, which states, "The compounder is solely responsible for the finished preparation."

While compounding in the pharmacy lab, safety, accuracy, and proper record keeping are essential. These safety precautions are used both in the lab setting and in practice. You must wear gloves throughout all compounding procedures in order to protect (1) yourself from exposure to the medication, (2) the medication from degradation caused by skin cells and oils, and (3) the patient from potentially contaminated medications. Depending on the ingredients used to prepare the compound, you may also be required to wear safety glasses, a face mask, and/or a protective smock. Refer to the individual recipe for safety requirements. Accuracy is crucial in drug measurement and dose calculations. Some compounding lab procedures provide one or more **recipes**, which list the exact quantity of each ingredient and the processes required to compound a particular prescription. Other procedures provide dosage information and require your calculations to prepare the final product. Finally, you must keep careful and precise records each time you compound a prescription, which is accomplished by creating a **compounding log**, an official, detailed record of the processes and materials used to compound a prescription. Because requirements for record-keeping may vary widely among states and individual facilities, you should check with your instructor about specific, local record-keeping procedures for compounded pharmaceutical products. An example of a compounding log is shown in Figure 23.1.

 © Paradigm Publishing, Inc.

TAKE NOTE

You must keep accurate records when preparing extemporaneous compounds. Each time you compound a prescription, even if it is a product you have previously prepared, you must create an entry in a compounding log. The compounding log contains detailed information and commonly includes the name of the final compound; the quantity prepared; a copy of the patient label, recipe, or instructions; the name, lot number, and quantity of all products and ingredients used; and a record of the steps followed to prepare the prescription. In addition, the compounding log will require you to create a unique lot number and expiration date to easily identify the compounded product. The process for record keeping in a compounding log may vary widely among states and individual facilities.

FIGURE 23.1 **Pharmacy Compounding Log Sheet**

Product Label ______________________

Date Prepared ______________________

Pharmacy Lot Number ______________________

Strength ______________________

AFFIX PHARMACY LABEL HERE

Quantity Prepared ______________________

Quantity Packaged ______________________

	Manufacturer's Lot Number	Ingredient Name	Amount Needed	Measured By	Verified By
1					
2					
3					
4					
5					
6					
7					
8					

Directions for Preparation:

Completion Time: ______________________

Prepared By ______________________

Auxiliary Labeling

Approved By ______________________

Date ______________________ Expiration Date

Many liquids and suspensions for oral use are supplied as commercially prepared powders that must be **reconstituted** (changed into liquid form by having water or another fluid added to them) before they can be dispensed to the patient. When reconstituting a powder medication, you should take special care to measure the proper amount of **diluent** (the liquid that is added to the powder)to ensure the correct concentration of medication. Manufacturers may vary in using distilled water or sterile water for reconstitution.

Reconstituting powder medications requires particular equipment. Some facilities might have you use a graduated cylinder or similar product to measure diluent volumes. Easy and accurate diluent measurements can be made with a Reconstitube, a modified graduated cylinder with two tubes attached. The upper tube connects the cylinder to a supply of water or other liquid, and the lower tube, which is open-ended, enters the medication bottle.

When you open a small clamp on the upper tube, diluent flows from the liquid source into the graduated cylinder of the Reconstitube. Opening the lower tube allows the liquid to flow from the cylinder into the powder. You must add the diluent to the powder in two stages, shaking the solution at both stages to thoroughly mix the powder into an oral solution. To complete the reconstitution process, affix a medication label and appropriate auxiliary labels to the oral solution bottle.

In some instances, after preparing an amount of liquid medication, you will be asked to take the next step in getting the medication ready for patients: performing calculations to determine the volume of an individual dose. You will use the equations, as given below. Always start with the information that is provided on the label. In this case, Augmentin will have a concentration of 125 mg/5 mL once it has been diluted. Given that information, determine how many milliliters you would need to give a patient for the following doses: Augmentin 200 mg and Augmentin 250 mg.

Use the following equations to calculate the doses:

$$\frac{125\text{ mg}}{5\text{ mL}} = \frac{200\text{ mg}}{x\text{ mL}} \qquad \frac{125\text{ mg}}{5\text{ mL}} = \frac{250\text{ mg}}{x\text{ mL}}$$

In order to solve for x, the unknown volume, you will cross multiply and then divide. (To review the cross multiplication process, refer to Lab 19, Preparing Oral Syringes.) In these two examples, your calculations will show you that a 200 mg dose of Augmentin is 8 mL, and a 250 mg dose is 10 mL.

Procedure

In this lab, you will use a Reconstitube (or similar device) to reconstitute a bottle of Augmentin powder for oral use. You will measure an appropriate amount of diluent (in this case, water), add it to the suspension, prepare the powder medication for dispensing, and practice related dose calculations.

© Paradigm Publishing, Inc.

Prepare a compounding log, if directed by your instructor, to record the steps and ingredients that you use.

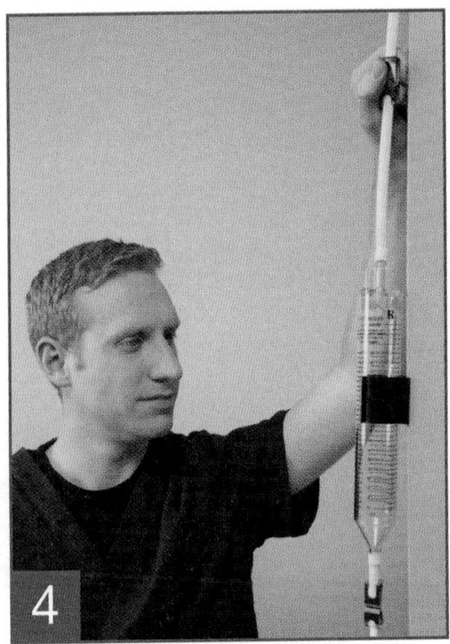

Pharmacy technician opening the upper clamp of a Reconstitube.

1 Gather the supplies listed for this lab, set them on the workspace, and arrange them in an easily accessible and organized manner.

2 Wash your hands thoroughly. If directed to do so by your instructor, put on gloves, and wear them throughout the procedure.

3 Bring the Augmentin bottle to the area in the pharmacy where the Reconstitube is located. Ensure that the lower clamp on the Reconstitube is securely closed by pinching the clamp until it clicks shut.

For Good Measure

When reconstituting powder medications, read the accompanying package insert to verify the diluent amount prior to measuring it in the Reconstitube. The diluent volume will be different with each medication.

4 Open the upper clamp on the Reconstitube by pinching the clamp until it clicks open. You will see water from the storage container begin flowing into the tube. Allow the water to flow freely into the Reconstitube until it reaches approximately the 70 mL mark. (You will ultimately be filling the Reconstitube to the 90 mL mark.)

5 Grasp the upper clamp on the Reconstitube and squeeze softly such that the flow of water slows. While applying slight pressure to the upper clamp, allow water to continue slowly filling the Reconstitube. When the tube is filled to the desired volume of 90 mL, close the upper clamp by pinching it until it clicks shut. See Figure 23.2 for an illustration of this technique.

6 Ask for an instructor check of the diluent volume in the Reconstitube.

7 Grasp the Augmentin bottle and carefully tap it against your palm or a countertop so that the powder is dislodged from the bottom of the bottle and moves freely within the container. Remove the cap from the Augmentin bottle.

Safety Alert

To prevent cross-contamination, take care not to get any powder on the lower tube.

8 Place the tip of the lower tube of the Reconstitube into the mouth of the Augmentin bottle, and while holding the medication bottle in place, open the lower clamp and allow water to flow into the bottle, maintaining slight pressure on the lower clamp to control the flow of diluent.

© Paradigm Publishing, Inc.

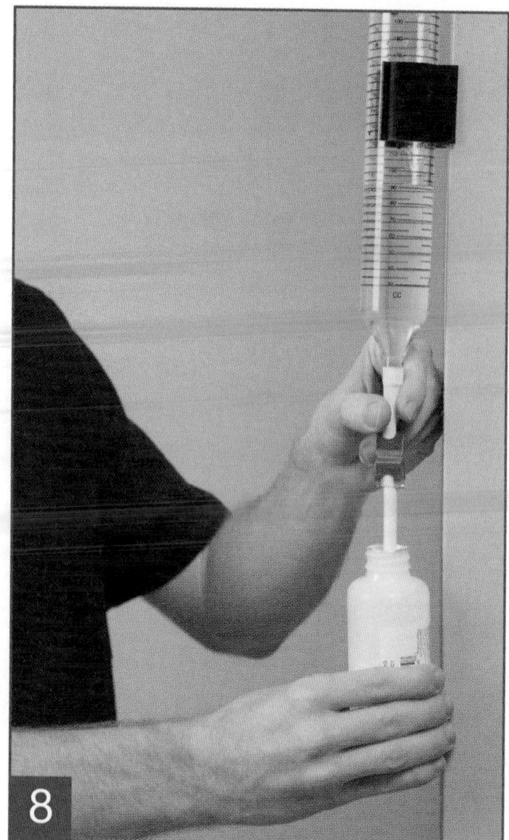

Pharmacy technician opening the lower Reconstitube clamp, which allows water to flow into the medication bottle

FIGURE 23.2 Reconstitube Components

Illustration of a Reconstitube containing 90 mL of diluent; notice that the lowest point of the meniscus rests on the 90 mL line.

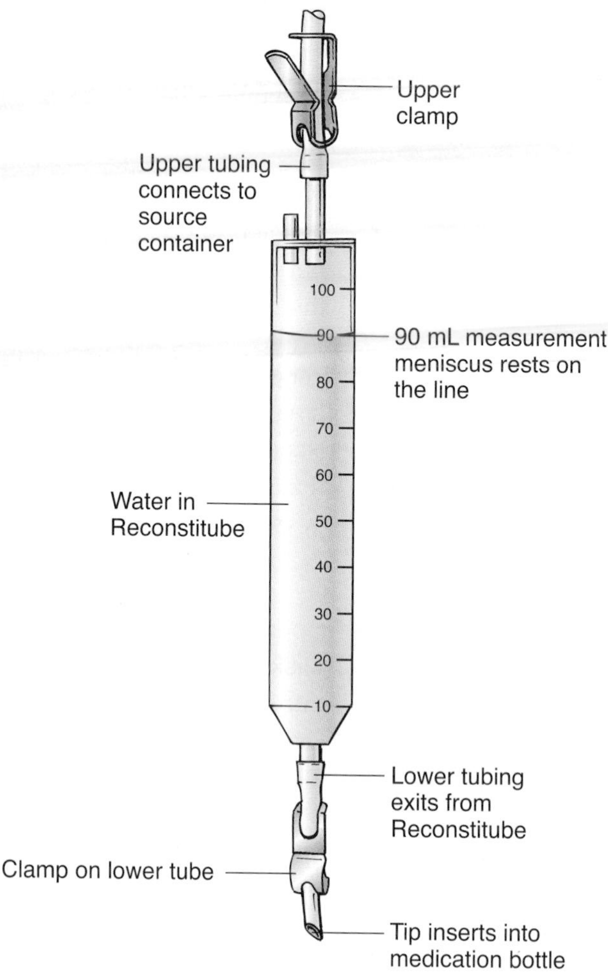

For Good Measure

You should add only one-third of the diluent to the medication bottle at first, allowing the powder to dissolve gradually in the diluent. If you add all the liquid at once, the powder medication would likely stick to the bottom of the medication bottle and resist dilution. In addition, the water could overflow and you would end up with lost medication.

9 When approximately one-third (or 30 mL) of the total volume of diluent has been added to the medication bottle, close the lower clamp.

10 Recap the medication bottle and shake it vigorously.

11 Once again, remove the cap of the medication bottle and place the tip of the lower tube of the Reconstitube into the mouth of the bottle. Open the lower clamp and allow all of the remaining diluent to flow freely into the medication bottle.

© Paradigm Publishing, Inc.

12 Tightly recap the medication bottle and again shake it vigorously. Verify that the powder has been fully incorporated into the diluent and that no powder remains stuck to the bottom of the Augmentin bottle. If you notice any undissolved powder, continue to shake the medication bottle until the drug is fully dissolved and the dilution is complete.

13 Affix the patient label to the medication bottle as directed by your instructor. Also affix "Shake Well" and "Refrigerate" labels to the medication bottle.

14 Prepare the compounding log, if directed by your instructor.

15 **Conclusion:** Present your log (if created), your calculations, and your final product to your instructor for a final check. Then go to the Course Navigator, answer all questions in the Lab Review section, and submit your answers to your instructor.

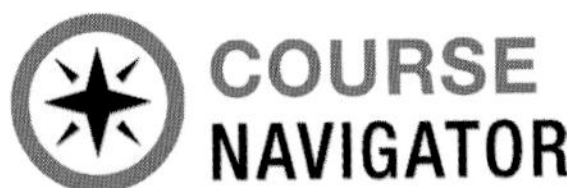

Access interactive chapter review exercises, practice activities, flash cards, and study games.

© Paradigm Publishing, Inc.

24

Filling Capsules

Learning Objectives

1 Demonstrate proficiency in the process of compounding capsules from other dosage forms.

2 Demonstrate skill in the punch method of filling empty capsules.

3 Demonstrate skill in the use of laboratory equipment used in compounding.

4 Become familiar with the compounding log as a means of recording the measurements, ingredients, and procedures used in compounding nonsterile products.

Supplies

- 10 placebo or metronidazole 500 mg tablets
- 6 empty gelatin capsules, size 0
- Counting tray and counting spatula
- Mortar and pestle
- Glass ointment slab
- 8- or 10-inch stainless steel spatula
- Digital balance that provides metric unit weights and displays three decimal spaces (e.g., 1.001 g)
- Clean, dry gauze pad or cloth
- Prescription vial for packaging the compounded capsules
- Weighing boat or paper

Access additional chapter resources.

Although the practice of filling capsules in today's pharmacies is uncommon, it is still sometimes used. One method of filling capsules is known as the **punch method**, which gets its name from the filling technique used—punching the capsules into a leveled cake of drug powder. Filling capsules using the punch method can be messy, because you are dealing with large amounts of powder. Despite this challenge, you must maintain accuracy. When preparing the compounded prescription, work carefully, and take your time.

To create the powder, you will use a mortar and pestle to **triturate** (break up or grind into smaller pieces) tablets into a fine, uniform **particulate** (a powder or fine-textured material). Adding and removing small amounts of powder from the capsules and weighing and reweighing them may be frustrating. However, you may also find it rewarding, because you are preparing a specific product for a specific patient using essential ingredients.

Procedure

In this lab, you will practice using the punch method to prepare the number of capsules requested by a prescription. For example, consider this scenario:

> Metronidazole is a manufactured product, but it is produced in tablet form. Because some patients have a difficult time swallowing tablets, a physician has asked your pharmacy to compound tablets into capsules. You can help by filling five capsules to the requested weight (and preparing a compounding log, if directed by your instructor, to record the steps and ingredients that you use).

In this case, a compounding formula is not needed; you will simply be given the recipe as the steps proceed.

1 Set your supplies on the workspace, and arrange them in an easily accessible and organized manner. Visually inspect them to ensure that they are clean. If they are not, wash and dry them before use.

2 Wash your hands thoroughly, put on gloves, and wear them throughout the procedure.

3 Using the counting tray, count 10 tablets from the stock bottle and place them into the mortar. Use the pestle to triturate the tablets into a fine, uniform particulate.

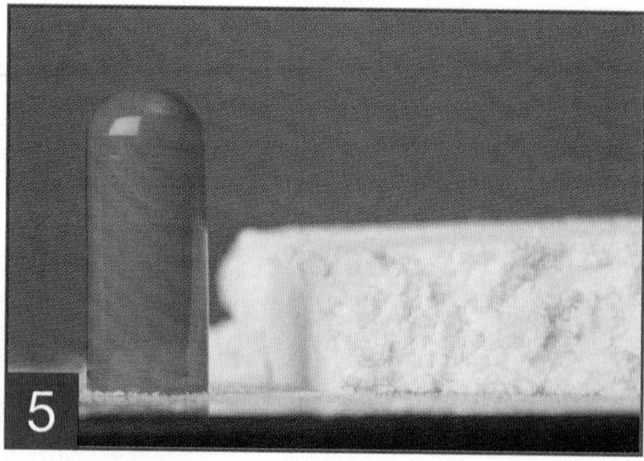

Powder leveled into a cake approximately one-half the height of the empty capsule body

4 Pour the contents of the mortar onto the ointment slab, and with the spatula, scrape the sides of the mortar to get as much powder as possible out of the vessel and onto the slab.

5 Using the spatula, form the powder into a leveled cake approximately one-half the height of the empty capsule body.

© Paradigm Publishing, Inc.

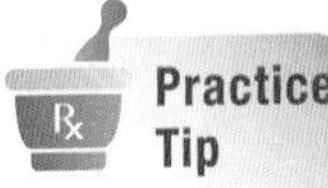

Practice Tip

Do not use a scooping motion when removing the capsule body. Rather, be sure to pull it straight up and out of the powder cake.

6 Remove the capsule cap (the smaller section of the empty capsule) from five of the empty capsules and set them aside. Place the five capsule bodies (the larger sections of the empty capsules) on the ointment slab. Leave the sixth capsule intact.

7 Grasp the larger section of an empty capsule, open side down, with the thumb and forefinger. Punch the open capsule into the cake of powder (7a). When you reach the bottom of the powder, rotate the capsule slightly (7b), gently pinch the open end of the capsule, and withdraw the capsule from the powder (7c).

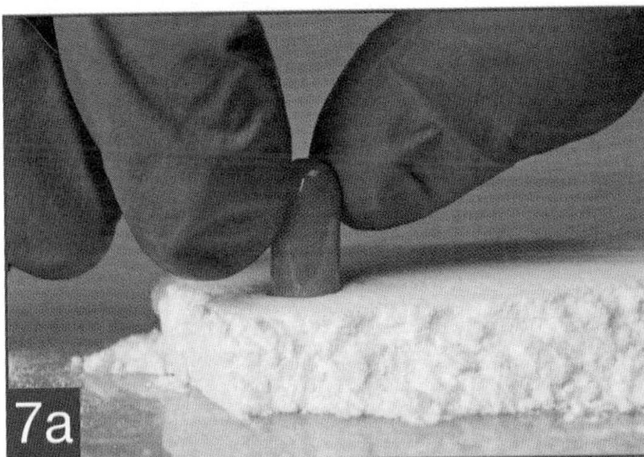

8 Punch the capsule into the powder a second time, keeping the open end of the capsule pinched until you reach the top of the powder cake. Open the capsule just as you reach the cake, pushing into the powder. When you reach the bottom of the powder, rotate the capsule slightly, gently pinch the open end of the capsule, and withdraw the capsule from the powder.

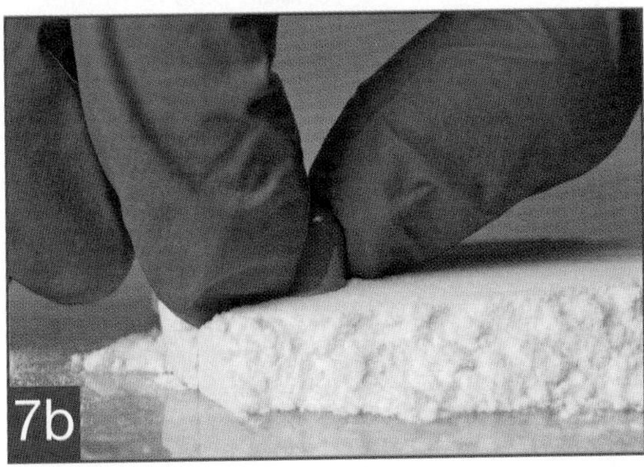

7c

The punch method of capsule preparation.

TAKE NOTE

Some capsules have smooth bodies that allow for easy removal and application of the capsule top. Others, however, have a ridge in the middle of the capsule that acts as a locking mechanism. If you have ridged capsules, be careful not to reattach the capsule too tightly. You may not be able to reopen the capsule to adjust the weight of the capsule contents without damaging it. The pharmacy cannot dispense a damaged capsule.

© Paradigm Publishing, Inc.

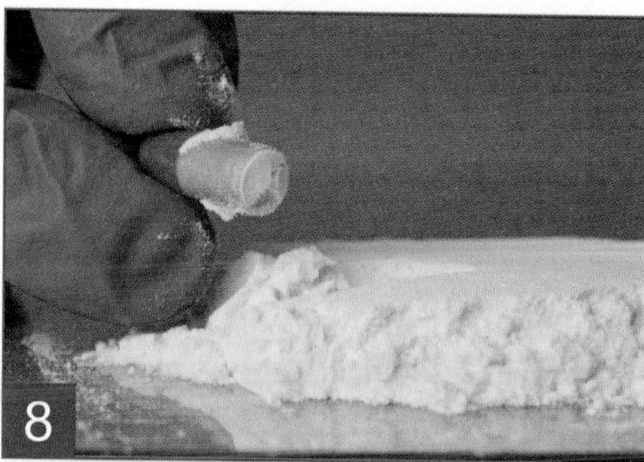

Filled capsule being withdrawn from powder

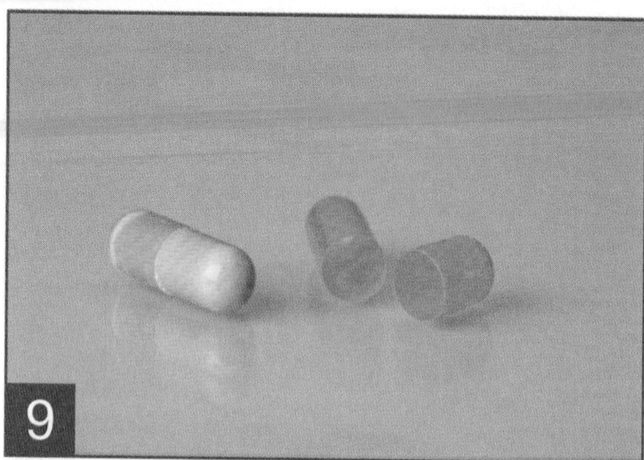

Filled capsule (left) and empty capsule (right). Both capsules will be weighed in the next several steps

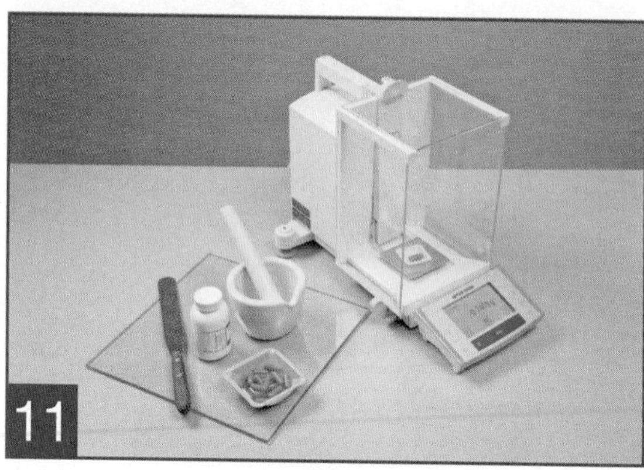

Empty capsule being weighed on a digital scale

9 Hold the capsule body with the open end upward, being careful not to spill any powder from the capsule. Place the cap of the capsule back onto the body of the capsule and set it aside.

10 Ensure that the digital scale is on a flat surface and set it level, following the directions in the scale's user manual. Turn it on, and allow it to zero.

11 Place the intact, empty capsule (the sixth capsule) on the weighing pan, and allow the scale to stabilize and provide a reading.

12 Press the **tare** or zero button. Pressing tare or zero resets the scale to zero and accounts for the weight of the capsule itself when weighing a capsule plus contents. The scale is now set to display only the weight of the capsule contents.

13 Remove the empty capsule from the scale pan. Gently wipe the exterior of the filled capsule with the gauze pad or cloth to remove excess powder. Place the filled capsule on the pan and take the reading.

14 If this initial weight is *greater than* the required amount of 500 mg (the amount indicated by the prescription), open the capsule, and gently tap out some powder onto the powder cake. Reseal, wipe, and reweigh the capsule, repeating the process until the desired weight is reached.

However, if the initial weight of the capsule is *less than* the required amount, reshape the powder into a leveled cake (as in Step 5), open the capsule, and repeat the punching process. Reseal, wipe, and reweigh the capsule. Repeat the process until the desired weight is reached.

© Paradigm Publishing, Inc.

For Good Measure

You should do your best to fill the capsule to the exact amount of 500 mg. However, a margin of error of 1 or 2 mg is allowable for this lab.

15 Reshape the powder into a leveled cake (Step 5), and perform the punching, weighing, and quantity-adjusting process (Steps 7–14) for the remaining four capsules.

16 Gently wipe the exterior of the five filled capsules with the gauze pad or cloth one more time to remove excess powder. Ask for an instructor check; he or she will verify the weight of each capsule. Once they are approved, place the five compounded capsules into a vial.

17 Wash, dry, and put away all supplies, and clean up the work area. Prepare the compounding log, if directed by your instructor.

18 **Conclusion:** Present your log (if created) and your final product to your instructor for verification. Then go to the Course Navigator, answer all questions in the Lab Review section, and submit your answers to your instructor.

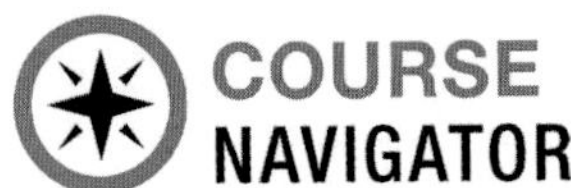

Access interactive chapter review exercises, practice activities, flash cards, and study games.

© Paradigm Publishing, Inc.

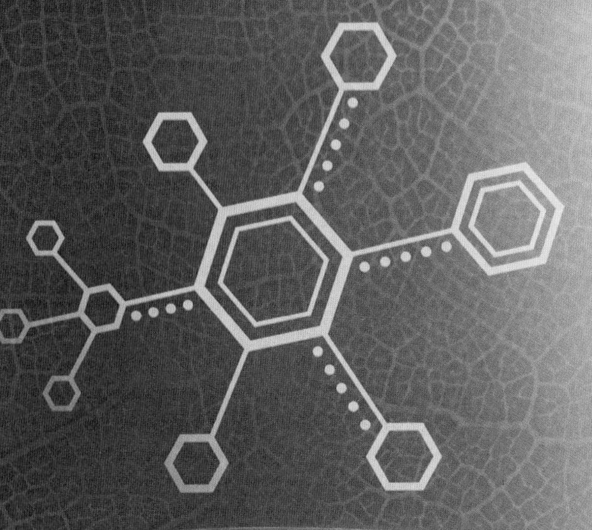

25 Preparing Suspensions from Tablets

Learning Objectives

1. Demonstrate proficiency in the process of compounding an oral suspension from tablets.
2. Demonstrate competence in mathematical calculations related to the preparation of an oral suspension from tablets.
3. Discuss the procedure and rationale for compounding oral suspensions from tablets.
4. Become familiar with the compounding log as a means of recording the measurements, ingredients, and procedures used in compounding nonsterile products.

Supplies

- A balance or scale (digital or analog)
- 2 weighing boats
- Mortar and pestle
- Compounding spatula
- Beaker or Erlenmeyer flask (250 mL or larger)
- Stirring rod
- Gloves
- Metronidazole 500 mg tablets (bulk bottle) or placebo
- Syrpalta 200 mL (or similar)
- Amber bottle for liquid medications (8 oz or larger)
- "Shake Well" auxiliary label
- Calculator

Access additional chapter resources.

Many oral liquid medications are readily available as a **suspension** (a dispersion of fine solid particles in a liquid), which may be administered to the patient with a spoon, an oral syringe, or a dosing cup. However, at times you may be required to compound such an oral suspension pursuant to a medication order, or because a manufactured suspension may not be available.

To compound a suspension, you will begin with a medication manufactured in either tablet or capsule form. (In this lab, you will use tablets as your starting material, and in Lab 26 you will use capsules as your starting material.) The original medication form is then reduced to a fine powder, either through **tablet trituration** (diluting a drug powder with an inert diluent powder) or by releasing the medication from the capsules. The required amount of powder is weighed and then is checked by the pharmacist. The liquid component, a suspending agent that is often a solution such as Syrpalta, is also measured as required and then is checked by a pharmacist. Compounding oral solutions requires a digital balance for powder measurement and a beaker for solution measurement. In addition, oral solutions compounded from tablets will require the use of a mortar and pestle. Once combined, the powder and solution must be shaken well to ensure that the medication particles are thoroughly dispersed throughout the mixture.

Procedure

In this lab, you will prepare metronidazole oral suspension 500 mg/5 mL from tablets. You must prepare an amount that provides enough medication to supply the following prescription in its entirety: Metronidazole 500 mg qid × 10 days.

You will need to perform calculations to determine how many tablets are required to prepare the final product. The tablets will be triturated, weighed, and then mixed with a suspending agent such as Syrpalta. If directed by your instructor, you will also prepare a compounding log to record the steps and ingredients that you use.

1. Set your supplies on the workspace and arrange them in an easily accessible and organized manner. Visually inspect them to ensure that they are clean. If they are not, wash and dry them before use.

2. Wash your hands thoroughly, put on gloves, and wear them throughout the procedure.

3. Complete the calculations provided below to determine the amount of metronidazole necessary to prepare the entire product ordered by the physician:

   a. First, determine the **amount of medication** needed for **one day** of the prescription by setting up this statement:

      500 mg (number of milligrams per tablet) × 4 (number of doses per day) = 2,000 mg (needed per day)

   b. Second, determine the **number of tablets** needed to deliver that daily medication quantity **for one day** of the prescription. Do this by setting up a ratio and proportion problem.

© Paradigm Publishing, Inc.

Place the number of milligrams in one tablet over the words "1 tablet" (similar to writing down a fraction). Next to that item, place the number of milligrams in one day's prescription over the words "*x* tablets" (again, creating a fraction). Place an equals sign between the two fractions.

To solve this (and all ratio and proportion problems), cross multiply and then divide:

$$\frac{500 \text{ mg}}{1 \text{ tablet}} = \frac{2{,}000 \text{ mg}}{x \text{ tablets}}$$

Solve by cross multiplying: 2,000 mg × 1 tablet = 2,000 mg-tablet

And then divide: 2,000 mg-tablet ÷ 500 mg = 4 tablets

The answer to this problem is: 4 tablets (needed to compound one day's worth of prescription)

c. Third, determine the **number of tablets** needed to compound the **entire prescription** by multiplying your answer from b (above) times the total number of days for the prescription.

In this case, the prescription is for 10 days:

4 tablets (per day) × 10 days (duration of the entire prescription) = 40 tablets (for the entire prescription)

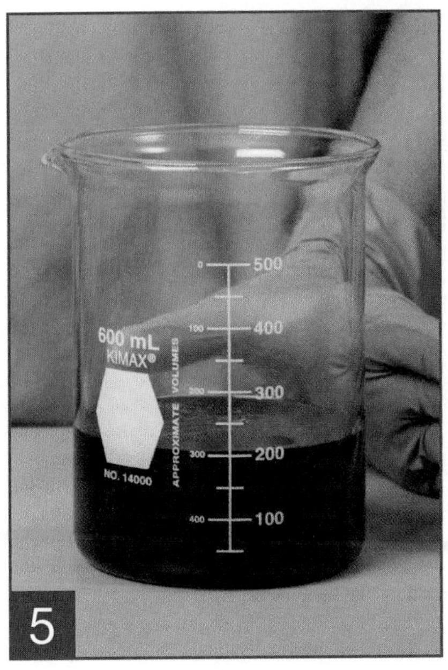

Beaker filled with 200 mL of Syrpalta

4 Place the number of tablets needed for the entire prescription (calculated above) into a weighing boat and temporarily set the boat aside.

5 Pour 200 mL of Syrpalta into a beaker and temporarily set it aside.

6 If necessary, calibrate the balance according to standard procedures. Place an empty weighing boat on the balance and tare or zero it. If you have questions about this process, see Steps 10–12 in Lab 24, or ask your instructor for specific directions.

7 Remove the empty weighing boat, and place the boat containing the metronidazole tablets onto the balance. Record the weight of the tablets here: _______. This is the amount you will need for the final product that you are going to compound.

Practice Tip

In this and other situations where you want to reduce the product to a very fine powder with the mortar and pestle, it is most effective to use a forceful, back and forth, grinding motion rather than a stirring or pounding motion.

8 Ask for an instructor check on the weight of tablets and the volume of Syrpalta.

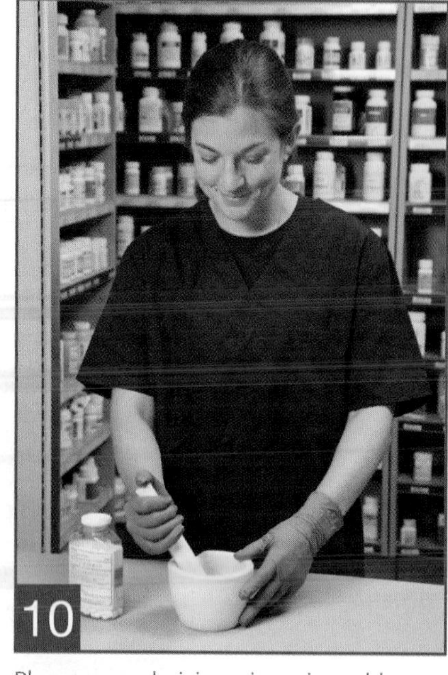

Pharmacy technician triturating tablets with a mortar and pestle

9 Place the metronidazole tablets into the mortar. Add an additional three tablets of metronidazole to the mortar. Adding this extra amount will allow for the powder loss that results from the medication adhering to the mortar and pestle and will ensure that you have adequate powder to measure for the final product.

For Good Measure

While the standard margin of error is ±5%, the allowed margin may vary in the case of medications used in chemotherapy treatments, neonate or geriatric medications, and other unique situations.

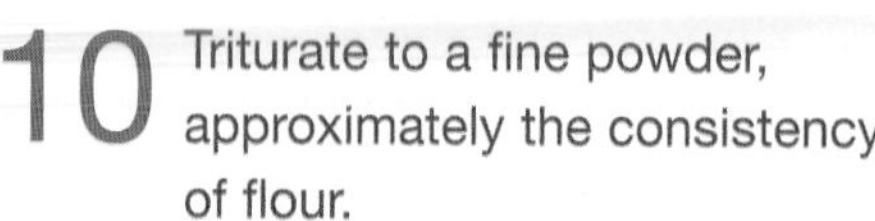

10 Triturate to a fine powder, approximately the consistency of flour.

11 Place an empty weighing boat onto the scale and tare it. Using the spatula, transfer from the mortar into the weighing boat an amount of powder equal to the weight of the tablets you recorded previously (in Step 7). The amount transferred to the boat must be no more than ±5% of the target amount.

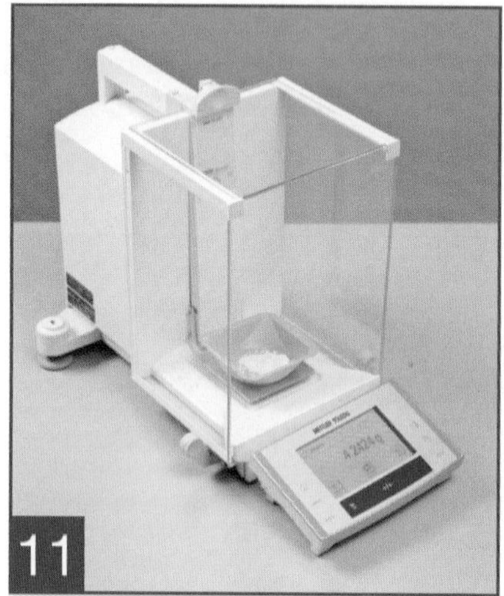

Drug powder being weighed on a digital scale

12 Ask the instructor to verify the weight of the triturated metronidazole.

For Good Measure

Always get an instructor to check your ingredient quantities (weights, volumes, or other measurements) before you begin mixing.

13 After both ingredients have been checked, use a spatula to transfer a small amount of powder from the weighing boat into the beaker that contains the Syrpalta. Stir the suspension until that small amount of powder is dissolved in the Syrpalta.

© Paradigm Publishing, Inc.

Practice Tip

Stir continuously as you add the rest of the powder, to promote uniform consistency. Be sure to scrape the metronidazole completely from the weighing boat into the Syrpalta so that the proper concentration of drug is contained in the final product.

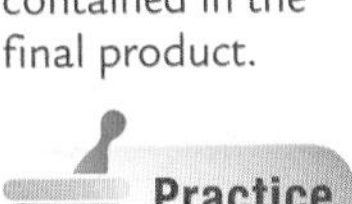

Practice Tip

To ensure that all of the medication is transferred into the final container, swirl the final product in the beaker as you gradually pour it into the amber bottle.

14 Gradually add more metronidazole until it has all been incorporated into the Syrpalta.

15 Carefully pour the suspension from the beaker into the amber bottle.

16 Label the product according to your instructor's directions, place a "Shake Well" auxiliary label on the bottle, and ask your instructor for a final check.

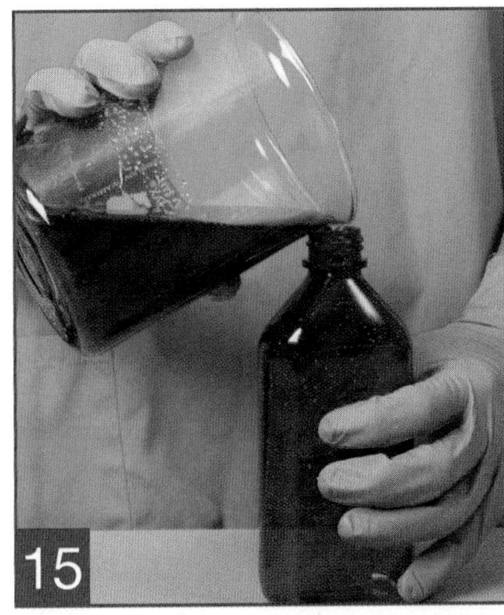

Syrpaltra being poured into the amber bottle

17 Wash, dry, and put away all supplies, and clean up the work area. Prepare the compounding log, if directed by your instructor.

18 **Conclusion:** Present your log (if created) and your final product to your instructor for verification. Then go to the Course Navigator, answer all questions in the Lab Review section, and submit your answers to your instructor.

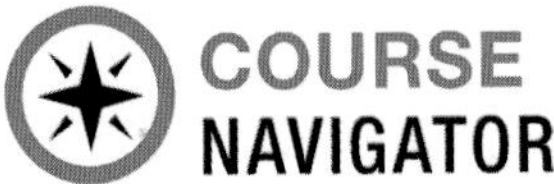

COURSE NAVIGATOR

Access interactive chapter review exercises, practice activities, flash cards, and study games.

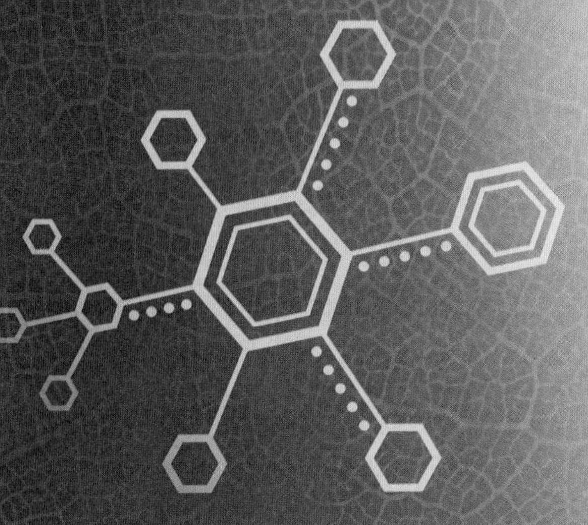

26 Preparing Suspensions from Capsules

Learning Objectives

1. Demonstrate proficiency in the process of compounding an oral suspension from capsules.
2. Demonstrate competence in calculations related to the preparation of an oral suspension from capsules.
3. Discuss the procedure and rationale for compounding oral suspensions from capsules.
4. Become familiar with the compounding log as a means of recording the measurements, ingredients, and procedures used in compounding nonsterile products.

Supplies

- Weighing boat
- Beaker or Erlenmeyer flask (250 mL or larger)
- Stirring rod
- Gloves
- Amoxicillin 250 mg capsules (bulk bottle)
- Syrpalta 200 mL (or similar)
- Amber bottle for liquid medications (8 oz or larger)
- Calculator

Access additional chapter resources.

Many oral liquid medications are readily available as a **suspension** (a dispersion of fine solid particles in a liquid), which may be administered to the patient with a spoon, an oral syringe, or a dosing cup. However, at times you may be required to compound such an oral suspension pursuant to a medication order, or because a manufactured suspension may not be available.

To compound a suspension, you will begin with a medication manufactured in either tablet or capsule form. (In this lab, you will use capsules as your starting material, whereas in Lab 25, tablets are your starting material.) The original medication form is then reduced to a fine powder, either through **tablet trituration** (diluting a drug powder with an inert diluent powder) or by releasing the medication from the capsules. The required amount of powder is weighed and then is checked by the pharmacist. The liquid component, a suspending agent that is often a solution such as Syrpalta, is also measured as required and then is checked by a pharmacist. Compounding oral solutions from capsules requires a weighing boat, to provide a temporary receptacle for the capsules, and a beaker, for solution measurement. Once combined, the powder and solution must be shaken well to ensure that the medication particles are thoroughly dispersed throughout the mixture.

Procedure

In this lab, you will compound an oral suspension from capsules in order to prepare amoxicillin 250 mg/5 mL, an oral liquid medication. You must prepare enough medication to supply the following prescription in its entirety: Amoxicillin 250 mg qid × 10 days.

You will need to perform calculations to determine how many capsules are required to prepare the final product. Before mixing the medication with a suspending agent such as Syrpalta, you will open the capsules and remove the powder from within the capsule shell. If and as directed by your instructor, you will also prepare a compounding log to record the steps and ingredients that you use.

1. Set your supplies on the workspace and arrange them in an easily accessible and organized manner. Visually inspect them to ensure that they are clean. If they are not, wash and dry them before use.

2. Wash your hands thoroughly, put on gloves, and wear them throughout the procedure.

3. Use the following calculations to determine the amount of amoxicillin necessary to prepare the entire product ordered by the physician:

a. First, determine the **amount of medication** needed for **one day** of the prescription by setting up this statement:

250 mg (number of milligrams per capsule) × 4 (number of doses per day) = 1,000 mg (needed per day)

b. Second, determine the **number of capsules** needed to deliver that daily medication quantity **for one day** of the prescription. Do this by setting up a ratio and proportion problem.

 © Paradigm Publishing, Inc.

Place the number of milligrams in one capsule over the words "1 capsule" (similar to writing down a fraction). Next to that item, place the number of milligrams in one day's prescription over the words "*x* capsules" (again, creating a fraction). Place an equals sign between the two fractions.

To solve this (and all ratio and proportion problems), cross multiply and then divide:

$$\frac{250 \text{ mg}}{1 \text{ capsule}} = \frac{1000 \text{ mg}}{x \text{ capsules}}$$

Solve by cross multiplying: 1,000 mg × 1 capsule = 1,000 mg-capsule

And then divide: 1,000 mg-capsule ÷ 250 mg = 4 capsules

The answer to this problem is: 4 capsules (needed to compound one day's worth of prescription)

c. Third, determine the **number of capsules** needed to compound the **entire prescription** by multiplying your answer from b (above) times the total number of days for the prescription.

In this case, the prescription is for 10 days:

4 capsules (per day) × 10 days (duration of the entire prescription) = 40 capsules (for the entire prescription)

4 Pour 200 mL of Syrpalta into a beaker or Erlenmeyer flask and temporarily set it aside.

5 Place the number of capsules (calculated above) needed for the entire prescription into a weighing boat and temporarily set it aside.

6 Ask your instructor to check the number of capsules and the volume of Syrpalta.

7 Carefully open a capsule and empty it into the beaker containing the Syrpalta. All of the powder must be transferred into the Syrpalta, so examine the inside of both capsule halves and if any powder remains, tap the capsule shell gently against the inside of the beaker so the powder is dislodged and enters the Syrpalta.

For Good Measure

Always have your instructor check your ingredients (capsules, volumes, other measured quantities) before you begin mixing.

8 Continue the process until all of the contents of all of the capsules have been emptied into the Syrpalta. Stir the suspension until the powder is thoroughly incorporated into the Syrpalta.

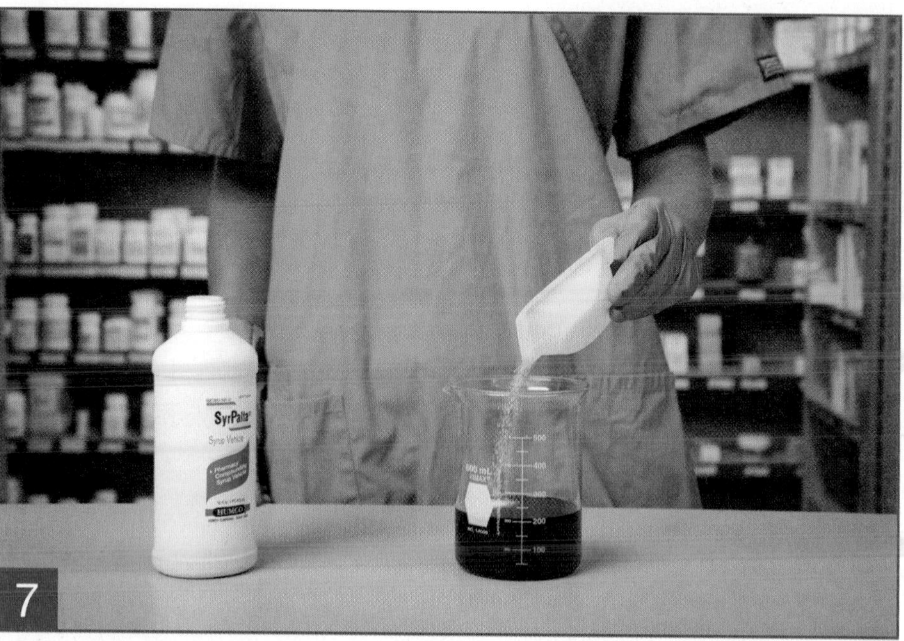

Pharmacy technician emptying capsules into a beaker of Syrpalta

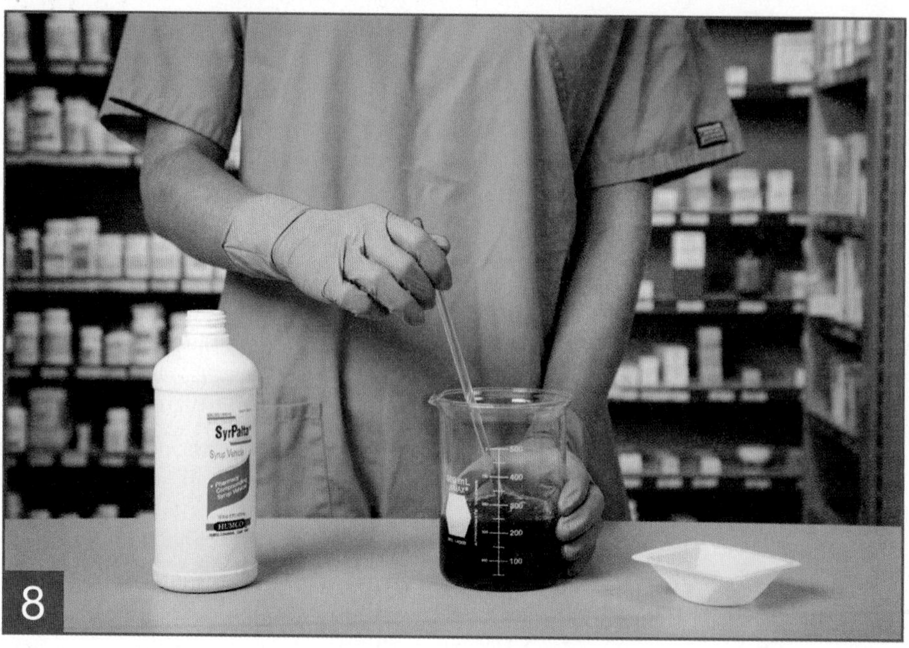

Pharmacy technician mixing powder and Syrpalta in a beaker

Practice Tip

While you are pouring, swirl the final product in the beaker to ensure that all of the medication remains in suspension and is transferred into the final container.

9 Carefully and gradually pour the suspension from the beaker into the amber bottle.

10 Consult your instructor for labeling instructions, and place a "Shake Well" auxiliary label on the bottle. Ask your instructor for a final check of the finished product.

 © Paradigm Publishing, Inc.

11 Wash, dry, and put away all supplies, and clean up the work area. Prepare the compounding log, if and as directed by your instructor.

12 **Conclusion:** Present your log (if created) and your final product to your instructor for verification. Then go to the Course Navigator, answer all questions in the Lab Review section, and submit your answers to your instructor.

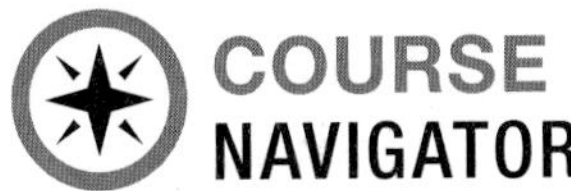

Access interactive chapter review exercises, practice activities, flash cards, and study games.

27

Preparing Creams, Ointments, Gels, and Pastes

Learning Objectives

1 Demonstrate proficiency in the process of nonsterile compounding, specifically in the preparation of a topical gel.

2 Discuss the procedure and rationale for compounding nonsterile creams, ointments, gels, and pastes.

3 Become familiar with the compounding log as a means of recording the measurements, ingredients, and procedures used in compounding nonsterile products.

Supplies

- A balance or scale (digital or otherwise)
- Two weighing boats
- Mortar and pestle
- Two compounding spatulas
- Ointment slab
- Small ointment jar
- Gloves
- Thirteen aspirin 325 mg tablets (without film coating)
- One tube of surgical lubricant (minimum 15 g)

Access additional chapter resources.

Most topical preparations are readily available as premade creams, ointments, gels, or pastes. However, there are times when you may be required to compound nonsterile topical products pursuant to a prescription or medication order. In such compounding, a base ingredient is combined with an active ingredient. The **base ingredient** is an inert delivery vehicle such as a cream, ointment, gel, or paste. The required amount of base is carefully weighed by a pharmacy technician and then verified by a pharmacist. The **active ingredient**, the medication that is added to the base ingredient, is commonly provided by the manufacturer in either tablet or capsule form. The original form is then reduced to a fine powder, either through tablet trituration or by releasing the medication from the capsules. The required amount of powder is also carefully weighed by the pharmacy technician and then checked by the pharmacist.

Compounding of a topical preparation is performed on an ointment slab, using compounding spatulas to mix the preparation. With this compounding method—often referred to as **spatulation**—the powder should slowly be incorporated into the base to ensure that the final product is prepared to a uniform consistency and concentration. While there are some differences in the consistency and uses of creams, ointments, gels, and pastes, the basic compounding process, which you will practice in this lab, is the same.

Procedure

In this lab, you will compound a gel for topical application, using aspirin tablets as the active ingredient and surgical lubricant as the base gel (and prepare a compounding log, if directed by your instructor, to record the steps and ingredients that you use). In this case, a compounding formula is not needed; you will simply be given the recipe as the steps proceed.

1. Set your supplies on the workspace, and arrange them in an easily accessible and organized manner. Visually inspect them to ensure that they are clean. If they are not, wash and dry them before use.

2. Wash your hands thoroughly, put on gloves, and wear them throughout the procedure.

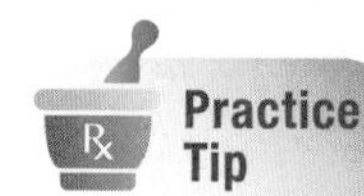

Practice Tip

It is most effective to use a forceful, back-and-forth, grinding motion when using a mortar and pestle, not a stirring or pounding motion.

3. Crush 13 (10 for the compound, plus 3 additional tablets to allow for some extra powder, as some of the product may be lost during the trituration and pouring processes) aspirin 325 mg tablets with a mortar and pestle. Triturate to a fine powder, approximately the consistency of flour.

4. If necessary, calibrate the balance according to standard procedures, place an empty weighing boat on the balance, and tare (zero) it.

5. Weigh out 2.5 g of the finely ground aspirin powder into the empty boat. Set the boat filled with powder to the side.

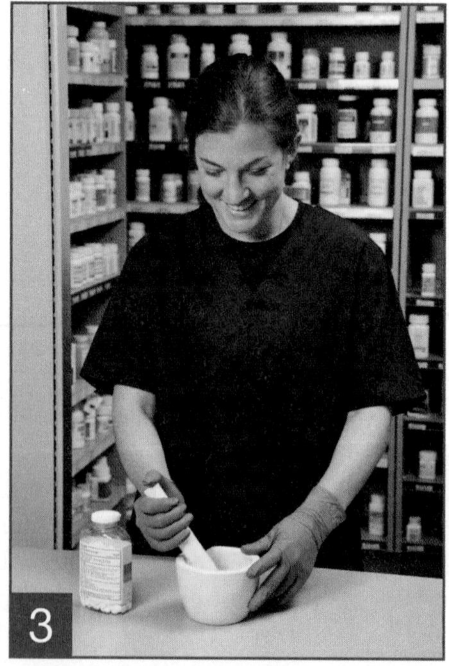

Pharmacy technician triturating tablets with a mortar and pestle

 © Paradigm Publishing, Inc.

For Good Measure

Always get an instructor to check your ingredient quantities (mass, volumes, or other measurements) before you begin mixing.

6 Repeat the process for the next ingredient using a second, empty weighing boat: place it on the scale, tare the scale, and weigh out your quantity—here, 10 g of the surgical lubricant.

7 Ask the instructor to verify the weight of the aspirin and the surgical lubricant.

8 Once the two ingredients have been checked, you will put them onto different parts of a single ointment slab. Using the spatula, carefully scrape the contents of the first boat into a small pile at one upper corner of the ointment slab, being sure to scrape any remnants from the boat onto the slab.

9 Then, using the spatula, carefully scrape the contents of the second boat into a small pile at the upper corner of the *opposite side* of the slab, being sure to scrape out the remnants.

10 To begin the mixing process, use the spatula to drag a small amount (approximately one-fifth of the total amount) of powder to the center of the slab.

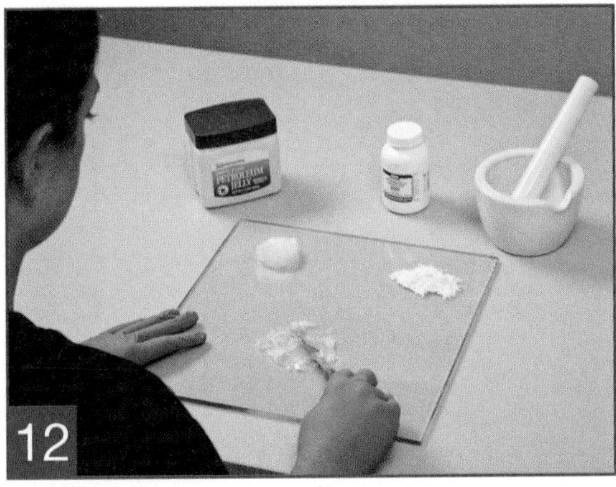

Pharmacy technician mixing a small amount of powder and base on an ointment slab

11 Using the same spatula, drag a small amount (again, approximately one-fifth of the total amount) of surgical lubricant to the center of the slab.

12 Mix the two ingredients together by using the flat surface of the spatula against the flat surface of the slab. You should apply a downward force and move the spatula back and forth in a sideways "S" pattern, as illustrated in Figure 27.1. The motion is similar to the hand motion you might use to frost a cake.

FIGURE 27.1 The "S" method of spatulation

Powder and gel are mixed together in an "S" motion against the slab, similar to the motion used to frost a cake.

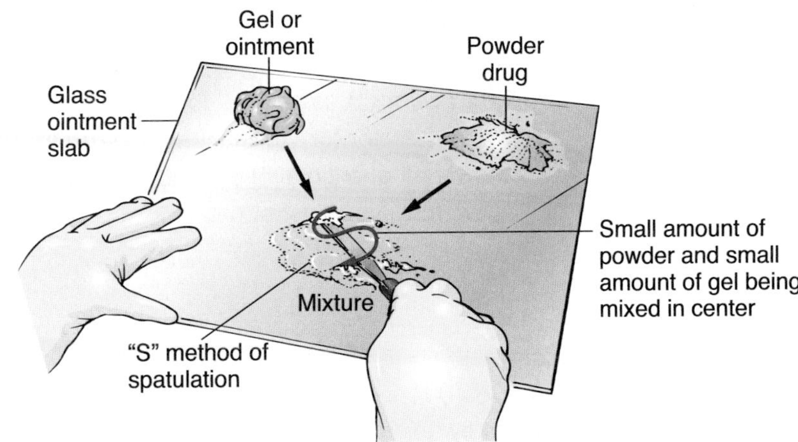

13 Gradually mix the small amounts of the two ingredients together by continuing to apply downward pressure as the mixture takes on a smooth, uniform texture.

14 Now use the spatula to drag an additional, similarly small amount of both ingredients into the center of the slab. Using the same process, blend the ingredients together while incorporating them into the portion that you have already mixed.

15 Continue this process, gradually adding more of each ingredient until both piles of ingredients have been moved from the corners to the center of the slab, and the entire product has a smooth and uniform texture.

16 Ask your instructor to check the consistency of your product.

17 Once your product is approved, scrape everything off the slab and into an ointment jar.

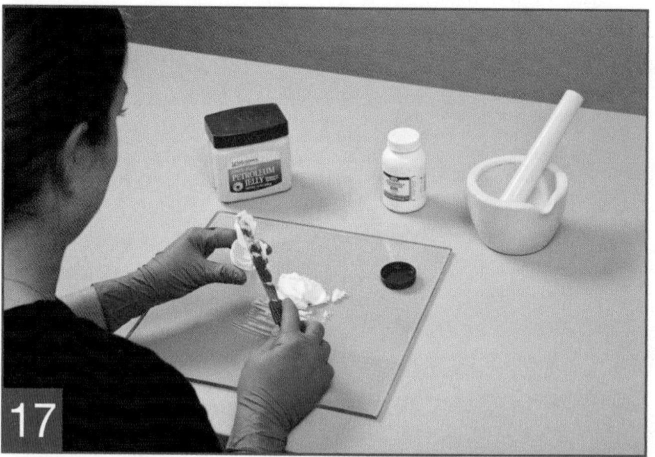

Pharmacy technician placing finished topical preparation into an ointment jar

18 Wash, dry, and put away all supplies, and clean up the work area. Prepare the compounding log, if directed by your instructor.

19 **Conclusion:** Present your log, if created, and your final product to your instructor for verification. Then go to the Course Navigator, answer all questions in the Lab Review section, and submit your answers to your instructor.

Access interactive chapter review exercises, practice activities, flash cards, and study games.

© Paradigm Publishing, Inc.

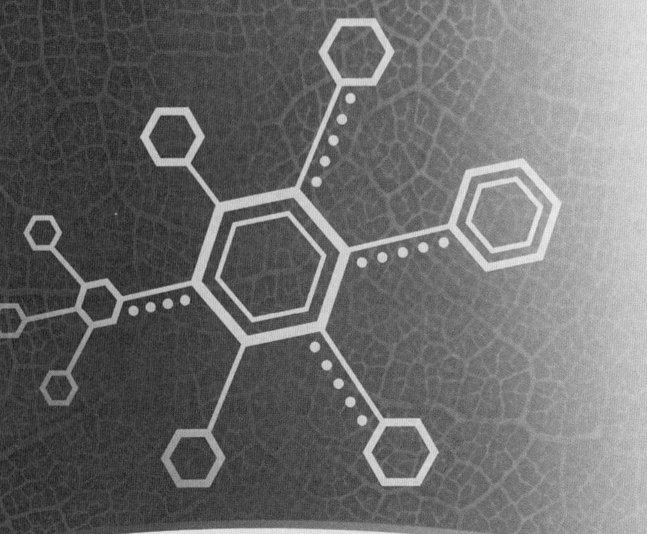

28

Preparing Lozenges

Learning Objectives

1 Demonstrate proficiency in the preparation of compounded, custom-made lozenges.

2 Demonstrate skill in the use of laboratory equipment required for compounding.

3 Become familiar with the compounding log as a means of recording the measurements, ingredients, and procedures used in compounding nonsterile products.

Supplies

- Balance/digital scale
- Thermometer capable of reaching 155°C (311°F); a candy thermometer is best
- Hot plate capable of generating temperatures of 155°C (311° F)
- Can of cooking spray (canola or olive oil)
- Glass stirring rod
- 100 mL or 125 mL beakers × 2
- Beaker tongs or one pair of heat-resistant gloves
- Set of protective eyewear
- 0.25 oz lozenge mold (20 lozenges per mold)
- 20 individual aluminum wrappers or aluminum foil pieces cut into 3 × 3 inch squares
- Access to a freezer
- Lozenge ingredients:
  - 77 g granular sugar, powdered sugar, or Splenda® or other equivalent sugar substitute (for diabetic patients)
  - 50 g light corn syrup
  - 33 mL distilled water
  - Bottle of food flavoring (per customer/prescriber request)
  - Bottle of food coloring
  - 9 g benzocaine powder, USP

Access additional chapter resources.

The hard **lozenge** is another common dosage form created by compounding. Also known as a **troche** (pronounced "tro-shay" or "tro-kee") or **pastille** ("pas-teel"), a lozenge is a hard-candy-like dosage form that contains an active ingredient and may contain flavoring, sugar, or another form of sweetener. Hard lozenges are administered orally, and patients suck on the lozenge until it dissolves, like hard candy; patients are *not* to swallow the lozenge. These dosage forms come in a variety of sizes, colors, and flavors, depending on the manufacturer, preparer, and patient preference.

The lozenge is often used to increase patient adherence, especially in pediatric patients, as its sweetened contents are more palatable to children. While compounding is, in general, rather rare, it does occur, and you may be asked to compound hard lozenges—especially in a compounding pharmacy.

Procedure

In this lab, you will compound lozenges. Imagine the following scenario:

> Your pharmacy has received a prescription for a 7.5% benzocaine lozenge compound to soothe a child's sore throat. Using the following steps, compound the product (and prepare a compounding log, if directed by your instructor, to record the steps and ingredients that you use). In this lab, a compounding formula is not needed; you will simply be given the recipe as the steps proceed.

1. Set your supplies on the workspace and arrange them in an easily accessible and organized manner. Visually inspect them to ensure that they are clean. If they are not, wash and dry them before use.

2. Wash your hands thoroughly, put on gloves and protective eyewear, and wear both throughout the procedure.

3. Using the balance or digital scale, carefully weigh out each of the four weighed ingredients in the recipe (70 g [2.5 oz] of sugar or one of the suggested alternatives, 45 g [1.5 oz] of light corn syrup, 30 mL [1 fl oz] of distilled water, and 9 g of benzocaine powder). Clearly label each ingredient and have each weight verified by your instructor. Once the ingredients are weighed, labeled, and verified, set them aside for use later in the recipe.

4. Set out the lozenge mold and lightly spray it with cooking spray to prevent the hardened lozenges from sticking to the mold.

5. Switch on the hot plate, and set the temperature to 155°C (311°F) or high.

© Paradigm Publishing, Inc.

6 Add the powdered sugar (or sugar substitute), corn syrup, and distilled water to the beaker and carefully place the beaker on the hot plate.

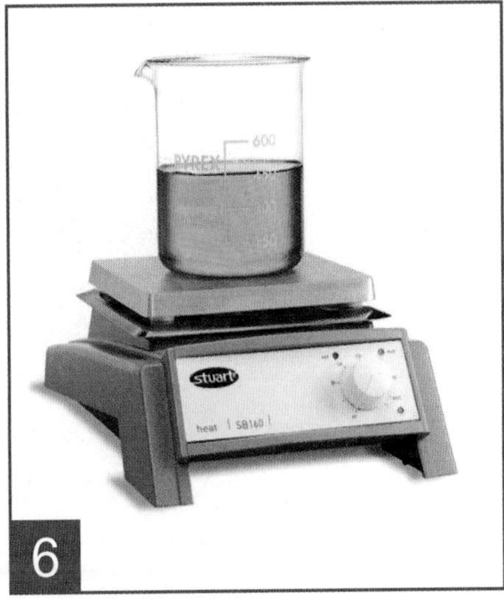

The lozenge preparation heats to 149°C (300°F).

7 Using the glass stirring rod, stir the contents of the beaker until the contents form a homogeneous solution. Constantly check the solution's temperature as it approaches 149°C (300°F). *Do not allow the solution to go above 155°C (311°F), or the sugar may caramelize.*

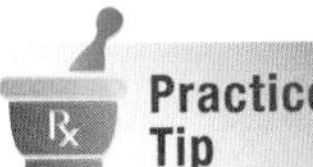

Practice Tip

When sugar reaches 149°C (300°F), the sugar molecules restructure and will cool into a hard candy (or hard crack) substance.

8 At 149°C (300°F), add the desired flavoring (according to the manufacturer's specifications), and stir.

9 Stir in food coloring until desired color is reached.

10 Use the beaker tongs or heat-resistant gloves to hold the beaker, and pour its contents into the unused beaker to a volume of 120 mL.

11 Add 9 g of benzocaine to the solution, and stir until it is completely dissolved and homogeneous.

12 Pour 5 mL of the solution into each cup of the lozenge mold and allow the lozenges to cool and firm up in the mold for approximately 5 to 8 minutes. Then place the lozenges in the freezer, where they will take approximately 120 minutes to harden completely.

13 Once the lozenges have hardened, remove them from the mold, and individually wrap them in aluminum wrappers to prevent them from sticking to each other.

14 While the lozenges cool, prepare the compounding log, if directed by your instructor. Wash, dry, and put away all supplies, and clean up the work area.

© Paradigm Publishing, Inc.

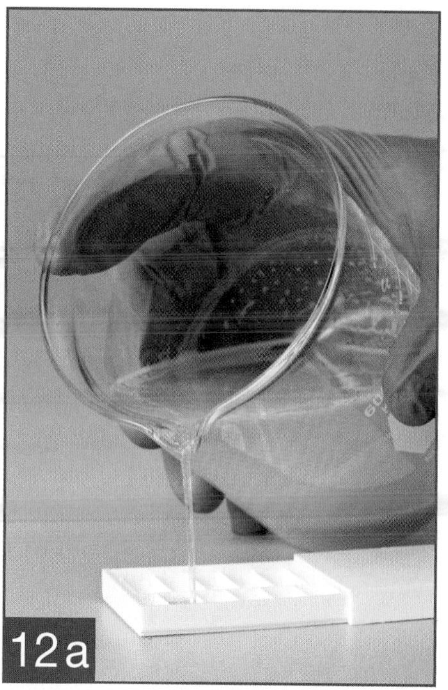

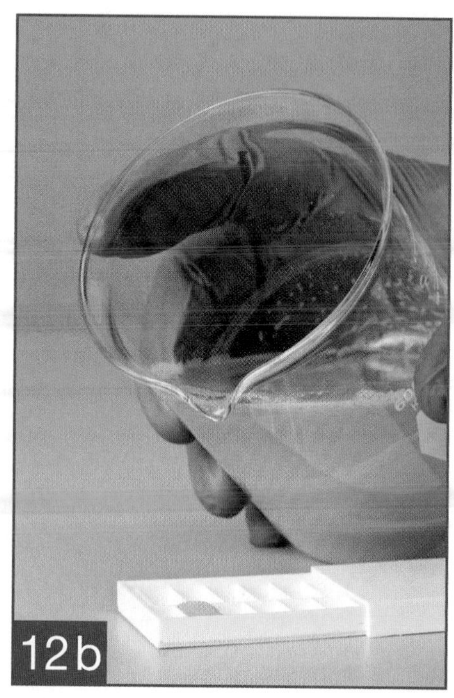

Pharmacy technician pouring finished solution into molds

15 **Conclusion:** Package and label the product, and submit it with the compounding log (if created) to your instructor for final verification. Then go to the Course Navigator, answer all questions in the Lab Review section, and submit your answers to your instructor.

Access interactive chapter review exercises, practice activities, flash cards, and study games.

© Paradigm Publishing, Inc.

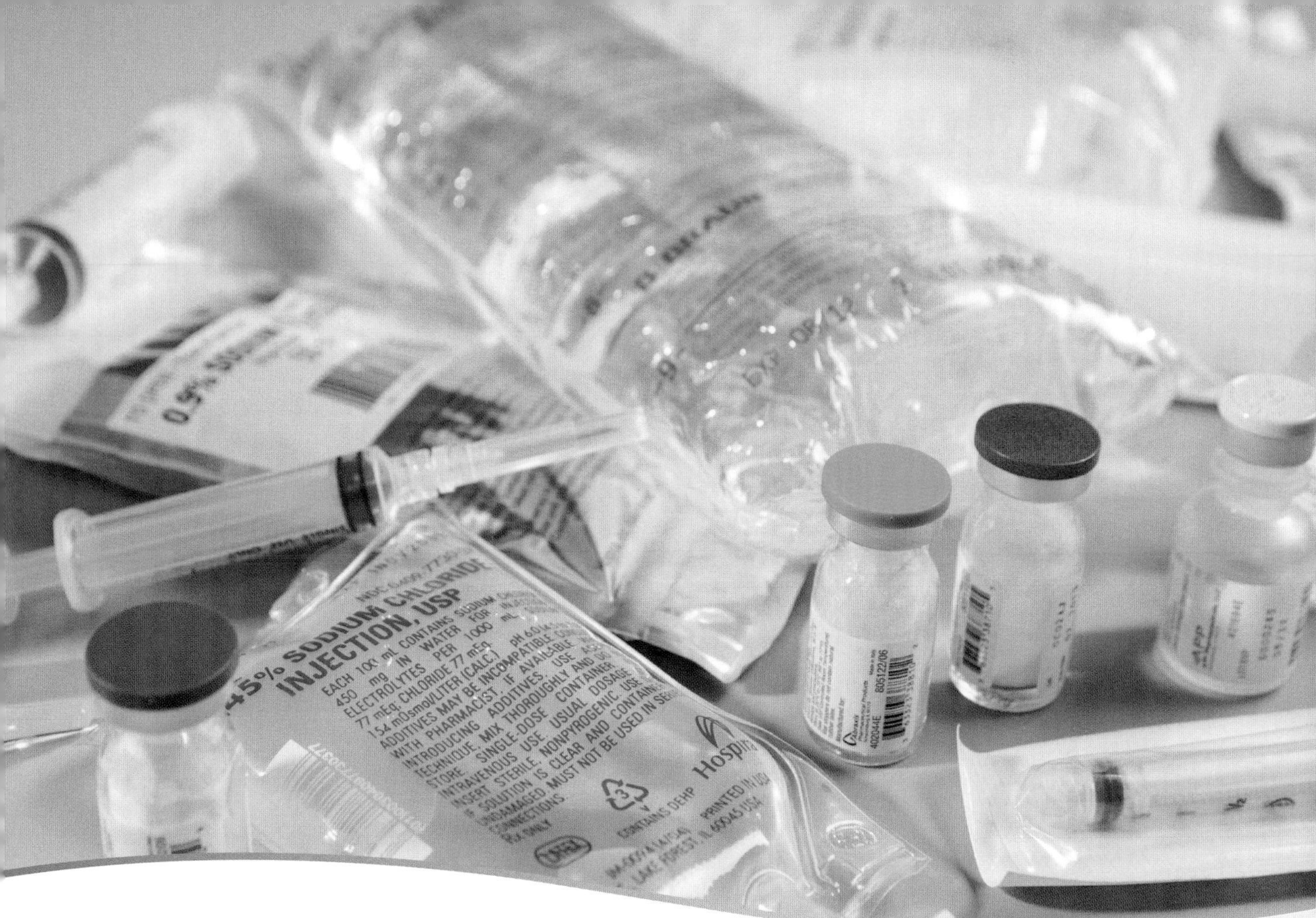

UNIT 5 Aseptic Technique

A day in the life of a pharmacy technician...

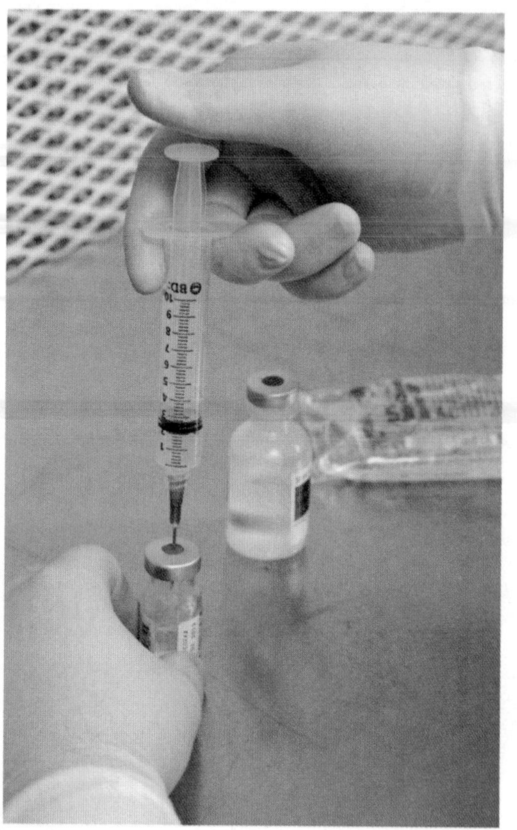

The stack of labels for the IV batch has grown to two inches high, there are four total parenteral nutrition (TPN) solutions ready to be prepared, there is a new order for an investigational medication that is due in 30 minutes, and the pharmacist has just handed you three STAT IV medication labels.

Are you prepared to work in the fast paced, high stress environment of sterile compounding?

Pharmacy technicians with special training in sterile compounding and aseptic technique prepare intravenous and other types of parenteral medications for hospitalized patients. Patients requiring parenteral medications are often very sick and depend on these lifesaving medications for survival. Pharmacy technicians who prepare compounded sterile preparations (CSPs) must have excellent aseptic technique in compliance with the guidelines set forth in Chapter <797> of the United States Pharmacopeia (USP Chapter <797>).

This unit will guide you through the essential tasks of the sterile compounding technician, including aseptic garbing and hand washing, hood cleaning, and large- and small-volume parenteral preparations. These tasks are the foundational aspects of sterile compounding and aseptic technique.

While speed and accuracy are essential when preparing CSPs, you must also perform each step with careful adherence to USP Chapter <797> requirements in order to ensure that safe and effective medication is dispensed to the patient.

TAKE NOTE

The aseptic technique labs in the *Pharmacy Labs for Technicians*, Third Edition provide only a basic introduction to sterile compounding and aseptic technique. Students should refer to Paradigm's *Sterile Compounding and Aseptic Technique*, by Lisa McCartney, for in-depth instruction and training in sterile compounding and aseptic technique.

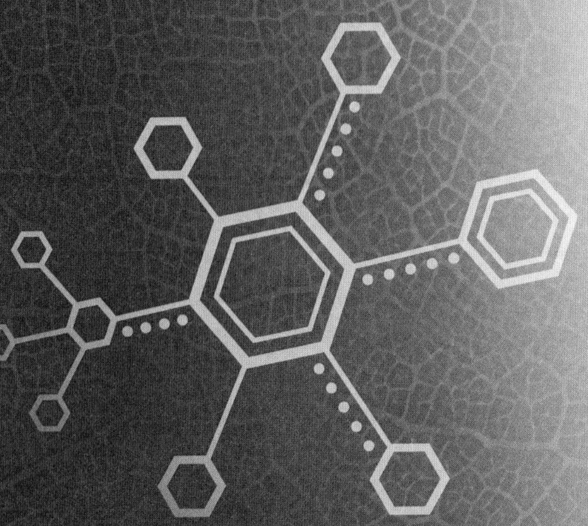

Garbing According to USP Chapter <797> Standards

29

Learning Objectives

1 Demonstrate proficiency in the processes and procedures related to garbing as defined in USP Chapter <797>.

2 Discuss the procedures and rationale of the garbing procedures and related technique testing outlined in USP Chapter <797>.

3 Understand how USP Chapter <797> affects the institutional pharmacy technician.

Supplies

- Sterile gown
- Sterile, powder-free gloves
- Hair cover or bouffant cap
- Shoe covers
- Face mask, beard cover (if applicable)
- Foamed alcohol or similar hand sanitizer
- Agar plates appropriate for gloved fingertip testing X 2
- Access to a tabletop or other surface that has been disinfected with sterile, 70% isopropyl alcohol or another suitable cleansing agent

Access additional chapter resources.

The United States Pharmacopeia (USP) is the official public standards-setting authority for all prescription and over-the-counter medicines, dietary supplements, and other healthcare products manufactured and sold in the United States. USP sets standards for the quality of these products and works with healthcare providers to help them reach the standards, according to Chapter <797> of the USP as approved by the United States Pharmacopeial Convention.

The USP establishes policies regarding medication quality, patient safety, and healthcare personnel training and sets the standard of care to which all pharmacies in the United States conform. In 2008, the USP revised Chapter <797>, the section of the book that outlines standards for pharmaceutical compounding of sterile preparations. USP <797> is currently undergoing revision, which will update, clarify, and reinforce the standards outlined in the chapter.

USP <797> affects your work as a pharmacy technician because it addresses many issues related to the preparation of compounded sterile preparations (CSPs), including personnel training and evaluation in aseptic technique, environmental quality and control, verification of automated compounding devices such as total parenteral nutrition (TPN) compounders, medication storage, beyond-use dating, patient monitoring, and adverse events.

The sections of USP <797> that most directly affect the pharmacy technician address proper cleaning and preparation of the aseptic compounding environment and related products. This includes preparing your body and donning aseptic garb (according to procedures specified in the chapter), prior to entering the aseptic compounding area. Another area of USP <797> that will directly affect you concerns the training and testing of your skills and abilities as a qualified pharmacy technician.

Procedure

You will now garb according to strict USP <797> standards and undergo gloved fingertip sampling to verify that you have properly performed the procedure.

While a body piercing cannot itself be removed, you should remove the jewelry from all body piercings that are visible outside your clothing.

1 Read the instructions for agar plate gloved fingertip testing prior to beginning this lab. Instructions are included in the agar plate package and will be provided to you by your instructor.

2 According to USP <797>, you should be free of cosmetics, jewelry, and visible body piercings, and your natural nails should be kept trimmed and clean (i.e., no false nails or nail polish). If you need to address these issues, do so now.

3 Remove your outer garments (e.g., coats, hats, sweaters, or jackets). If you haven't already done so, don clean medical scrubs or other clean, nonshedding garments appropriate for working in a clean room.

4 Apply foamed alcohol to your hands or thoroughly wash them with soap and water before beginning this lab.

TAKE NOTE

It is considered "best practice" to apply foamed alcohol or another appropriate hand sanitizer to your hands after donning each shoe cover and after donning a hair cover. See Step 10 for directions on the use of foamed alcohol.

© Paradigm Publishing, Inc.

Practice Tip

You do not have to worry about "left" and "right" shoe covers because they are interchangeable.

5 Don each shoe cover by first identifying the toe end (the longer end) of the cover and then slipping it over the toe of the shoe. Pull the shoe cover around the bottom of the shoe and up onto the heel. The shoe cover should completely envelop the shoe. Repeat this procedure with the other shoe.

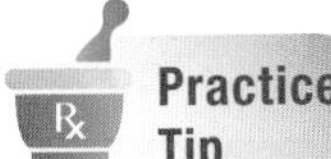

Practice Tip

People with long hair may find it helpful to put hair in a ponytail or otherwise tie it back prior to donning the hair cover.

6 Put on the hair cover by gathering any loose hair and placing it into the hair cover so that the back of the hair cover contains the majority of the hair, and the elastic at the back of the hair cover is positioned against the back of the neck. Pull the front of the cap over the head until the elastic on the front of the hair cover is positioned against the forehead. Tuck any remaining hair under the hair cover. All hair must be covered by the hair cover.

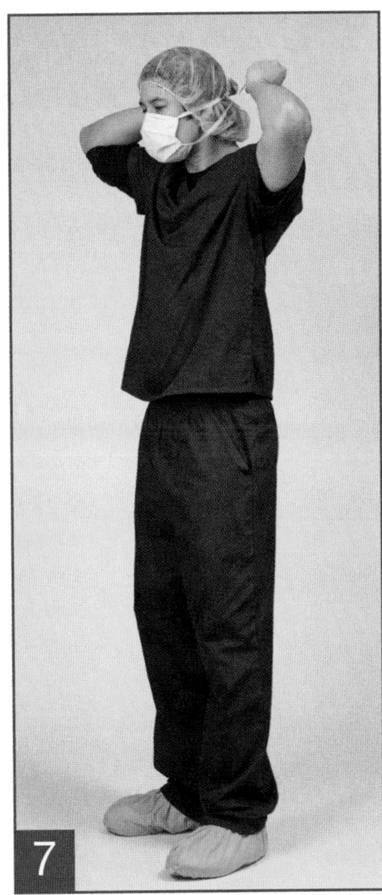

Pharmacy technician donning a face mask

7 Don a face mask by positioning it over the face with the top of the mask at the bridge of the nose. Pull the two uppermost ties around the sides of the face and then tie them behind the head so that the ties rest just above the ears. Grasp the two lower ties and tie them behind the back of the neck. Adjust the mask so that it is positioned securely over the nose, mouth, and chin.

TAKE NOTE

At this point in the procedure, USP <797> requires that the technician complete a full, aseptic hand-washing procedure (as taught in Lab 30) before donning a sterile gown. Due to time constraints, your instructor may have you forgo that step during this training lab, instead having you use foamed alcohol to sanitize your hands. Be aware that in practice, you will be required to complete a full, aseptic hand washing at this step in the garbing procedure.

8 Open the package containing a sterile gown, ensuring that the gown does not touch the floor or any other surface at any time.

© Paradigm Publishing, Inc.

9 Insert one arm into the sleeve of the gown, and pull it up onto the shoulder of that arm. Insert the other arm into the other sleeve, and pull the gown up to the neck. Tie the neck ties of the gown behind the neck. Wrap the waist ties of the gown around the body, and tie them behind the back.

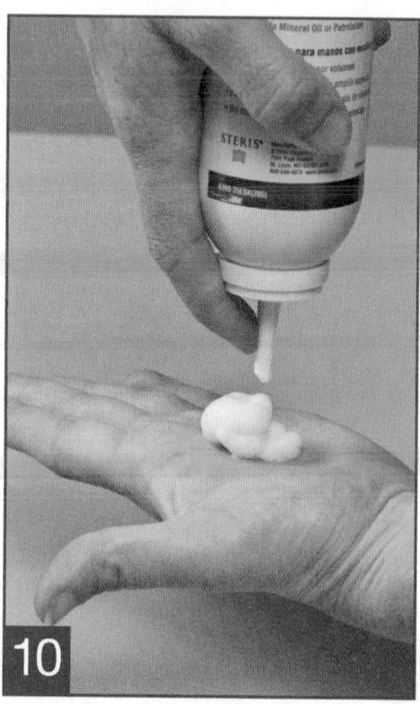
Proper procedure for dispensing foamed alcohol

10 Hold a can of foamed alcohol so that the tip is pointed down into the palm of the hand. Use the index finger of the hand that is holding the can to press against the tip of the dispenser, releasing a small (approximately golf ball-sized) amount of foamed alcohol onto the palm.

11 Rub the hands together, making sure that the alcohol coats each finger, the palms, the backs of the hands, and the areas between the fingers. Allow the alcohol to evaporate until the hands are dry.

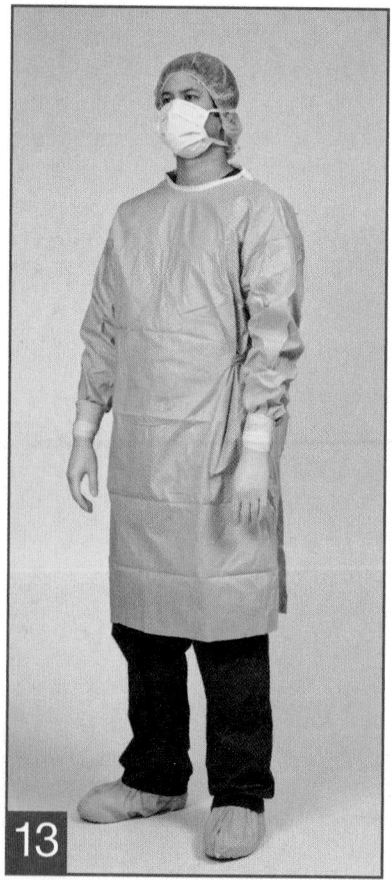
Fully gowned and gloved pharmacy technician

12 Open the outer wrapper of the package of sterile gloves. Place the inner package on a clean surface, such as a table or countertop that has been disinfected with sterile, 70% isopropyl alcohol.

13 The gloves will be labeled "left" and "right." Do not touch the outer surface of the gloves at any time. Place the right glove on the right hand by grasping the inner part of the cuff (it will be folded over for easy access) with the left hand and carefully pulling it onto the right hand and up to the wrist. Pull the glove over the cuff of the gown. Repeat the procedure with the other glove using the opposite hand.

© Paradigm Publishing, Inc.

14 Remove the top from the agar plate and place it onto an aseptic surface, such as a table or countertop that has been cleaned with sterile, 70% isopropyl alcohol.

15 Carefully press the gloved forefinger of the right hand onto the agar plate. Press the gloved right thumb onto a different section of the agar plate. Replace the cover on the agar plate.

16 Using a new agar plate, repeat Steps 14 and 15 with the left hand.

17 Label the plates as instructed, and give both plates to your instructor for processing.

18 Unless otherwise instructed, remove the garb in this order: gloves, gown, face mask, hair cover, and shoe covers. All items should be disposed of in the pharmacy waste receptacle or designated area.

19 **Conclusion:** Go to the Course Navigator, answer all questions in the Lab Review section, and submit your answers to your instructor.

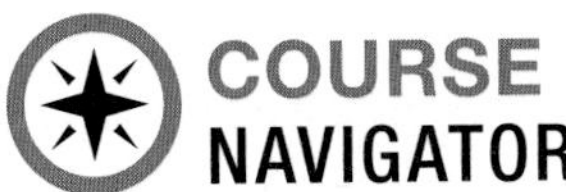

Access interactive chapter review exercises, practice activities, flash cards, and study games.

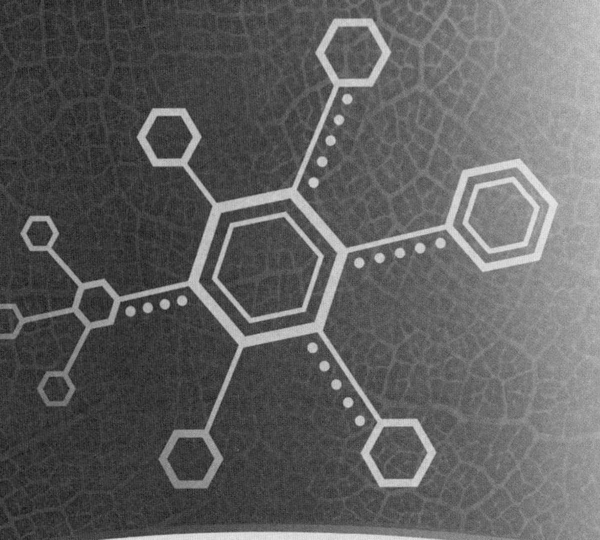

30

Aseptic Hand Washing

Learning Objectives

1 Demonstrate excellence in aseptic hand-washing procedures.

2 Discuss the procedures for and rationale behind aseptic hand washing.

Supplies

- Prepackaged surgical scrub sponge/brush containing a suitable antimicrobial solution, such as chlorhexidine 4%
- Sink appropriate for aseptic hand washing
- Aseptic, nonshedding, disposable towels dispensed from a container that does not compromise the cleanliness or integrity of the towels
- Garb (as required by your instructor)
- Sterile, powder-free gloves

Access additional chapter resources.

Proper hand cleansing is the foundation of good aseptic technique. The word **aseptic** means “without infection; free of pathogens,” and aseptic hand washing is vital to keeping sterile products free from potentially infectious microorganisms. Pharmacy technicians must master aseptic hand washing, which is an essential skill when preparing sterile parenteral products such as intravenous (IV) solutions, total parenteral nutrition (TPN) solutions, and injectable solutions. Policies and procedures regarding hand washing vary slightly among hospitals. For example, you will sometimes do only a basic aseptic hand washing and at other times you will perform a complete aseptic hand washing, which requires the use of a surgical scrub sponge/brush.

A basic aseptic hand washing is achieved by vigorously washing both hands and forearms (spanning from the wrist to the elbow) for at least 30 seconds with an appropriate antimicrobial agent. Extra attention must be paid to areas with higher concentrations of microorganisms, such as under the fingernails and in skin creases. A basic hand washing follows the same steps (outlined in this lab) as a complete aseptic hand washing; however, a surgical scrub sponge/brush is not used. You may perform a basic hand washing—using antimicrobial soap or another hand-cleansing product such as foamed alcohol—any time there is the potential for **minor contamination** (a small amount of contamination of the washed and scrubbed aseptic area), such as after using a calculator or pen or inadvertently spilling a few drops of drug onto your hand.

Basic aseptic hand washing is an acceptable form of hand cleansing and meets all of the requirements set forth by USP Chapter <797>. However, many facilities that prepare parenteral products, including compounded sterile preparations (CSPs), often require a more thorough type of aseptic hand washing that uses a surgical scrub sponge/brush. While basic aseptic hand washing is used upon minor hand contamination, in these facilities there are circumstances in which a complete aseptic hand washing is desirable.

In particular, all personnel must perform a complete aseptic hand washing upon first entering the sterile compounding area; when reentering the area; after eating, using the restroom, sneezing, or coughing; or upon experiencing **major contamination** (a large amount of contamination of the washed and scrubbed aseptic area), such as a large (greater than 5 mL) drug spill or a needlestick. A complete aseptic hand washing should take a *minimum* of 30 seconds. Spending 2 to 4 minutes is preferred, since the procedure contains many specific steps within these main categories: preparing the body; preparing the soap; scrubbing the nails; washing the fingers, palms, backs of the hands, and forearms; rinsing the hands and forearms; drying the hands and forearms; and gloving the hands.

Complete aseptic hand washing requires rigorous technique but only simple tools: a sink and a few items kept nearby, including aseptic, nonshedding, disposable towels or an aseptic, hot-air hand dryer; sterile, powder-free gloves; and a surgical scrub sponge/brush presaturated with an appropriate antimicrobial solution. The sink itself should be located in the anteroom or ante-area, located just outside the door of the sterile compounding area, and the sink's use should be restricted to aseptic hand-washing procedures only. The sink should be deep, have a gooseneck faucet with hot and cold running water, and preferably be controlled by foot pedals. It should be clean and free of anything that might cause splashing.

A surgical scrub sponge/brush (which usually has both a sponge side and a brush side) is required for the complete aseptic hand-washing technique and is a very effective tool. Many facilities, especially those preparing medium-risk CSPs, and high-risk parenteral products compounded from nonsterile ingredients, prefer using a sterile, prepackaged surgical scrub sponge/brush that is presaturated with an approved antimicrobial soap.

 © Paradigm Publishing, Inc.

Although the surgical scrub sponge/brush is a simple tool to use, you must take several precautions to ensure a contamination-free procedure. Do not use the brush side when scrubbing the skin. While the brush side of the tool is effective for scrubbing under the nails and around the cuticles, using it on the skin may cause skin particles to flake off into the clean environment. Do not reuse the scrub sponge/brush; it is intended for one-time use only and should be thrown away immediately after use. Do not touch the sink or faucet with your fingers, hands or arms, or with the scrub sponge/brush at any time. Do not apply lotion to your hands after completing the washing procedure. If you inadvertently do any of these things, you must repeat the entire hand-washing procedure with a *new* surgical scrub sponge/brush.

Procedure

In this lab, you will perform a complete aseptic hand-washing procedure using a sterile, presaturated surgical scrub sponge/brush.

1. Remove all jewelry. Because jewelry, makeup, nail polish, and false nails may not be worn in the compounding area, you should make adjustments as needed to comply with these rules.

2. Check with your instructor for guidance regarding garbing, and garb accordingly.

TAKE NOTE

According to USP <797>, you should don hair cover, shoe covers, and a mask prior to proceeding with this lab, and you should don a sterile gown and gloves after completing the hand-washing procedure. However, because this is a training lab with time constraints, your instructor may have you eliminate one or more of these steps. In actual practice, all of the steps are mandatory.

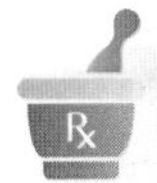

Practice Tip

If your sink is not equipped with foot pedals, you must let the water run throughout the entire hand-washing procedure and ignore any steps asking you to turn the water back on.

3. Prior to opening the scrub sponge/brush packet, squeeze it several times to activate the soap suds. Carefully open the packet, remove the scrub sponge/brush and nail pick, and throw away the outer wrapper.

4. Press the foot pedals to begin the flow of water and, when the water is warm, wet your hands and forearms.

5. Without setting down the scrub sponge/brush, use the nail pick included in the scrub packet to clean under your fingernails. Throw away the pick when finished.

Practice Tip

Throughout this lab's entire hand-washing procedure, you should squeeze the scrub sponge/brush or add a small amount of water as needed to maintain a good, soapy lather.

6 Apply a small amount of water to the scrub sponge/brush, and then squeeze it several times so that it has an ample, soapy lather. Manipulate the scrub sponge/brush so that you are using the brush side of the scrub, not the sponge side.

7 Scrub under the thumbnail with the scrub brush. Scrub under the nail of the next finger with the scrub brush, and proceed until you have scrubbed under all of the fingernails on the initial hand.

8 Use the brush to clean under the thumbnail on the opposite hand, and continue scrubbing under the nail of each finger until you have cleaned under all the nails on that hand.

Safety Alert

Remember not to use the brush side of the scrub sponge/brush on your skin, because doing so may introduce skin cells into the environment, contaminating the aseptic procedure.

9 Manipulate the scrub brush to switch to its sponge side. Beginning with the thumb on the initial hand, clean each of the four surfaces of the thumb (the two sides and the top and bottom surfaces) with the sponge.

10 Clean the webbing between the thumb and forefinger.

11 Proceed to clean all four surfaces of the forefinger and the webbing between it and the next finger. Continue this process of cleaning on the next finger, the following webbing, the next finger, and so on until you have cleaned all fingers and webbings on that hand.

12 Move to the opposite hand and repeat Steps 7–11, beginning with the thumb and continuing through all the fingers and webbings on that hand.

13 Move back to the initial hand and clean the palm with the sponge. Repeat the palm cleaning on the opposite hand.

14 Move back to the initial hand and clean the back of the hand with the sponge. Repeat the cleaning process on the back of the other hand.

15 Return to the initial hand and start at the wrist, cleaning in a circular pattern, moving around the forearm as you work toward the elbow, where you stop. Repeat the procedure on the other forearm. This procedure is illustrated in Figure 30.1.

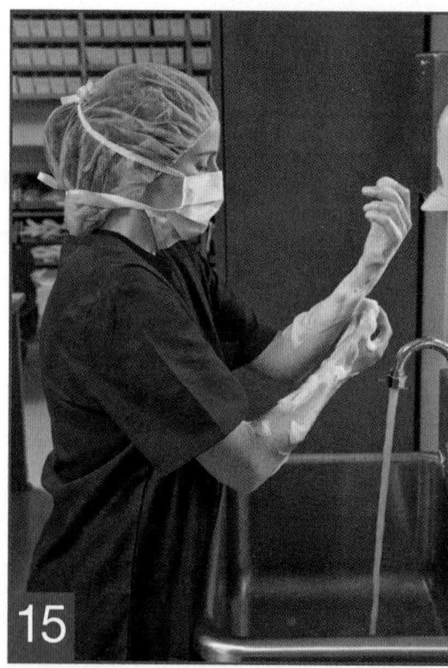

Pharmacy technician performing complete aseptic hand-washing procedure

© Paradigm Publishing, Inc.

FIGURE 30.1 Proper Aseptic Hand-Washing Technique for Forearms

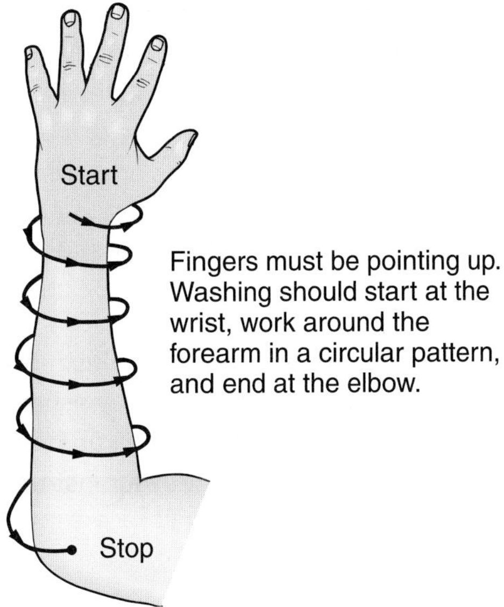

Keep your fingers pointing upward throughout the entire rinsing and drying procedure. Do not allow the water to run down toward your fingers, because this directional change will compromise the aseptic nature of the process.

16 Throw away the scrub sponge/brush.

17 Run the water until the flow is warm. On the side on which you began the hand-washing procedure, rinse the hand and forearm, starting with the fingers and keeping them pointing upward so that the water runs down toward the elbow.

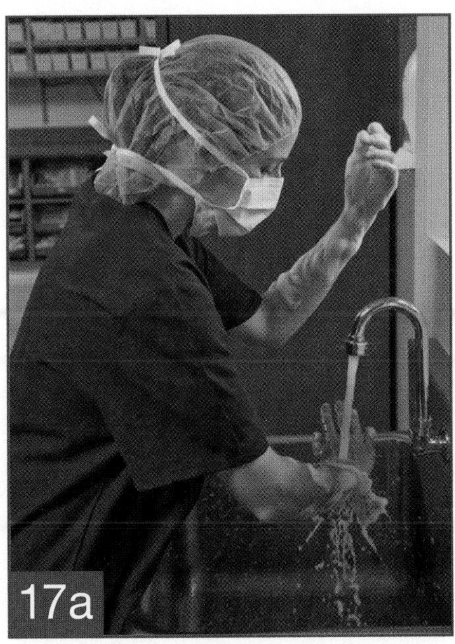

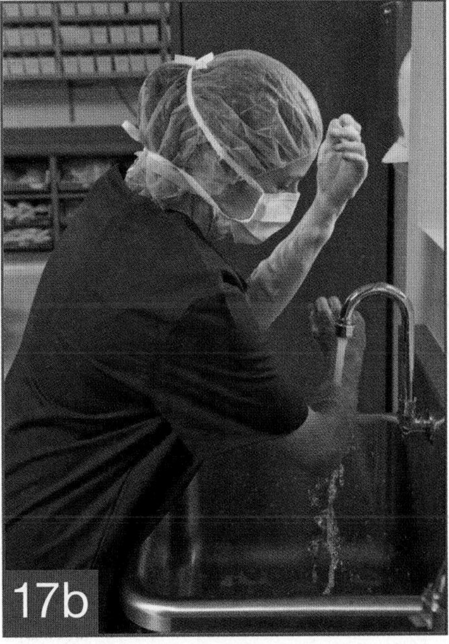

Pharmacy technician rinsing hands and forearms after aseptic hand washing

Practice Tip

If you do not have foot pedals at your sink, use a nonshedding, disposable towel to turn off the faucet before throwing away the towel.

18 Repeat the hand and forearm rinsing process on the other side. Using aseptic, nonshedding, disposable towels, dry your hands first and then throw away the towels. Using new towels, dry the forearms and throw away the towels. If using a hot air hand dryer, skip Step 18 and instead dry hands and arms with air from the dryer.

19 Check with your instructor about gowning and gloving (as noted in the Practice Tip for Step 2), and proceed accordingly.

20 **Conclusion:** Ask for instructor verification that you have properly completed the hand-washing procedure. Then go to the Course Navigator, answer all questions in the Lab Review section, and submit your answers to your instructor.

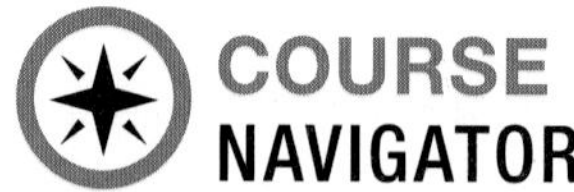

Access interactive chapter review exercises, practice activities, flash cards, and study games.

© Paradigm Publishing, Inc.

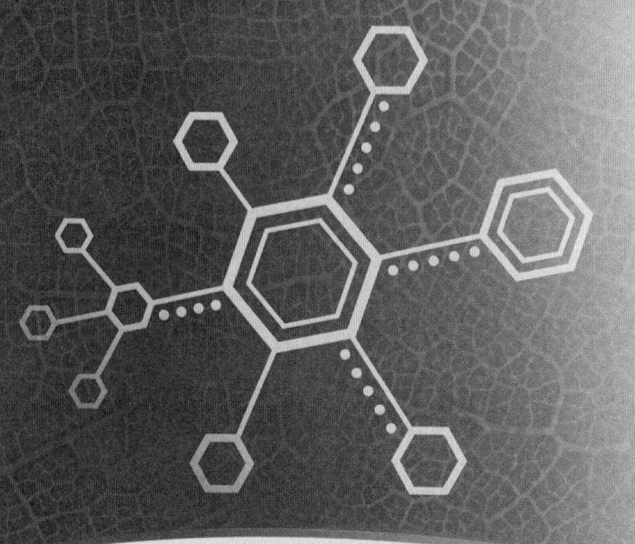

31

Hood Cleaning

Learning Objectives

1 Demonstrate proficiency in the cleaning of a standard horizontal laminar airflow hood.

2 Explain the rationale and procedures for basic hood cleaning.

Supplies

1 Sterile water for irrigation (in a pour bottle holding 250 mL or more)

2 Sterile, 70% isopropyl alcohol (in a pour bottle holding 250 mL or more)

3 Aseptic, lint-free, and nonshedding hood-cleaning wipes

4 A hood appropriate for this procedure (any size horizontal laminar airflow hood in which the HEPA filter is contained in the back wall of the cabinet)

5 Hood-cleaning log sheet (kept nearby inside of a plastic sheet protector)

Access additional chapter resources.

Laminar airflow hoods are constructed to provide a constant flow of sterile air across a work surface that has been aseptically cleaned. The air is sterilized by being blown through a high-efficiency particulate air (HEPA) filter. As a pharmacy technician, you will probably work with several types of hoods, including the **vertical laminar airflow hood** (known as a *biological safety cabinet*, or *BSC*), the self-contained laminar airflow barrier isolator hood, and the horizontal laminar airflow hood. All of these hoods are used to compound sterile preparations for parenteral administration using strict aseptic technique.

The vertical laminar airflow hood is primarily used to prepare chemotherapy drugs, chemotherapy medications, and other **antineoplastic agents**. (An antineoplastic agent inhibits or prevents the growth or development of malignant cells.) You will likely use this hood at some time in your work, but you must first receive specialized training. The self-contained laminar airflow barrier isolator hood, sometimes called a "glove box," is primarily used in environments where a relatively small number of sterile products are prepared at one time. Glove boxes are also sometimes used in small, rural hospitals that do not have a dedicated pharmacy compounding room. However, pharmacies that prepare a large number of compounded sterile preparations (CSPs) usually use a standard horizontal laminar airflow hood because of its ease of use. Also referred to as a "workbench" or "cabinet," the standard horizontal laminar airflow hood is the hood most frequently used in both hospital and compounding pharmacies and is the hood you will probably use most often as a pharmacy technician.

Because of the critical nature of the products prepared in a laminar airflow hood, the hood must be cleaned properly. Be aware that airflow in the hood should be left running at all times. If airflow in the hood is somehow turned off, you must turn it back on and run it for a minimum of 30 minutes prior to using or cleaning the hood. Proper cleaning of the horizontal laminar airflow hood is generally performed with sterile, 70% isopropyl alcohol and aseptic, nonshedding wipes. Most facilities start the cleaning process by wiping down the interior surfaces of the cabinet using sterile water. Because some drugs are not soluble in alcohol, using water first allows those drugs to be dissolved and removed from the work surface prior to cleaning it with alcohol. Proper hood cleaning requires several batches of cleaning wipes, because when you reach the outer edge of the hood, the pads become contaminated and must be discarded. The outer edge of the hood refers to the outer 6 inches of the hood working surface. This is considered the "dirty edge," because it is where sterile air mixes with room air.

At times it may be appropriate to clean only the work surface of the hood, such as when a few drops of drug solution are spilled. However, a complete cleaning of the cabinet is usually required, such as when you begin each shift and every 30 minutes during continuous compounding periods. A complete hood cleaning should also be done when a large amount (greater than 5 mL) of drug is spilled, when drug has been aspirated into the hood, when the prefilter is changed or the HEPA filter is recertified, or any time that major contamination (resulting from a needlestick or inadvertently sneezing or coughing into the hood) is suspected.

The hood-cleaning procedure requires strict record keeping for quality assurance. Thus, you should find a **hood-cleaning log sheet** for each hood, which is maintained inside a plastic sheet protector and is generally kept near the hood or in the anteroom. You must initial, date, and record the time on the log sheet each time you clean the hood. These records are kept for a minimum of 2 years, and completed sheets may be reviewed by investigators from The Joint Commission, the state board of pharmacy, and other regulatory agencies. The hood-cleaning log sheet should reflect that the

© Paradigm Publishing, Inc.

hood is being cleaned, at minimum, at the beginning of every shift, every 30 minutes during continuous compounding periods, and upon any major contamination. You will likely need to clean each hood multiple times during your shift. Despite this frequency, it is imperative that you fill out the hood-cleaning log sheet every time you perform this task.

Procedure

In this lab, you will clean a standard horizontal laminar airflow hood with sterile water and sterile, 70% isopropyl alcohol, according to standard USP Chapter regulations.

1 Garb, hand wash, gown, and glove as directed by your instructor.

2 Remove everything (vials, syringe caps, and all other objects) from the hood, including anything hanging inside the hood.

3 Place an approximately 2-inch stack of aseptic, lint-free hood-cleaning wipes on the work surface, at least 6 inches inside of the hood.

4 Pour sterile water onto the wipes so that the entire stack is lightly saturated (but not dripping) with water.

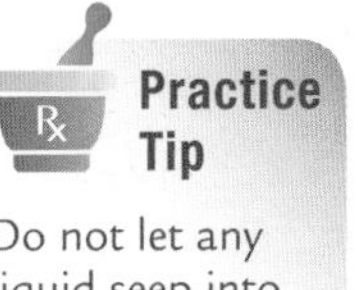

Practice Tip

Do not let any liquid seep into the HEPA filter, and do not touch the HEPA filter at any time.

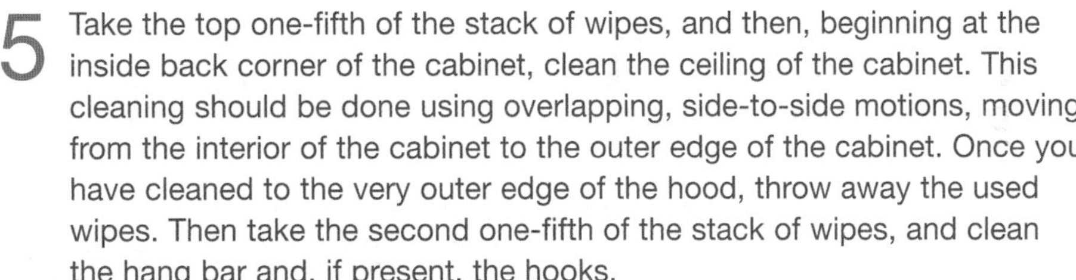

5 Take the top one-fifth of the stack of wipes, and then, beginning at the inside back corner of the cabinet, clean the ceiling of the cabinet. This cleaning should be done using overlapping, side-to-side motions, moving from the interior of the cabinet to the outer edge of the cabinet. Once you have cleaned to the very outer edge of the hood, throw away the used wipes. Then take the second one-fifth of the stack of wipes, and clean the hang bar and, if present, the hooks.

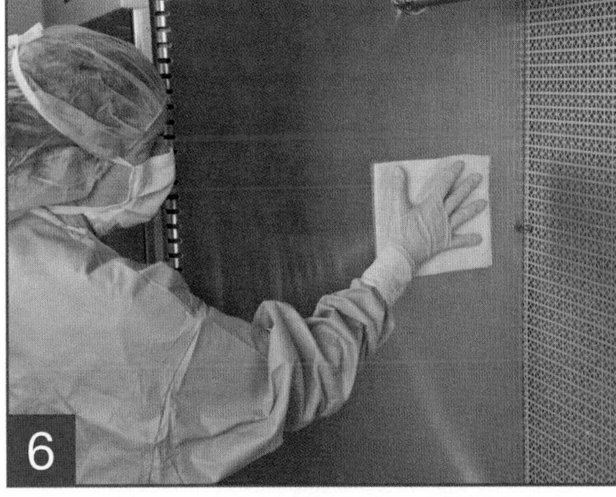

Pharmacy technician cleaning a side panel of a hood

6 To begin cleaning the side panels, pick up the third one-fifth of the clean, water-saturated stack of wipes. Beginning with the interior upper corner of one side panel, clean using overlapping, down-and-up motions. Move from the interior upper corner of the cabinet toward the outer edge. This procedure is illustrated in Figure 31.1 on the next page. Once you have cleaned to the outer edge of the hood, throw away the used wipes.

© Paradigm Publishing, Inc.

FIGURE 31.1 Horizontal Laminar Airflow Hood: Proper Cleaning of Side Panels

Cleaning of the side panels starts at the interior upper corner (X), close to the HEPA filter, and proceeds in sweeping, overlapping, down-and-up motions that move toward the outer edge of the hood.

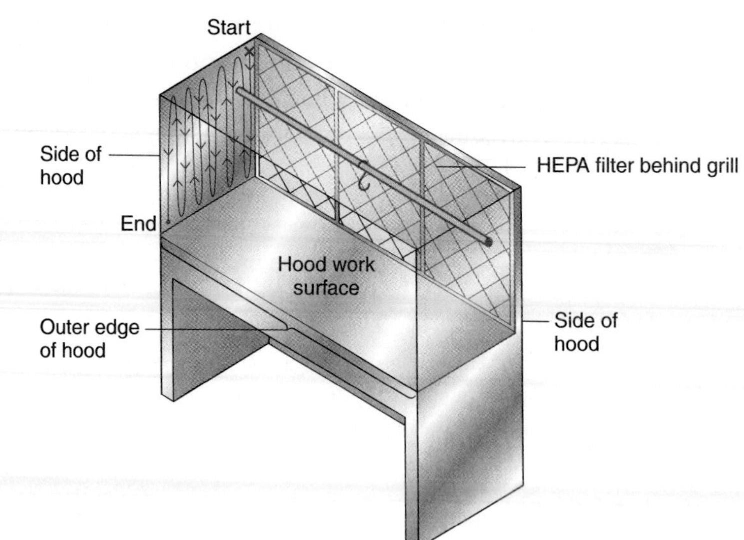

7 Pick up the fourth one-fifth of the clean, water-saturated stack of wipes and repeat Step 6 on the other side panel. Once you have cleaned to the outer edge of the hood, throw away the used wipes.

8 Take the remaining water-saturated wipes and clean the work surface. Start in the back corner, and clean with overlapping side-to-side strokes, working your way from the inside of the hood to the outer edge as illustrated in Figure 31.2. Once you have cleaned to the outer edge of the hood, throw away the used wipes.

FIGURE 31.2 Horizontal Laminar Airflow Hood: Proper Cleaning of Work Surface

Cleaning of the work surface starts at the interior back corner (X), close to the HEPA filter, and proceeds in sweeping, overlapping, side-to-side motions that move toward the outer edge of the hood.

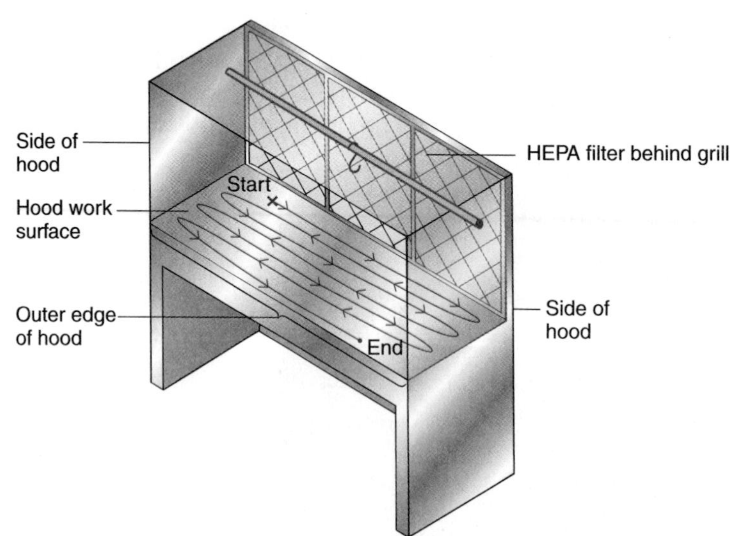

 © Paradigm Publishing, Inc.

9 Repeat Steps 3–8 in the same order, using a new, approximately 2-inch stack of hood-cleaning wipes saturated with sterile, 70% isopropyl alcohol.

10 Initial, date, and record the time on the hood-cleaning log sheet that is near the hood or in the antechamber. If you have questions about filling out this sheet, check with your instructor.

11 **Conclusion:** Go to the Course Navigator, answer all questions in the Lab Review section, and submit your answers to your instructor.

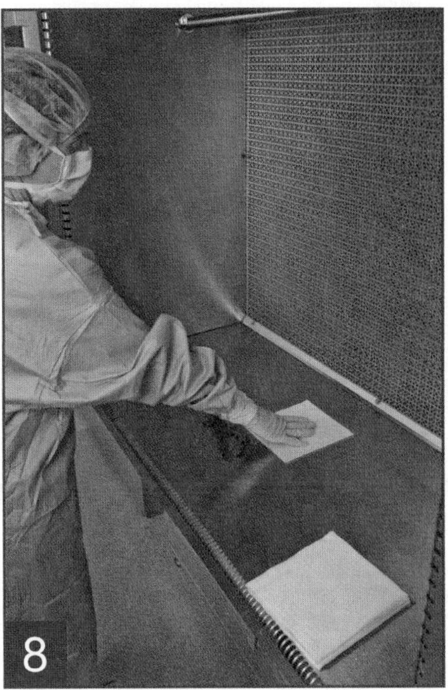

Pharmacy technician cleaning the work surface of a hood.

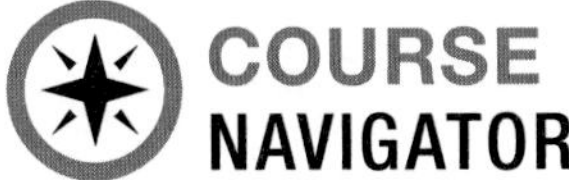

Access interactive chapter review exercises, practice activities, flash cards, and study games.

© Paradigm Publishing, Inc.

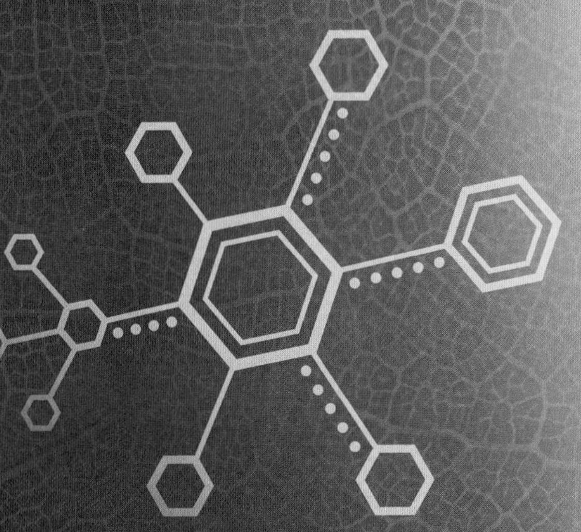

32 Preparing Large-Volume Parenteral Solutions

Learning Objectives

1. Demonstrate proficiency in aseptic technique as it relates to the preparation of large-volume parenteral products.
2. Demonstrate accuracy in basic calculations related to the preparation of large-volume parenteral products.
3. Discuss the procedures and rationale for the preparation of large-volume parenteral products.

Supplies

- Potassium chloride 2 mEq/1 mL, multi-dose, bulk vial 250 mL
- 0.9% sodium chloride 1,000 mL IV bag (with injection port)
- Sterile dispensing pin
- 20 mL syringe
- Regular needle × 1 (a regular needle has no filter and no vent)
- Sharps container (dedicated for IV room use only)
- Trash container (dedicated for IV room use only)
- Sterile Alcohol swabs × 3
- Calculator

Access additional chapter resources.

Introduction to Sterile Compounding for Labs 32–35

Previous labs in this aseptic technique unit provided you with background and practice in garbing by USP <797> standards, aseptic hand washing, and hood cleaning. In the final four labs of this book, Labs 32–35, you will employ these techniques while preparing sterile products. Your instructor may provide you with more detailed guidelines for following aseptic technique, and you should ask for clarification on any points about which you are unsure.

You will find Labs 32–35 to be considerably longer than many others in the textbook. However, sterile compounding and aseptic technique skills are essential in pharmacy work and important to the healthcare field. In fact, this work is frequently performed by the pharmacy's sterile compounding technician. Therefore, as you encounter a long series of steps in these labs, please take your time and follow each step to completion. Once you become familiar with the technique, the processes go very quickly.

The following list contains basic terms that apply generally to sterile product preparation labs:

- **Aseptic technique:** A clean, "without infection" technique that is free of pathogens.
- **Clean room:** A space where sterile parenteral products are prepared. This space is often referred to as the "buffer area or room," "IV room," or the "sterile compounding room." This is the room where the laminar airflow hoods are located. Clean rooms incorporate specialized HVAC systems that utilize high-efficiency particulate air (HEPA)-filtered airflow to sustain a specified room pressure and number of air exchanges that maintains air cleanliness standards as specified in USP <797>. Access to the clean room is restricted to trained and properly garbed personnel. Professional conduct is required in the clean room: eating, drinking, and chewing gum are prohibited. Only certain supplies are allowed, and they must first be wiped down with an antimicrobial solution.
- **Compounded sterile preparations (CSP):** A parenteral product that is produced by mixing various components and ingredients using aseptic technique, and which is intended to be sterile upon administration to the patient.
- **Coring:** An undesired event that occurs when a needle is inserted incorrectly into a rubber stopper atop a solution vial, causing a small bit of the stopper to tear off and contaminate the solution inside the vial.
- **Critical sites:** Parts of equipment or supplies that must never be touched and to which airflow from the HEPA filter should never be interrupted. These parts include the vial top, needle, hub of the needle, hub of the syringe, tip of the syringe, ampule neck, dispensing pin spike, and IV bag injection port.
- **Dilution:** Injection of a liquid medication into an IV solution such as sterile water or normal saline, which results in a more dilute concentration of the drug.
- **Direct compounding area (DCA):** The critical area within the PEC where sterile compounding takes place, and where critical sites receive unidirectional HEPA-filtered first air.
- **First air:** Clean air that exits the HEPA filter and which flows in a unidirectional air stream.
- **Milking technique:** A process used to ease the negative pressure in a vial or other closed container by adding positive pressure to the system. This technique involves inserting a needle attached to a syringe into the vial or container, adding a small amount of air to the vial, and then adding and removing small quantities of fluid and air as many times as necessary.

© Paradigm Publishing, Inc.

- **Negative pressure:** A quality inherent to vials and some other closed systems, wherein a pressure differential prohibits the withdrawal of fluid from a vial into a syringe. This situation is altered by equalizing the pressure inside of the vial through the use of a dispensing pin, a vented needle, or the milking technique.
- **Parenteral:** Refers to medications administered by any route other than through the alimentary canal (the digestive tract), thus including every method of dispensation other than by mouth or rectum. The parenteral route of administration includes intravenous, intramuscular, transdermal, intraocular, or intrathecal dispensation of drugs.
- **Pathogen:** An infectious agent that can cause disease or illness in a patient.
- **Primary engineering control (PEC):** Equipment such as a laminar airflow hood that is used to provide an environment suitable for sterile compounding.
- **Positive pressure:** This situation occurs when a small amount of air is introduced into a vial or other closed system, thereby easing the withdrawal of fluid from the vial and into a syringe. (See the entry on *milking technique* for additional explanation.)
- **Shadowing:** A form of contamination that results when a worker's hands or their supplies on the hood are incorrectly placed, disrupting sterile airflow from the HEPA filter to the critical site. Figure 32.1 shows airflow in a hood.
- **6-Inch rule:** Standard procedure whereby technicians must not work within the outer 6 inches of the hood's work surface. This area is considered the "dirty edge," because it is where sterile air mixes with room air. However, for ease of access, prewrapped objects that are to be used shortly, such as needles, syringes, and alcohol swabs, are often placed in this outer 6-inch area.
- **Touch contamination:** A form of contamination that results when a critical site, or the hood surface itself, is contaminated through incorrect technique, needlestick, sneezing, or coughing.

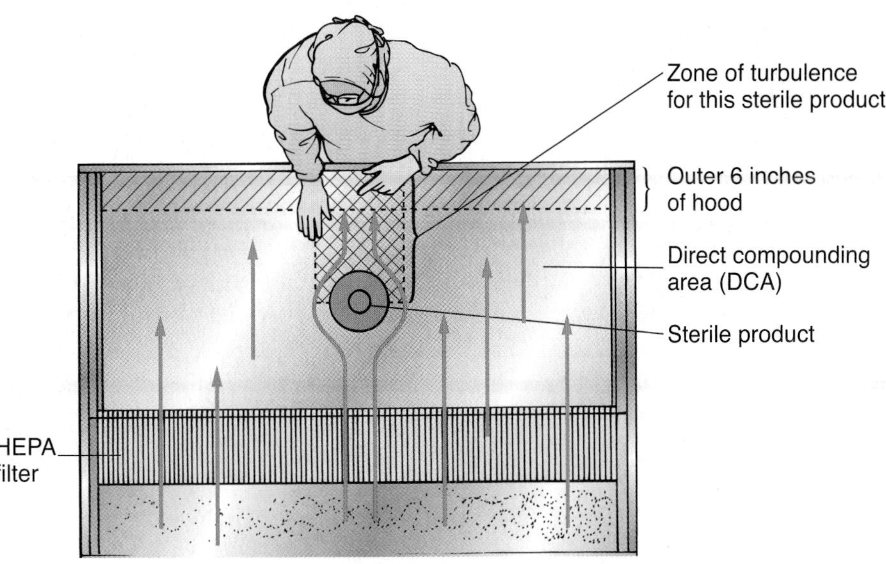

FIGURE 32.1 Airflow in a Horizontal Laminar Airflow Hood

This is a downward view onto the hood work surface; items should be placed in the hood so as to receive uninterrupted airflow.

- **Zone of turbulence:** The area behind any item (e.g., a vial, IV bag, or syringe) on the hood where sterile airflow is interrupted; this zone or area is contaminated. Sterile parenteral products should never be prepared within a zone of turbulence.

TAKE NOTE

As a pharmacy technician, you are required to adhere to strict aseptic technique when compounding sterile preparations. This is crucial because medications that are administered directly into the patient's bloodstream, internal organ, or internal tissue are considered to be the most dangerous to the patient; they are certainly more dangerous than enteral (nonparenteral) products. Danger exists for a few reasons. First, because parenteral medications are administered directly into the bloodstream, organ, or tissue, the patient's only defense against potential pathogens is his or her immune system, which is already compromised by fighting a primary infection or recovering from injury or surgery. In contrast, enteral products go through the digestive tract, where an abundance of flora defends against many pathogenic organisms. Second, once a medication is injected into the bloodstream, there is little to no chance of reversal; enteral medications can be reversed with ipecac or activated charcoal if a mistake is made (i.e., an incorrect drug or dose is administered). Third, parenteral agents introduce 100% of the drug into the bloodstream, whereas with enteral administration, only a portion of the drug reaches the bloodstream.

Large-volume parenteral preparations are sterile solutions with volumes of 250 mL or more that are administered parenterally. Many of the procedures performed while working in the sterile compounding room involve the aseptic preparation of large-volume parenteral (LVP) products that are administered intravenously. A large-volume IV solution is most often referred to as a "main" IV line, providing hydration for the patient and delivering electrolytes, such as potassium, directly into the patient's vein.

The most common large-volume parenteral preparations are IV solutions based on a standard solution such as 0.9% sodium chloride (which is called "normal saline"), dextrose 5% in water, dextrose 5% in normal saline, and lactated Ringer's solution. You will commonly see these base solutions referred to in abbreviated form (NS, D_5W, D_5NS, and LR, respectively) and will find that they are kept on hand at all times in the floor stock area of most hospitals. The most common volumes for large-volume IV solutions are 250 mL, 500 mL, and 1,000 mL.

© Paradigm Publishing, Inc.

These base solutions are frequently a component of the compounded sterile preparations that are assembled by pharmacy technicians. As a technician, you will compound large-volume parenteral solutions by aseptically injecting a medication into an IV base solution. Prior to preparing the solutions, however, you must execute the calculations most commonly used in sterile compounding—those based on ratio and proportion. Compounding large-volume parenteral solutions also requires familiarity with a dispensing pin, a syringe, and a needle. The **dispensing pin** is a specialized plastic device that includes a vent, a spike, and a syringe adaptor, and is inserted into the rubber stopper of a vial. The dispensing pin allows withdrawal of a large volume of fluid—in this lab, potassium chloride—without concern for air pressure.

Procedure

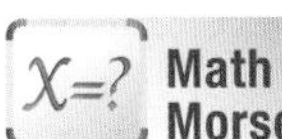

Math Morsels

"Eq" is the abbreviated form of "equivalent," a unit of concentration used in chemistry. Because the amount is often very small, it is described as a milliequivalent (mEq), with the prefix "milli" indicating that it is one one-thousandth of the base unit.

In this lab, you will perform a calculation related to the preparation of one large-volume parenteral product, demonstrate the correct use of a dispensing pin, and aseptically prepare a sterile solution for IV administration. The prepared IV solution will be composed of 1,000 mL of 0.9% sodium chloride (NS) and 25 mEq of potassium chloride (KCl).

1. In order to perform the necessary calculations for preparation of a 25 mEq dose of KCl solution, first verify the information provided on the KCl label. The KCl concentration should be stated as 2 mEq/1 mL.

2. Given this concentration, calculate how many milliliters you will need to withdraw from the vial in order to prepare the 25 mEq dose. Using the following formula, calculate the dose by cross multiplying and then dividing to solve for *x*, the unknown volume. When your calculations are complete, write your answer for *x* here: _______ mL. This is the amount you must draw up and add to the IV bag to create your solution.

$$\frac{2 \text{ mEq}}{1 \text{ mL}} = \frac{25 \text{ mEq}}{x \text{ mL}}$$

Safety Alert

In some instances you will be provided with a CSP label that tells you how much drug to draw up. However, it is important that you know how to perform these calculations, and that you verify that the correct amount was calculated prior to drawing it up.

3. Gather and wipe down necessary supply items, don aseptic garb, hand wash, don sterile gown and gloves, and clean the work area according to your instructor's directions.

4. Remove and discard the outer wrapper from the IV bag, and place the bag into the hood. Place the other necessary supplies in the hood, ensuring that supplies in an outer wrapper, such as syringes and needles, remain in the outer 6-inch zone closest to the edge of the hood until they are ready to be used.

Safety Alert

Potassium chloride is a commonly used electrolyte; however, it is also a "high alert" medication which, if administered incorrectly, can cause immediate cardiac cessation leading to death.

5 First, gently lift up the small pull tab on the top of the cap. Now grasp the pull tab, and pull it down toward the bottom of the vial, pulling all the way down and removing it. Take care not to twist the tab, so that it does not break. Once the entire tab has been removed, use it as a tool to pry off the aluminum ring encircling the rubber stopper and vial top. Then lift off and discard the coin-like aluminum circle resting atop the rubber stopper. This technique is illustrated in Figure 32.2 and the photograph accompanying Step 5.

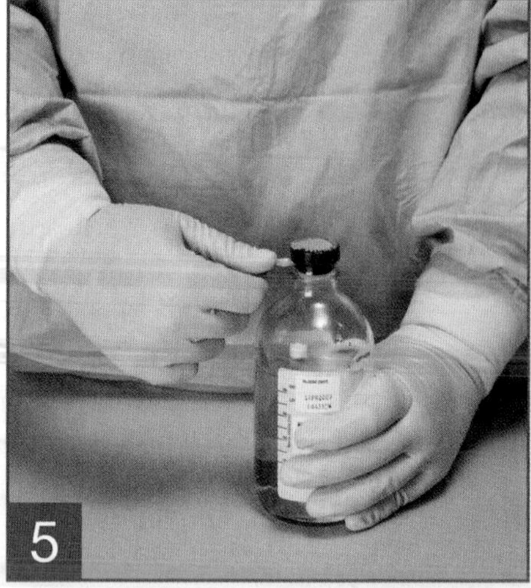

Pharmacy technician pulling the pull tab off of the aluminum cap on a bulk potassium chloride vial

Practice Tip

Be very careful in this step when removing the aluminum cap from the KCl bulk vial. The cap is quite sharp.

6 Clean the rubber stopper of the KCl vial with a sterile alcohol swab, and place the swab on the hood in an area that is free of airflow obstructions.

7 Remove and discard the outer wrapper of the sterile dispensing pin. Hold the top of the dispensing pin in the dominant hand, and with the other hand, take the cap off the spike of the dispensing pin and discard the cap.

FIGURE 32.2 Cap Removal from Bulk Vial

The correct technique for removing the aluminum cap from a bulk vial is demonstrated below.

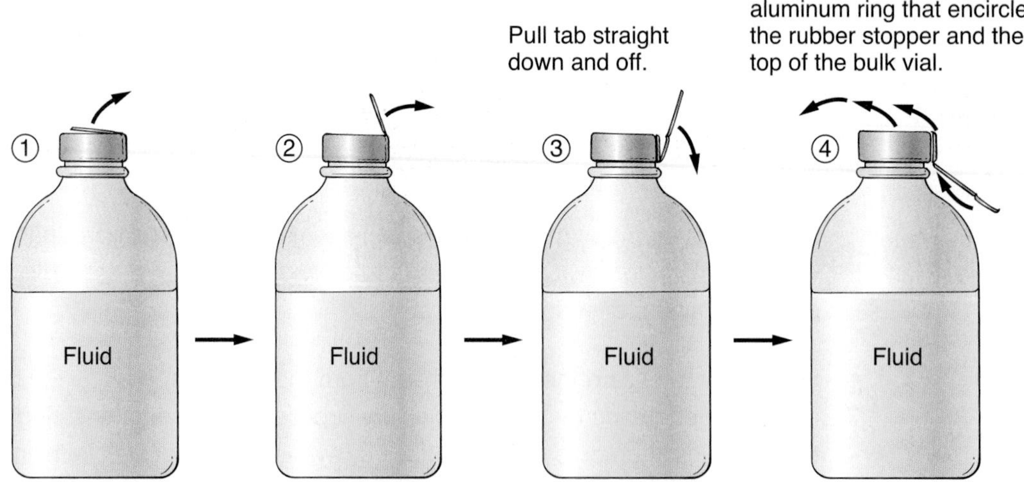

 © Paradigm Publishing, Inc.

Take care when removing the syringe from its outer wrapper. Some syringes have a cap on the tip; some do not. If there is a cap, it must be removed and discarded prior to attaching the syringe to the dispensing pin. If there is no cap, be careful not to shadow or otherwise contaminate the tip of the syringe. Never lay an uncapped syringe onto the work surface.

8 Hold the KCl vial steady against the hood work surface with the nondominant hand. Using the dominant hand, insert the spike of the dispensing pin straight into the rubber stopper of the KCl vial.

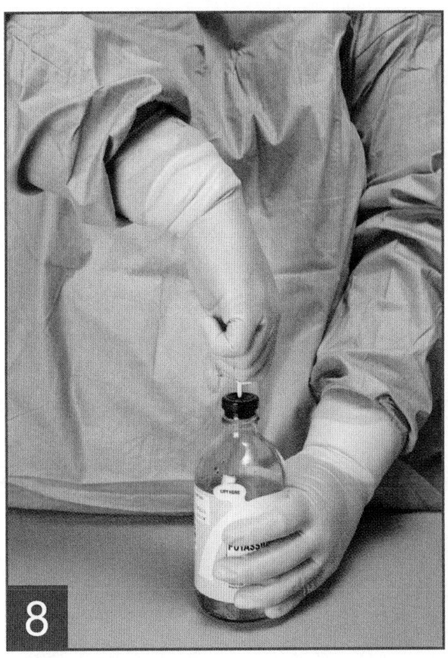

Correct technique for the insertion of a dispensing pin into a bulk potassium chloride vial

9 Remove the cap from the top of the dispensing pin, taking care not to shadow or otherwise contaminate the dispensing pin, the top of the KCl vial, or the cap itself. Place the cap onto the sterile alcohol swab.

10 Remove and discard the outer wrapper of the syringe. If necessary, remove and discard the cap from the tip of the syringe.

FIGURE 32.3
Critical Sites

Take care not to touch or shadow any of the critical sites.

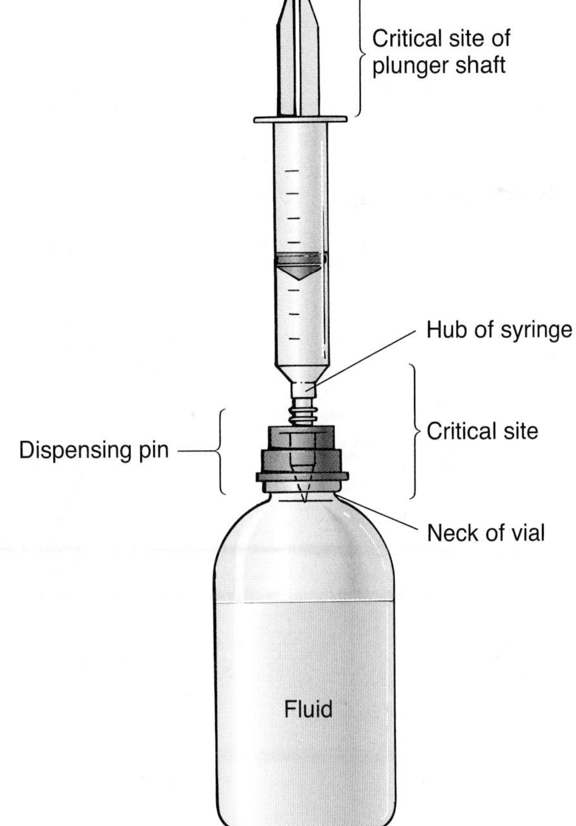

11 Without interrupting airflow to the KCl vial or the syringe, attach the tip of the syringe to the open port on the dispensing pin. Give the syringe a slight clockwise twist to ensure that it is firmly attached to the dispensing pin. Care must be taken to avoid contaminating the critical sites, shown in Figure 32.3

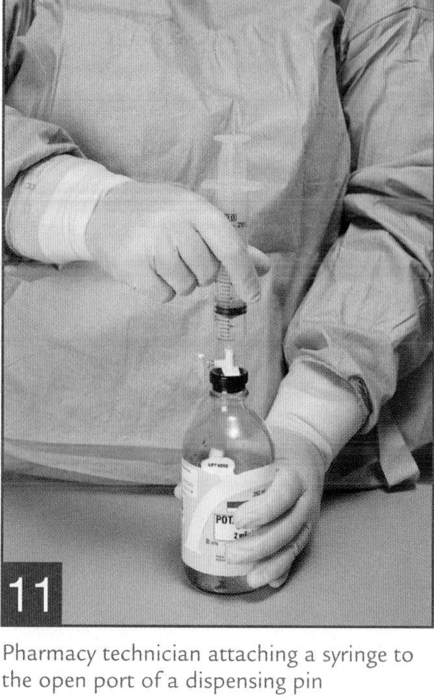

Pharmacy technician attaching a syringe to the open port of a dispensing pin

Practice Tip

Since the dispensing pin includes a vent, there is no need to add air to the vial when withdrawing fluid.

12 Invert the KCl vial such that the syringe is located underneath it.

13 Holding the KCl vial with the nondominant hand, pull down on the plunger of the syringe with the dominant hand until you reach approximately the 15 mL graduation mark on the syringe.

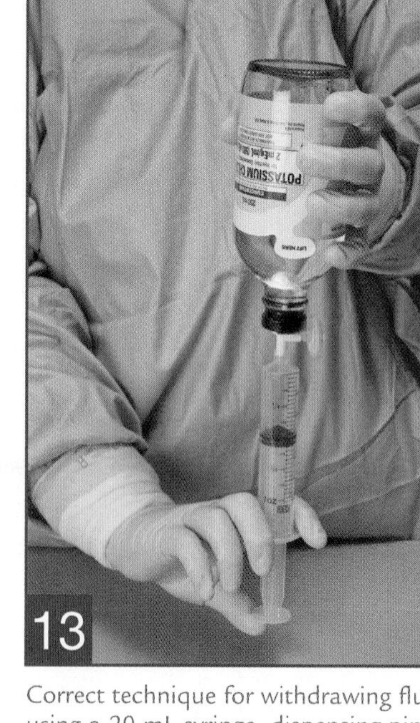

Correct technique for withdrawing fluid using a 20 mL syringe, dispensing pin, and inverted bulk vial

Practice Tip

Take care to hold the vial and syringe so that airflow to the critical sites (the syringe plunger shaft and the area from the hub of the syringe to the neck of the vial, including the entire dispensing pin and the rubber vial top) is unobstructed.

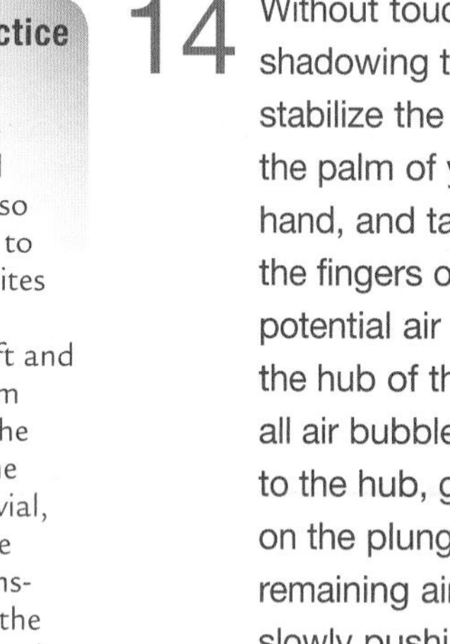

14 Without touching or shadowing the critical sites, stabilize the syringe against the palm of your nondominant hand, and tap the syringe with the fingers or palm to force potential air bubbles toward the hub of the syringe. When all air bubbles have risen to the hub, gently push up on the plunger to expel any remaining air, and continue slowly pushing up until the desired volume of 12.5 mL is reached. The configuration of the syringe and vial is shown in Figure 32.4.

© Paradigm Publishing, Inc.

FIGURE 32.4
Filling a Syringe from a Bulk Vial

Syringe measurement is taken where the shoulder of the rubber plunger meets the barrel of the syringe.

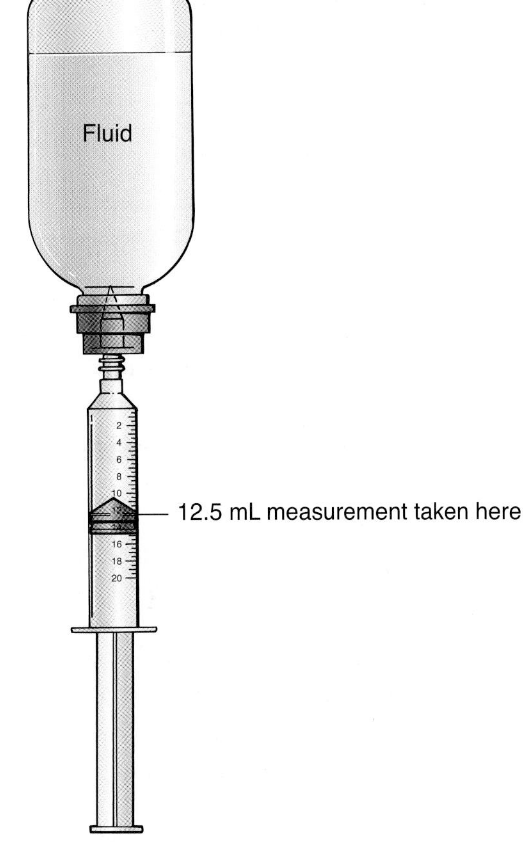

For Good Measure

Remember to take the syringe volume reading at the point where the shoulder of the rubber plunger meets the barrel of the syringe.

Practice Tip

Always keep the IV bag at least 6 inches from the outer edge of the hood.

15 Invert the vial-and-syringe unit, and return it to the work surface. Grasp the barrel of the syringe and twist counterclockwise to remove the syringe, from the dispensing pin, taking care not to interrupt airflow to either the KCl vial or the syringe.

16 Without laying the syringe down or shadowing the hub, and without touching the needle hub, aseptically attach a regular needle, with cap, to the syringe.

17 Place the syringe, with capped needle, onto the work surface next to the KCl vial and the IV bag.

18 Recap the top of the dispensing pin with the cap that was earlier placed on the alcohol swab, and ask for an instructor check.

19 Once your work has been approved, place the IV bag in a position to ensure that the injection port receives uninterrupted airflow. Clean the injection port of the IV bag with a new, sterile alcohol swab, and place the swab on the hood surface such that it receives uninterrupted airflow. This process is shown in Figure 32.5.

FIGURE 32.5
Critical Sites During IV Bag Preparation

Critical sites should not be touched or shadowed at any time.

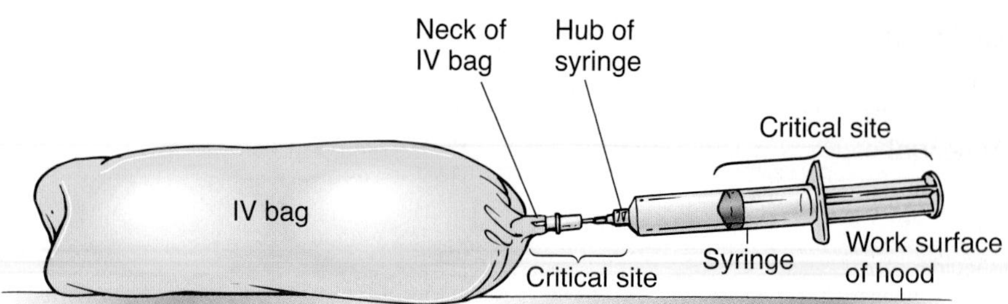

Safety Alert

The insertion should be smooth. If you encounter any resistance, the needle has likely entered the sidewall of the injection port stem, which is potentially dangerous. If this occurs, back out, and repeat the insertion process with the same needle.

20 Hold the barrel of the syringe in the dominant hand. Remove the cap of the needle and place it onto the alcohol swab used in Step 19. Hold the injection port steady with the nondominant hand and insert the needle straight into the injection port.

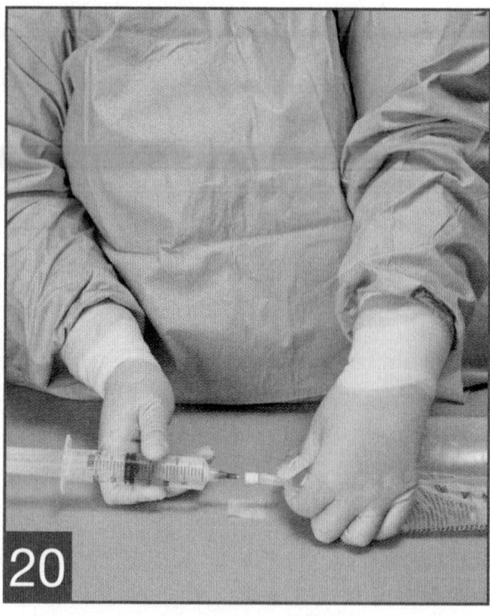

Correct technique for inserting a needle into the injection port of an IV bag containing a large-volume parenteral solution

21 Inject the medication into the bag by pressing on the plunger of the syringe.

22 Holding only the barrel of the syringe, carefully remove the needle-and-syringe unit from the IV bag. Place the unit into the sharps container.

Practice Tip

The waste container and the sharps container should be placed on the floor near the hood, but not within the hood itself.

23 Without removing the IV bag from the hood, squeeze the bag to check for leaks, and visually inspect the bag for precipitates.

24 **Conclusion:** Ask for a final check by the instructor. Then go to the Course Navigator, answer all questions in the Lab Review section, and submit your answers to your instructor.

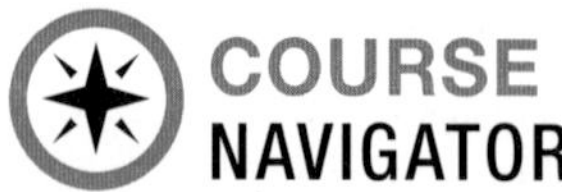

COURSE NAVIGATOR

Access interactive chapter review exercises, practice activities, flash cards, and study games.

© Paradigm Publishing, Inc.

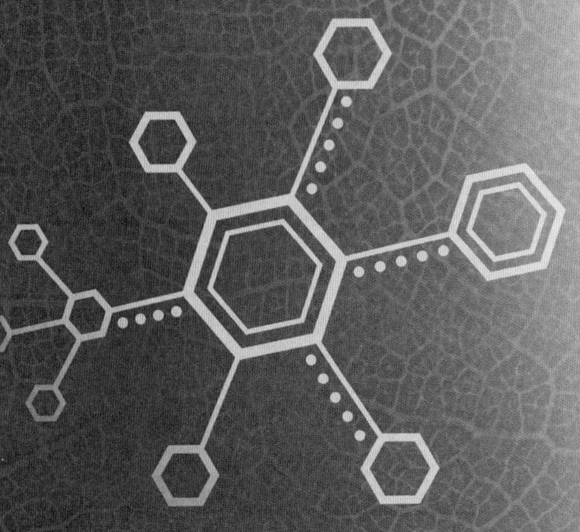

33 Preparing Small-Volume Parenteral Solutions

Learning Objectives

1. Demonstrate proficiency in aseptic technique as it relates to the assembly of small-volume compounded sterile preparations.
2. Demonstrate accuracy in basic calculations related to the preparation of small-volume parenteral products.
3. Discuss the procedures and rationale for the preparation of small-volume parenteral products.

Supplies

- Metoclopramide 10 mg/2 mL vials × 2
- D_5W 50 mL IV bags (with injection port) × 2
- Regular needles × 2 (a regular needle has no filter and no vent)
- 3 mL syringes × 2
- Sharps container (dedicated for cleanroom use only)
- Trash container (dedicated for cleanroom use only)
- Sterile alcohol swabs × 4
- Calculator

Access additional chapter resources.

Small-volume parenteral preparations are sterile solutions of 250 mL or less that are administered parenterally. The most common small-volume parenteral preparations compounded in the cleanroom are **intravenous piggyback (IVPB)** solutions, which are intermittent infusions containing a standard base solution plus an IV medication that are delivered, or "piggybacked," through a main IV line.

Sterile compounding of small-volume parenteral solutions requires that you first perform calculations to determine the amount of medication to add to the base.

Some of the most common IVPB base solutions are 0.9% sodium chloride (normal saline), dextrose 5% in water, and 0.45% sodium chloride (abbreviated as NS, D_5W, and 0.5 NS respectively). IVPB base solutions are most commonly supplied in 50 mL and 100 mL volumes.

Procedure

In this lab you will perform calculations related to small-volume parenteral preparation and then prepare two sterile solutions for IVPB administration using strict adherence to aseptic technique. The products you will prepare are as follows:

Metoclopramide 10 mg in 50 mL D_5W
Metoclopramide 7.5 mg in 50 mL D_5W

1 First, perform your necessary calculations based on the information provided on the metoclopramide label, which should indicate a concentration of 10 mg/2 mL. Given this concentration, separately calculate how many milliliters you need to withdraw from the vial in order to prepare the two doses (10 mg and 7.5 mg). Using the following equations, calculate the doses by cross multiplying and then dividing to solve for *x*, the unknown volume. When your calculations are complete, write your answers here: For the 10 mg dose, $x =$ _______ mL, and for the 7.5 mg dose, $x =$ _______ mL. These are the amounts you must draw up and add to the IV bags to create your solutions.

$$\frac{10\text{ mg}}{2\text{ mL}} = \frac{10\text{ mg}}{x\text{ mL}} \qquad \frac{10\text{ mg}}{2\text{ mL}} = \frac{7.5\text{ mg}}{x\text{ mL}}$$

Safety Alert

Take care when removing the syringe from its outer wrapper. Some syringes have a cap on the tip; some do not. If there is a cap, it must be removed prior to withdrawing fluid from the vial. If there is no cap, be careful not to shadow or otherwise contaminate the tip of the syringe. Never lay an uncapped syringe onto the work surface.

2 Don aseptic garb, hand wash, don sterile gown and gloves, and clean the hood according to your instructor's directions.

3 Remove the IVPBs from their outer wrappers. Place the wrappers in the trash, and place the IVPBs onto the hood surface, at least 6 inches inside the hood. Place the other supplies onto the outer 6-inch edge of the hood.

4 Remove the cap from the top of the metoclopramide vial, and clean the rubber stopper with a sterile alcohol swab. Place the swab on the hood in an area that is free of airflow obstruction.

5 Aseptically attach a regular needle to a 3 mL syringe. Details of a syringe are shown in Figure 33.1.

6 Prepare the syringe by adding an amount of air that is equal to the amount of diluent to be withdrawn. (When preparing your first dose, 2 mL will be withdrawn, and thus you should pull the plunger down to the 2 mL volume mark on the syringe.)

© Paradigm Publishing, Inc.

FIGURE 33.1 Critical Sites of Needle and Syringe

Always be cautious, and avoid touching or shadowing the critical sites.

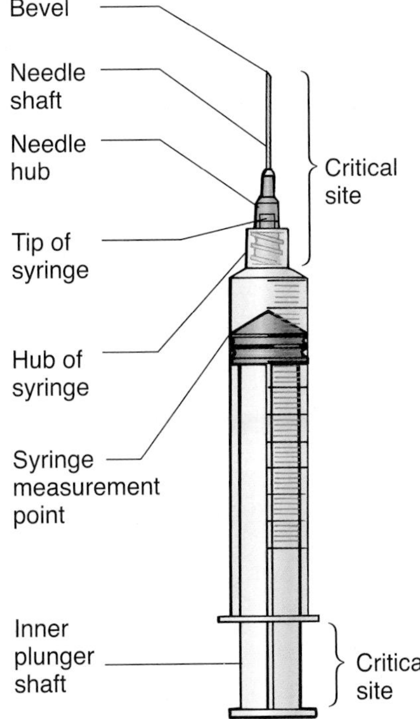

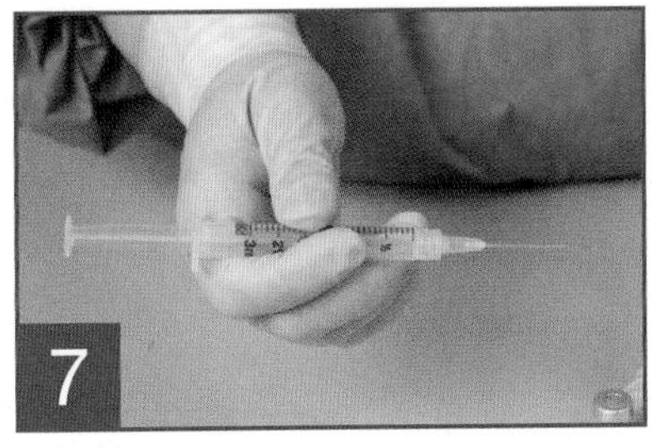

Correct technique for holding a syringe in preparation for insertion into a vial or bag

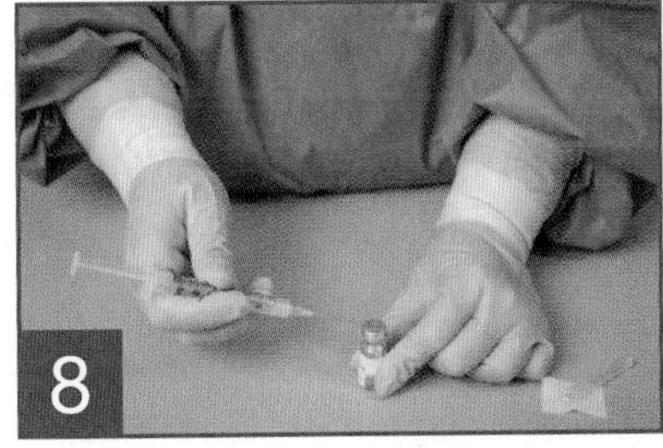

Correct placement of a needle onto the surface of the vial top. The beveled end of the needle should face upward

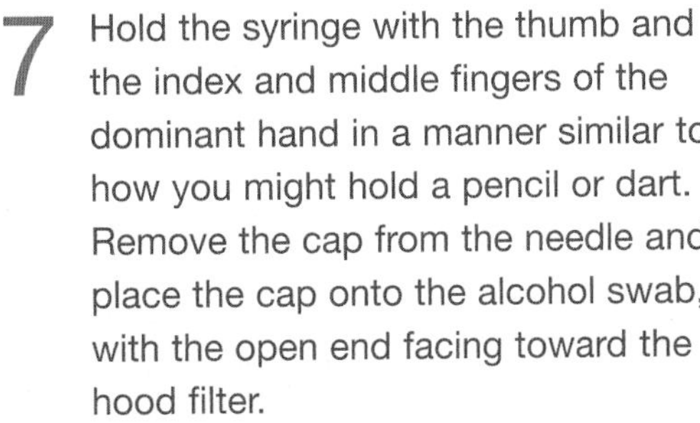

7 Hold the syringe with the thumb and the index and middle fingers of the dominant hand in a manner similar to how you might hold a pencil or dart. Remove the cap from the needle and place the cap onto the alcohol swab, with the open end facing toward the hood filter.

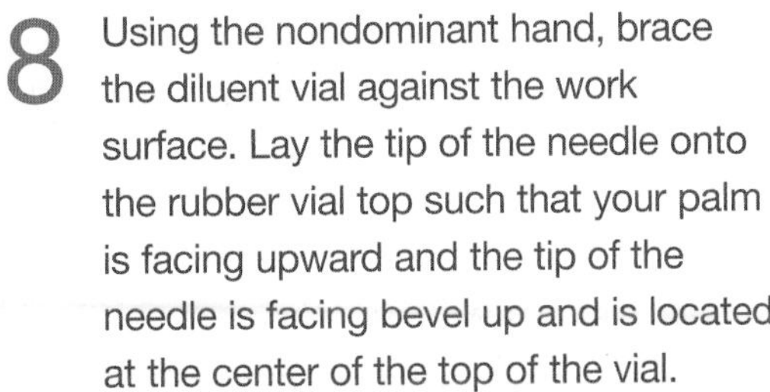

8 Using the nondominant hand, brace the diluent vial against the work surface. Lay the tip of the needle onto the rubber vial top such that your palm is facing upward and the tip of the needle is facing bevel up and is located at the center of the top of the vial.

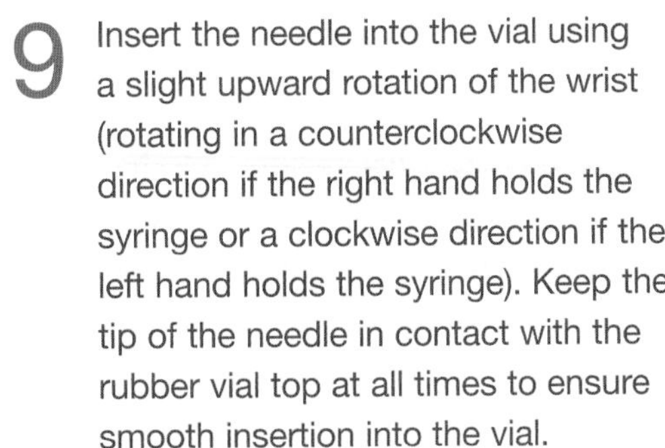

9 Insert the needle into the vial using a slight upward rotation of the wrist (rotating in a counterclockwise direction if the right hand holds the syringe or a clockwise direction if the left hand holds the syringe). Keep the tip of the needle in contact with the rubber vial top at all times to ensure smooth insertion into the vial.

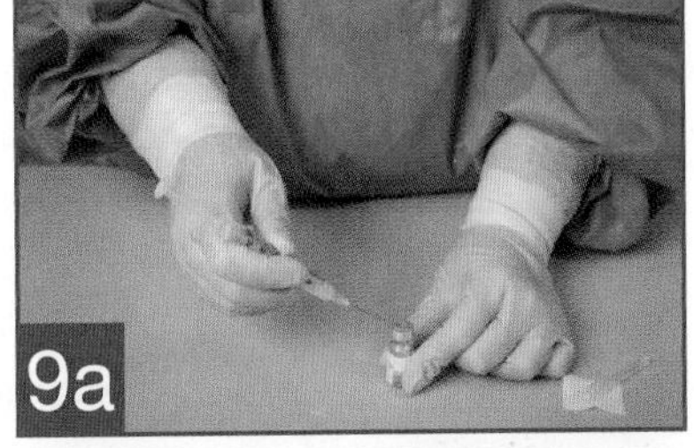

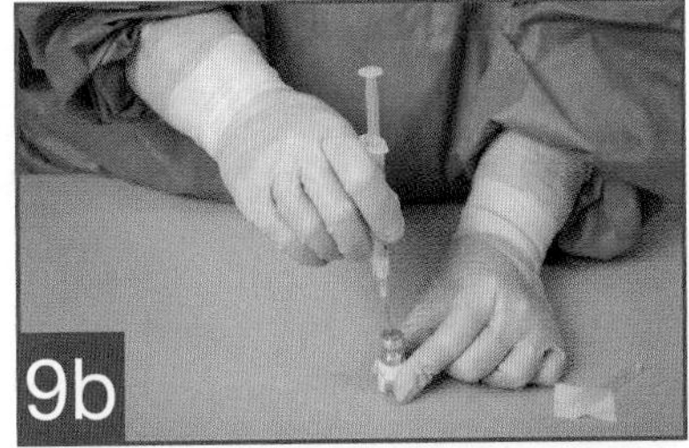

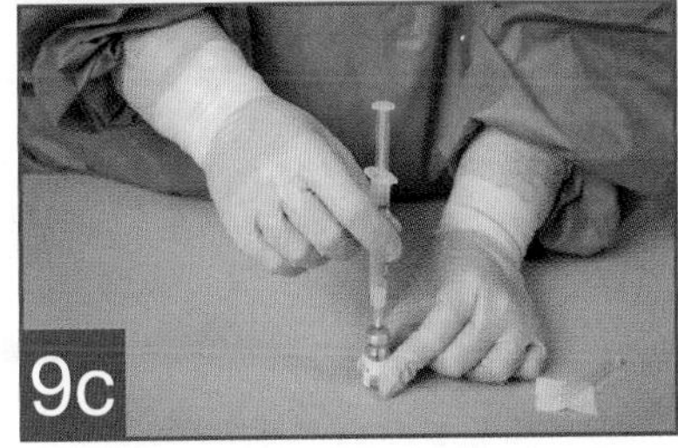

Correct technique for inserting a needle into a vial. Note the slight bending of the needle and the technician's arm motion (upward and toward the hand holding the vial) as the needle is inserted into the vial

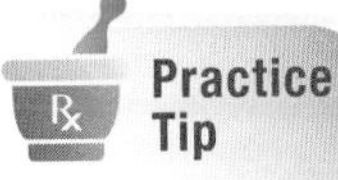

There should be a very slight—almost impercep-tible—bend in the needle from the gentle downward pressure as it enters the vial. Correct needle insertion will help to prevent coring of the vial's rubber top.

© Paradigm Publishing, Inc.

Take care to hold the vial and syringe so that airflow to the critical sites (the syringe plunger shaft and the area from the tip of the syringe to the neck of the vial, including the entire needle and the rubber vial top) is unobstructed.

10 Hold the metoclopramide vial in the nondominant hand and the barrel of the syringe in the dominant hand. While keeping the needle completely inserted into the vial, invert the vial so that the needle-and-syringe unit is now below the vial.

11 Gradually push up on the plunger to add a small amount (approximately 1 mL) of air to the vial. This addition creates a slight positive pressure environment within the vial and will assist you in withdrawing fluid from the vial. Release the plunger to allow some fluid to flow into the syringe. Repeat this process of adding a small amount of air and removing a small amount of fluid (often called the "milking technique") until all of the premeasured air has been added to the vial and an equal amount of diluent has been drawn into the syringe.

As you withdraw liquid from the vial, be sure to keep the tip of the needle within the fluid to avoid drawing air into the syringe.

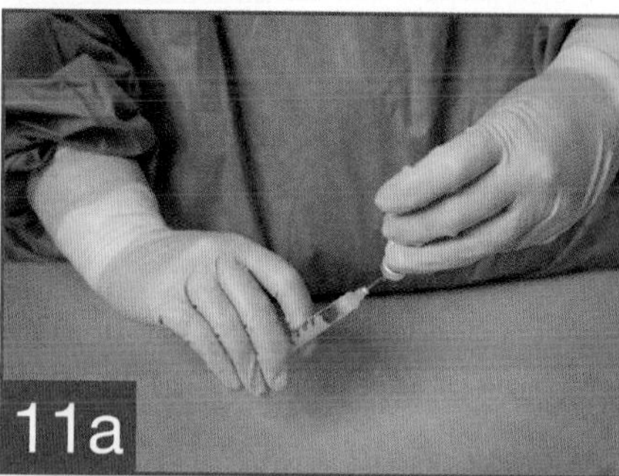

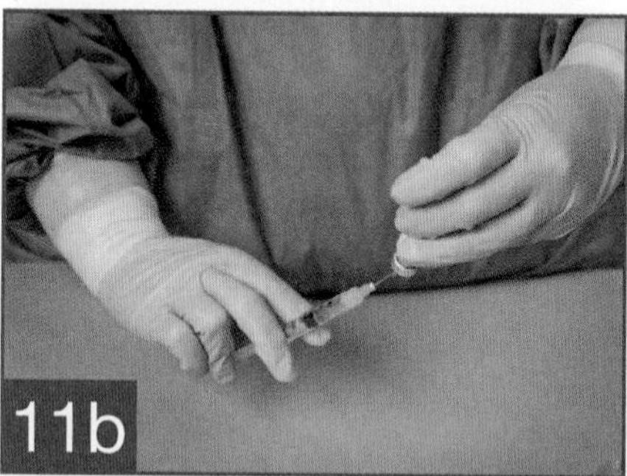

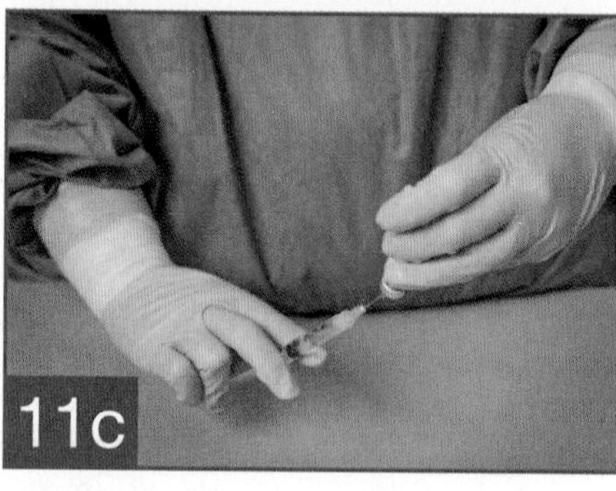

Creation of positive pressure within a vial using the milking technique. Notice the positioning of the technician's fingers and that the syringe volume changes from empty (top) to actively filling (middle) to mostly full (bottom)

Be sure that you have drawn up the correct amount of fluid and that there are no large bubbles in the syringe before proceeding to Step 13.

12 Verify that the syringe now contains the desired amount of medication (in the case of the first dose, 2 mL). If necessary, tap the syringe to force air bubbles to the tip of the syringe, and then expel any excess air by gently pressing upward on the plunger. Verify again that the desired amount of medication is present, and if it is not, pull down on the plunger to draw more fluid into the syringe.

13 While keeping the needle firmly inserted into the vial, return the vial and syringe to the original starting position, with the upright vial braced against the work surface and the dominant hand correctly holding the barrel of the inverted syringe. Slowly remove the needle-and-syringe unit from the medication vial. Remember to avoid touching the plunger of the syringe at any time while removing it from the vial.

© Paradigm Publishing, Inc.

14 Carefully recap the needle.

15 Repeat Steps 4–14 with the other 3 mL syringe, withdrawing the amount you calculated as necessary for the 7.5 mg dose.

16 Place both filled syringes, with capped needles, onto the work surface next to the metoclopramide vial and IVPBs, and ask for an instructor check.

17 Once your work has been approved, place the first IVPB (to which you will add the 10 mg dose) in a position to ensure that the injection port receives uninterrupted airflow. Clean the injection port of the IV bag with a new, sterile alcohol swab.

Safety Alert

The insertion should be smooth. If you encounter any resistance, the needle has likely entered the sidewall of the injection port stem, which is potentially dangerous. If this occurs, back out, and repeat the insertion process with the same needle.

Practice Tip

When inserting a needle into the injection port of an IV bag, it is not necessary to consider the direction of the bevel. The needle should be inserted straight into the bag, without angle and without bending the needle.

18 Place the swab on the hood surface such that it receives uninterrupted airflow.

19 Hold the barrel of the syringe in the dominant hand. Remove the cap of the needle and place it onto the alcohol swab.

20 Hold the injection port steady with the nondominant hand, taking care to avoid shadowing the injection port.

21 Insert the needle straight into the injection port.

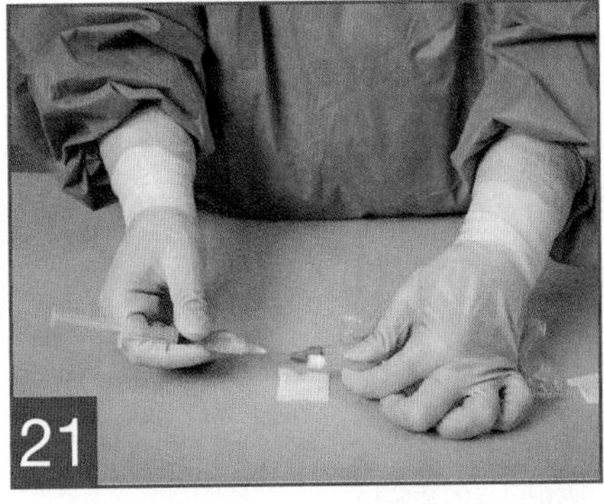

22 Inject the medication into the bag by pressing on the plunger of the syringe.

23 Holding only the barrel of the syringe, carefully remove the needle-and-syringe unit from the IV bag. Place the unit into the sharps container.

24 Repeat Steps 17–23 for the 7.5 mg dose, using the second IVPB.

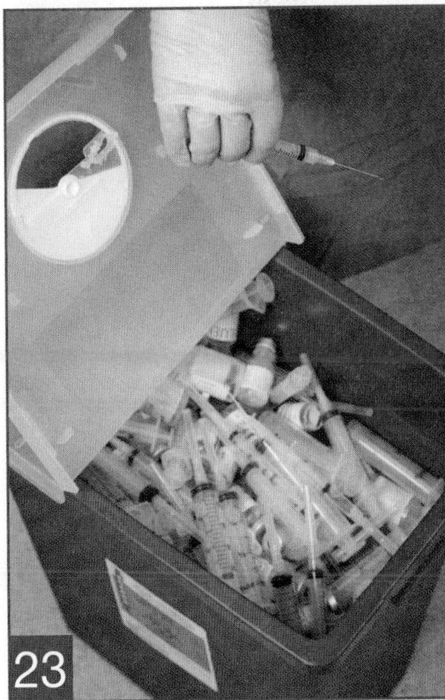

Technician placing a needle and syringe into the sharps container

25 Squeeze each IVPB to check for leaks, and visually inspect each bag for precipitates.

26 **Conclusion:** Ask for a final check from your instructor. Then go to the Course Navigator, answer all questions in the Lab Review section, and submit your answers to your instructor.

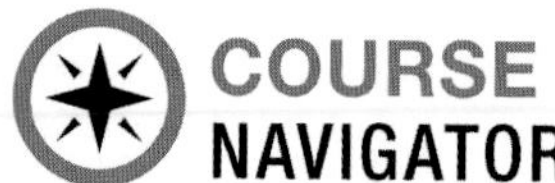

Access interactive chapter review exercises, practice activities, flash cards, and study games.

© Paradigm Publishing, Inc.

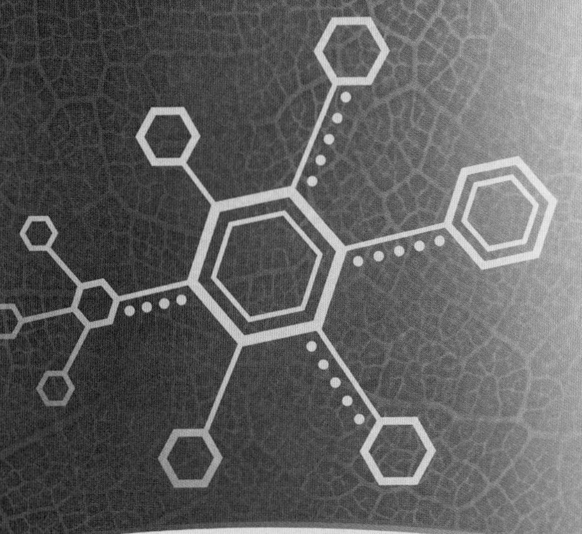

34

Preparing Sterile Powder Drug Vials

Learning Objectives

1. Demonstrate proficiency in aseptic technique as it relates to the preparation of sterile powder drug vials.
2. Demonstrate accuracy in basic calculations related to the preparation of sterile powder drug vials.
3. Discuss the procedures and rationale for the preparation of sterile powder drug vials.

Supplies

- Ampicillin 1 g vial (powder, for parenteral administration)
- Sterile water 10 mL vial for injection
- 10 mL syringe
- 5 mL syringe × 2
- Regular needle × 3 (regular needle has no filter and no vent)
- Vented needle
- Sharps container (dedicated for cleanroom use only)
- Trash container (dedicated for cleanroom use only)
- Sterile alcohol swabs × 3
- Calculator

Access additional chapter resources.

Working in the cleanroom often requires the pharmacy technician to prepare medications involving reconstitution of a sterile powder drug. While many medications for parenteral use are supplied by the manufacturer in the form of an injectable liquid, others are supplied in a powder form that requires reconstitution prior to use. Some medications are supplied in powder form primarily because the drug has a longer shelf life or stability as a powder than it would in liquid form. Reconstitution of sterile powder drugs demands strict adherence to aseptic technique and the execution of calculations commonly used in sterile compounding.

Hospital pharmacy technicians reconstitute many powder medications to be administered as intravenous, intravenous piggyback, and intramuscular injections. Many of these types of products are antibiotics that are given to the patient to treat infection from pathogenic microorganisms such as bacteria, protozoa, or fungi. Hospital inpatients are commonly too ill to take medications orally, either because of nausea or because of poor digestive system function. In addition, some infections require treatment by antibiotics that are available only in injectable form.

The two most common diluents used to reconstitute sterile powder drugs are sterile water and 0.9% sodium chloride (known as "normal saline"). Both of these diluents are available with or without preservatives. Diluents with preservatives are commonly referred to as **bacteriostatic**, indicating that they contain an agent that inhibits the growth of bacteria within the diluent vial. Two commonly used preservatives are methylparaben and benzyl alcohol, and diluents containing them are used to dilute most powders in the sterile compounding lab. Diluents without preservatives are referred to as "preservative-free" and are generally used only in special situations, such as for neonatal patients, for intrathecal administration, or upon a physician's request.

Procedure

In this lab you will perform calculations related to drug reconstitution, use correct venting technique to reconstitute a sterile powder drug, and aseptically prepare two syringes with the following antibiotic doses:

Ampicillin 450 mg	Ampicillin 375 mg

Preparatory Steps

1 Perform your calculations based on the following information: Once reconstituted, the vial will contain 1 g of ampicillin in 10 mL of solution. You need to draw up one dose of 450 mg and one dose of 375 mg. Use the following equations (cross multiply and then divide to solve for *x*, the unknown volume) to separately calculate how many milliliters you must withdraw from the vial in order to prepare the two doses. For the 450 mg dose, $x =$ _______ mL, and for the 375 mg dose, $x =$ _______ mL .

$$\frac{1000 \text{ mg}}{10 \text{ mL}} = \frac{450 \text{ mg}}{x \text{ mL}} \qquad \frac{1000 \text{ mg}}{10 \text{ mL}} = \frac{375 \text{ mg}}{x \text{ mL}}$$

2 Don aseptic garb, hand wash, don sterile gown and gloves, and clean the hood according to your instructor's directions.

 © Paradigm Publishing, Inc.

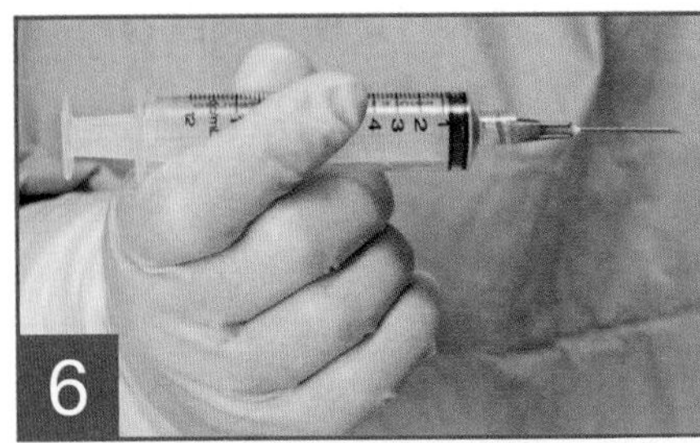

6

Correct technique for holding a syringe in preparation for insertion into a vial or bag

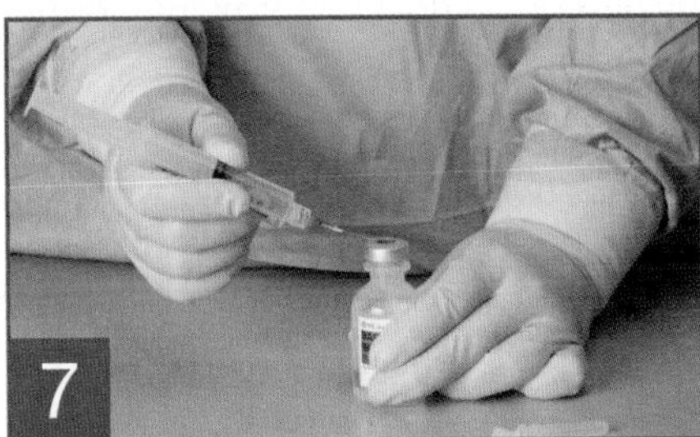

7

Correct placement of a needle onto the surface of the vial top. The beveled end of the needle should face upward

Drawing Up the Diluent

3 Remove the cap from the top of the diluent vials and clean the rubber stopper with a sterile alcohol swab. Place the swab on the hood in an area that is free of airflow obstruction.

4 Aseptically attach a regular needle to a 10 mL syringe.

5 Prepare the syringe by adding an amount of air that is equal to the amount of diluent to be withdrawn (in this case, 10 mL). Do this by pulling the plunger down to the 10 mL volume mark on the syringe.

6 Hold the syringe with the thumb and the index and middle fingers of the dominant hand in a manner similar to how you might hold a pencil or dart. Remove the cap from the needle, and place it onto the alcohol swab, with the open end of the cap facing toward the hood filter.

7 Using the nondominant hand, brace the diluent vial against the work surface. Lay the tip of the needle onto the rubber vial top of the diluent such that the tip of the needle is facing bevel up and is located at the center of the top of the vial.

8 Insert the needle into the vial using a slight upward rotation of the wrist (rotating in a counterclockwise direction if the right hand holds the syringe, or a clockwise direction if the left hand holds the syringe). Keep the tip of the needle in contact with the rubber vial top at all times to ensure smooth insertion into the vial.

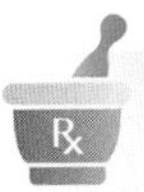

Practice Tip

There should be a very slight—almost impercep-tible—bend in the needle from the gentle downward pressure as it enters the vial. Correct needle insertion will help to prevent coring of the vial's rubber top.

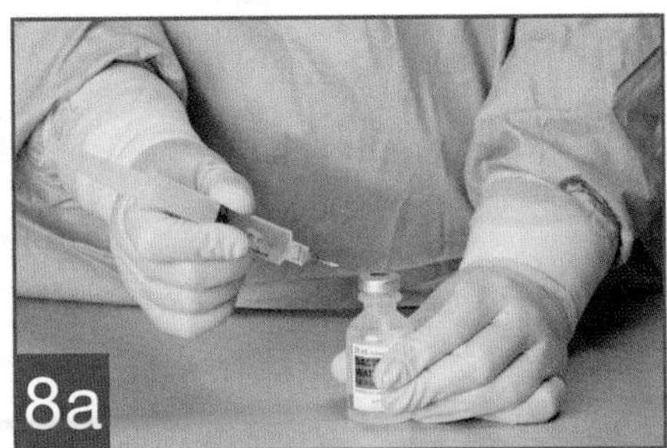

8a

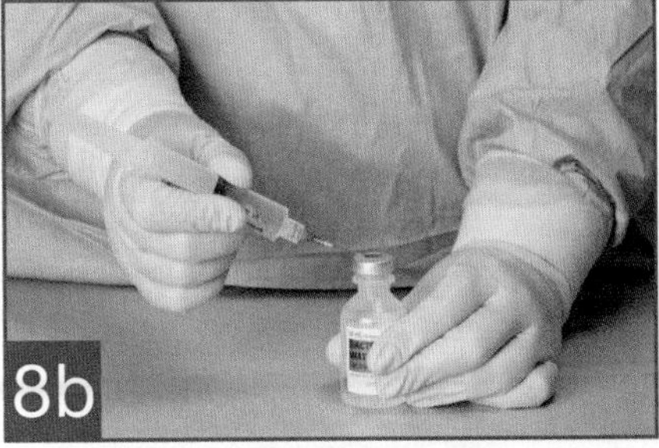

8b

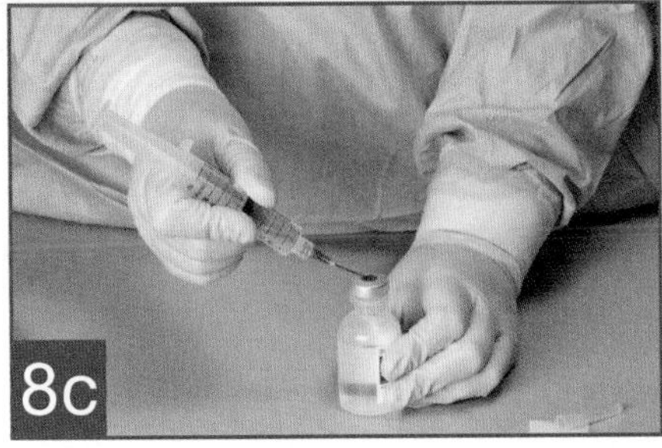

8c

Correct technique for inserting a needle into a vial. Note the slight bending of the needle and the technician's arm motion (upward and toward the hand holding the vial) as the needle is inserted into the vial

Safety Alert

Take care to hold the vial and syringe in such a manner that airflow to the critical sites (the syringe plunger shaft and the area from the tip of the syringe to the neck of the vial, including the entire needle and the rubber vial top) is unobstructed.

9 Hold the diluent vial in the nondominant hand and the barrel of the syringe in the dominant hand. While keeping the needle completely inserted into the diluent vial, invert the vial so that the needle-and-syringe unit is now below the vial, as shown in Figure 34.1.

10 Gradually push up on the plunger to add a small amount (approximately 2 mL) of air to the vial. This will create a slight positive pressure in the vial and will assist you in withdrawing the fluid. Release the plunger to allow some fluid to flow into the syringe. Repeat this process of adding a small amount of air and removing a small amount of diluent (often called the "milking technique") until all the air that was in the syringe has been added to the vial and the required amount of diluent has been drawn into the syringe. This technique is shown in the photos on the next page.

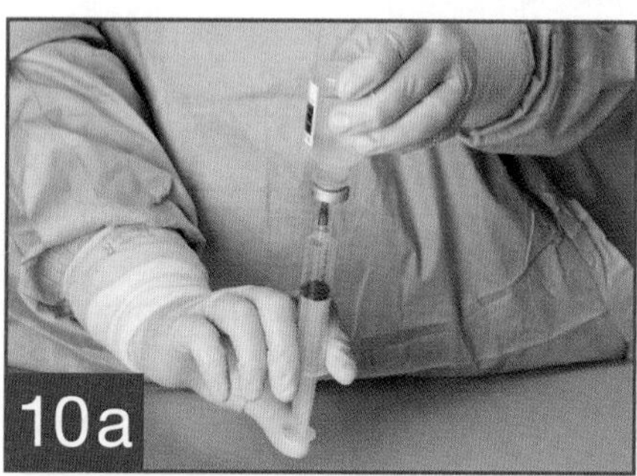

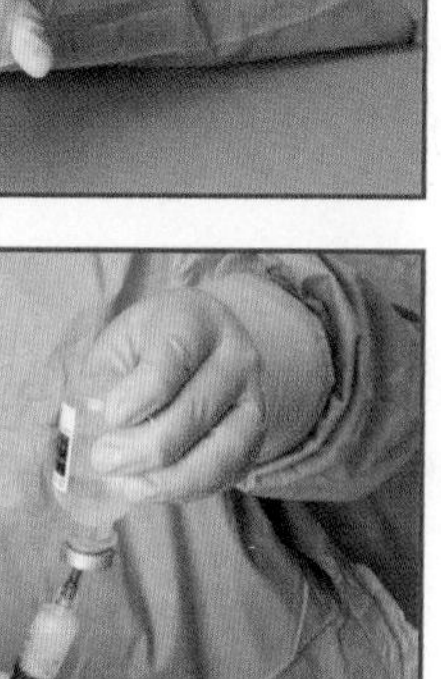

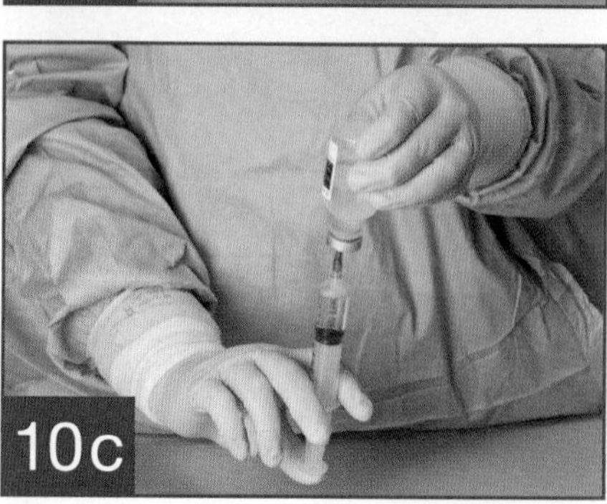

Creation of positive pressure within a vial using the milking technique. Notice the positioning of the technician's fingers and that the syringe volume changes from empty (top) to actively filling (middle) to mostly full (bottom)

FIGURE 34.1 Critical Sites of Vial, Needle, and Syringe

Take special care not to touch critical sites.

© Paradigm Publishing, Inc.

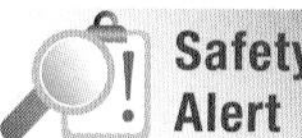

Safety Alert

Be sure to avoid touching the plunger of the syringe at any time while removing it from the vial. Also take care not to touch the needle to the work surface or other contaminant while recapping it.

11 Verify that the syringe now contains the desired amount of diluent (in this case, 10 mL). If necessary, tap the syringe to force air bubbles to the tip of the syringe, and then expel any excess air by gently pressing upward on the plunger. Verify again that the desired amount of diluent is present, and if it is not, pull down on the plunger to draw more fluid into the syringe.

12 While keeping the needle firmly inserted into the vial, return the vial and syringe to the original starting position, with the vial braced against the work surface and the dominant hand correctly holding the barrel of the syringe.

13 Slowly remove the needle-and-syringe unit from the diluent vial. Carefully recap the needle.

14 Hold the syringe so that the capped needle is pointing up, and gently pull the plunger down approximately 0.5 mL. This pulling action will draw fluid from the needle into the syringe.

15 Remove the capped regular needle and place it into the sharps container.

Attaching the Vented Needle and Diluting the Ampicillin

Practice Tip

Avoid getting fluid into the needle cap by always pulling down on the plunger to remove fluid from the needle *after* tapping the syringe to dislodge air bubbles. Pulling down must be the *last* thing you do before expelling the air from the syringe; do not tap the syringe again.

16 Aseptically attach a capped vented needle to the syringe. While holding the syringe with the needle pointing up, slowly push up on the plunger to expel any air that may be in the syringe. Tap the barrel of the syringe to dislodge air bubbles and move them up toward the needle (see Figure 34.2a). Pull down on the plunger to clear fluid from the needle (see Figure 34.2b). Gently push up on the plunger until the fluid enters the colored part of the needle hub, thus expelling the air pocket (see Figure 34.2c).

17 Place the filled syringe (with the capped vented needle) onto the work surface next to the diluent vial.

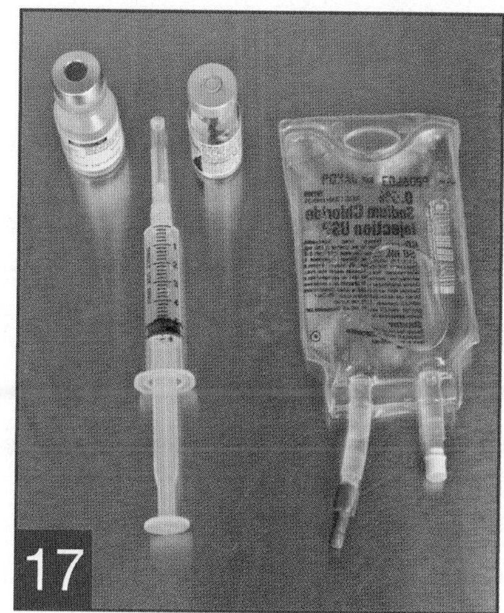

Filled syringe, capped vented needle, and vials set on the work surface, awaiting an instructor check

FIGURE 34.2 Bubble Expulsion from a Syringe

The procedure for expelling bubbles and air pockets from a filled syringe is detailed below.

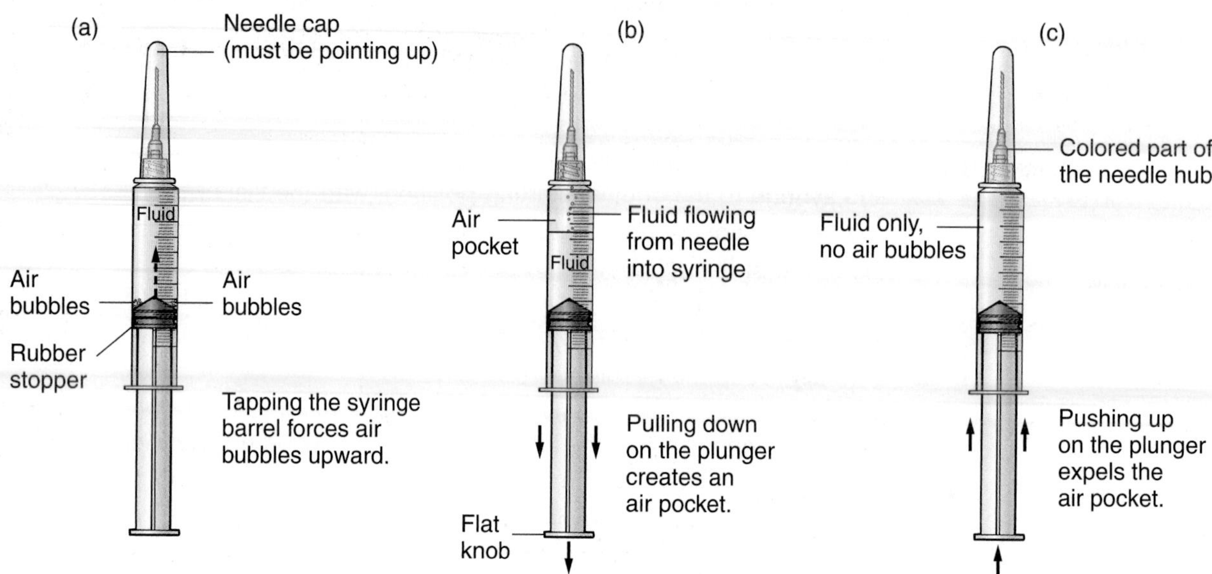

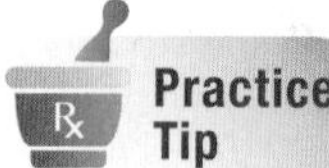

Practice Tip

Vented needles can be used *only to inject* a diluent into a vial containing a powder drug. Vented needles cannot be used to draw up fluid.

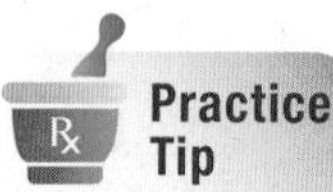

Practice Tip

Apply enough downward pressure so that the aluminum sheath surrounding the needle is firmly seated into the rubber vial top. If correctly inserted, the needle itself should be able to move up and down freely, while the sheath remains stuck in the rubber vial top.

18 Ask for an instructor check of the filled syringe, diluent vial, and calculations.

19 Once your work has been approved, remove the cap of the ampicillin vial, and clean the rubber stopper with a new, sterile alcohol swab.

20 Correctly grasp the barrel of the syringe, and remove the cap of the vented needle.

21 Use the nondominant hand to hold the ampicillin vial against the work surface. With the dominant hand, insert the vented needle directly into the top of the vial with a firm, downward motion (see Figure 34.3).

22 While keeping the needle in the vial at such a depth that the hub of the needle stays approximately one-eighth inch above the rubber vial top, inject the diluent into the ampicillin vial (see Figure 34.3).

© Paradigm Publishing, Inc.

FIGURE 34.3 Correct Use of a Vented Needle

The procedure for inserting a vented needle and diluting a powder drug vial is detailed below.

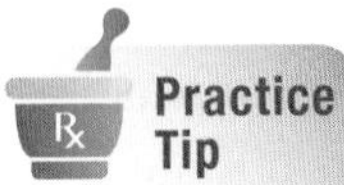

Practice Tip

While this lab procedure requires you to shake the vial in order to get the powder to dissolve, some drugs must not be shaken as it will compromise the strength, stability, or integrity of the drug. Be sure to read the package insert for specific instructions for that medication.

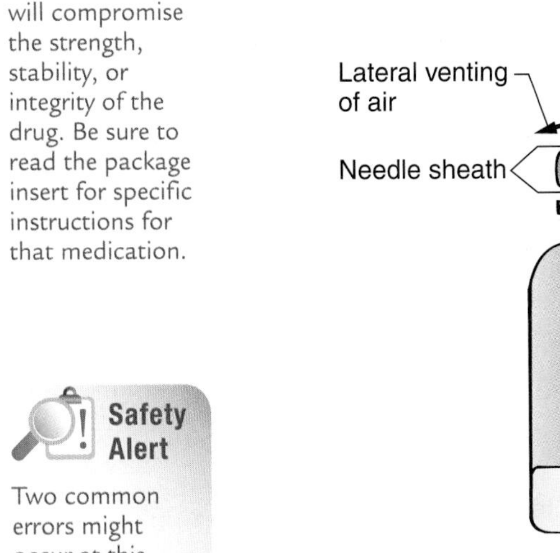

Safety Alert

Two common errors might occur at this point in the procedure. First, if there was a noticeable amount of fluid pooling on top of the rubber vial top while using the vented needle, it is likely that the syringe was held too far above the vial top. Second, if the vented needle failed to vent the vial adequately, it is likely that the syringe was held too close to the vial top, which prohibited adequate venting. If either of these errors occurs, notify your instructor.

23 Correctly grasp the barrel of the syringe, taking care not to touch the plunger, and remove the needle from the vial. Place the needle-and-syringe unit into the sharps container.

24 Shake the reconstituted ampicillin vial to dissolve the drug in the diluent. Continue shaking until the powder is completely dissolved, and then wait long enough for any foam or bubbles to dissipate.

Withdrawing the Correct Dose Volume

25 Aseptically attach a regular needle to a 5 mL syringe.

26 Clean the top of the ampicillin vial with a new alcohol swab, and place the swab on the hood surface such that it receives uninterrupted airflow.

27 Uncap the needle, and place it on top of the swab such that the cap faces the hood filter.

© Paradigm Publishing, Inc.

Take care to avoid inserting this needle into the hole left in the rubber vial top by the vented needle. Also, because the vial was previously vented by the vented needle, there is no need to add air to the vial or use the milking technique at this point in the procedure.

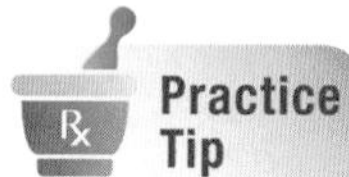

Be sure to keep the tip of the needle inside the fluid within the vial so that you do not withdraw from the air pocket within the vial.

28 Hold the barrel of the syringe according to standard procedure. Insert the needle with the bevel up, using appropriate technique to prevent coring.

29 Invert the vial and the needle-and-syringe unit, taking care to avoid blocking airflow, and withdraw 450 mg of diluted drug by pulling down on the plunger to the volume calculated earlier in the lab for the 450 mg dose.

30 Remove any bubbles or excess air using the technique mentioned earlier, in Step 11. Verify again that the desired amount of medication is present, and if it is not, pull down on the plunger to draw more fluid into the syringe.

31 Return the vial and needle-and-syringe unit to the original starting position, with the vial braced against the hood surface and the dominant hand holding only the barrel of the syringe.

32 Remove the needle-and-syringe unit from the ampicillin vial, and carefully recap the needle. Place the capped syringe on the work surface.

33 Repeat the withdrawal procedure (Steps 25–32), with the other 5 mL syringe, withdrawing the amount calculated for the 375 mg dose.

34 Place both filled syringes, with capped needles, on the work surface next to the ampicillin vial and ask for a final check by your instructor.

35 **Conclusion:** Go to the Course Navigator, answer all questions in the Lab Review section, and submit your answers to your instructor.

Access interactive chapter review exercises, practice activities, flash cards, and study games.

© Paradigm Publishing, Inc.

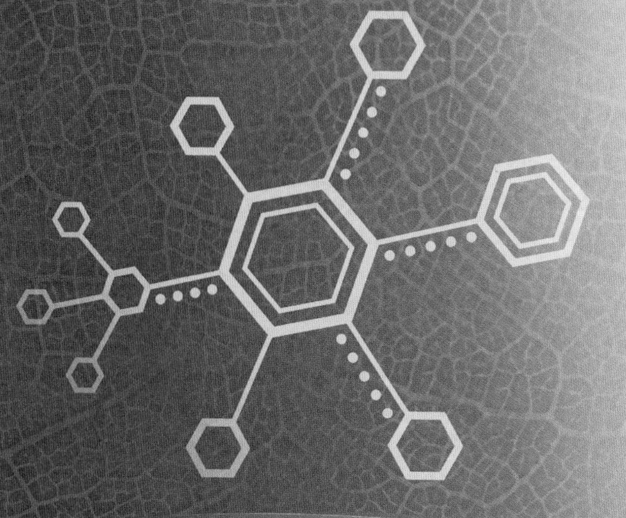

35 Using Ampules

Learning Objectives

1. Demonstrate proficiency in the aseptic preparation of an IV medication withdrawn from a glass ampule.
2. Demonstrate accuracy in basic calculations related to the preparation of an intravenous medication withdrawn from a glass ampule and then added to an intravenous piggyback.
3. Discuss the procedures and rationale for the use of medications supplied in ampule form.

Supplies

- Promethazine ampule
- 3 mL syringe × 1
- 1 mL syringe × 1
- Filter needle × 2
- Regular needle × 2 (a regular needle has no filter and no vent)
- Sterile alcohol swabs × 4
- Dextrose 5% in water 50 mL IVPB × 2
- Calculator
- Trash container (dedicated for cleanroom use only)
- Sharps container (dedicated for cleanroom use only)

Access additional chapter resources.

Historical records that verify the use of glass **ampules** (small, sealed glass vials) to hold important fluids began around the fourth century CE, though it is possible that ampules originated thousands of years earlier. For example, records indicate that some early Christians had a small ampule of their own blood entombed with them—a special ceremonial tradition originally reserved for martyrs. The association of ampules with ceremonies of death and honor carries on today in some areas of Europe, where religious pilgrims place ampules of oil next to the tombs of well-known saints and martyrs to honor them in annual ceremonies.

Your use of ampules links you, as a modern pharmacy technician, to ancient practices of careful storage, transport, and use of valuable liquids. Patients today receive life-sustaining liquid medications that you prepare by aseptically processing the contents of glass ampules into compounded sterile preparations. Although many of these medications are available in glass or plastic vials, some are provided only in ampule form, because they must be protected from air during storage. Ampules are airtight because they are flame-sealed after filling, which provides an optimum environment for certain drugs.

The most common motivation for drug manufacturers to supply a medication in ampule form is the drug's **incompatibility** with plastic, rubber, or polyvinyl chloride (PVC). In fact, most parenteral drug vials contain one of these components, and occasionally incompatibility arises from an undesired reaction between the medication and part of the drug vial. These undesired chemical reactions can affect the drug's composition or efficacy and can drastically reduce the medication's shelf stability. By using ampules made entirely of glass, compatibility problems are eliminated.

Ampule preparation requires excellent aseptic technique, with special attention focused on correctly breaking the ampule and on several specific processes for withdrawing and injecting its contents. Unlike other medications, drugs withdrawn from ampules must be filtered. A filter needle is used to prevent the transfer of tiny glass shards from the ampule to the patient. The same needle must not be used both to withdraw medication from an ampule and to inject it. Rather, you *must* change the needle prior to injecting the medication into the patient or the intravenous piggyback (IVPB). Once ampules are broken (and thus open to the air), you will not need to create a positive pressure environment, as is necessary when working with vials. You will use a syringe to withdraw liquid from ampules, and because air bubbles will float to the top of the liquid regardless of the direction in which the syringe is initially pointed, you must remove air bubbles from the syringe once you take it out of the ampule. Used ampules should be disposed of in the sharps container because of the risk of potential injury from the broken glass.

Procedure

In this lab you will perform basic calculations and aseptically prepare these two doses of intravenous medication from a glass ampule:

Promethazine 25 mg
Promethazine 10 mg

1 Perform calculations based on the concentration that is provided on the ampule label. For example, the label on the promethazine ampule states that it is 50 mg/2 mL. Based on this concentration, how many milliliters will you need to withdraw from the ampule to separately prepare the following two doses?

© Paradigm Publishing, Inc.

25 mg dose and **10 mg** dose

$$\frac{50 \text{ mg}}{2 \text{ mL}} = \frac{25 \text{ mg}}{x \text{ mL}}$$

Cross multiply, and then divide to solve for x, the unknown volume:

$$25 \times 2 = 50$$

$$\frac{50}{50} = \textbf{1 mL} \text{ required for the 25 mg dose}$$

$$\frac{50 \text{ mg}}{2 \text{ mL}} = \frac{10 \text{ mg}}{x \text{ mL}}$$

Cross multiply, and then divide to solve for x, the unknown volume:

$$10 \times 2 = 20$$

$$\frac{20}{50} = \textbf{0.4 mL} \text{ required for the 10 mg dose}$$

2 Don aseptic garb, hand wash, don sterile gown and gloves, and clean the hood according to your instructor's directions.

3 Gently tap or swirl the ampule so that the head and neck are free of fluid and all of the medication is in the body of the ampule. Clean the neck of the ampule with a sterile alcohol swab. A glass ampule is illustrated in Figure 35.1.

FIGURE 35.1
Glass Ampule

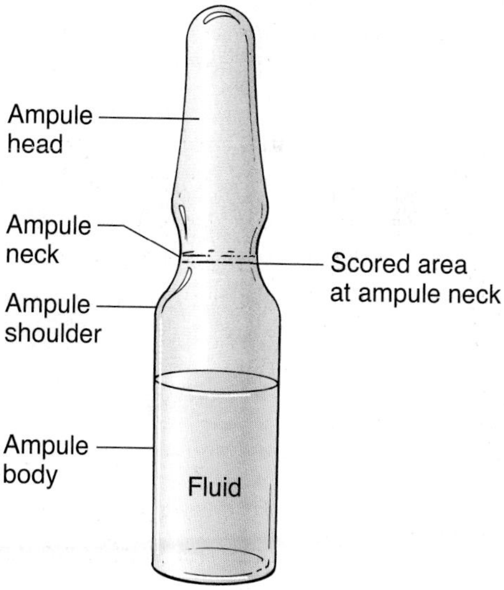

Ampule head
Ampule neck
Scored area at ampule neck
Ampule shoulder
Ampule body
Fluid

4 Prepare the syringe by aseptically attaching a regular needle.

Hold the ampule firmly, but avoid crushing it; the glass walls are quite thin.

5 Gently but firmly hold the body of the ampule with the thumb and index finger of the nondominant hand, curling the remaining three fingers around the body of the ampule to help stabilize it. Verify that the fingers of this hand are situated below the neck of the ampule.

© Paradigm Publishing, Inc.

Safety Alert

Because you will shortly be snapping the neck of the ampule, take care both to verify that the fingers of both hands are positioned away from the neck of the ampule, avoiding potential injury, and to aim toward the side of the hood rather than toward the back, avoiding damage to the hood filter from glass shards.

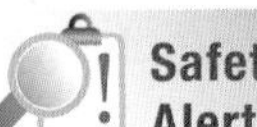

Safety Alert

Be sure to keep hold of the head of the ampule with the thumb and index finger of the dominant hand so that it does not dislodge when broken off. Keep your arms and fingers steady, and use a snapping motion at the wrist to break the ampule. Always snap away from your body, never toward yourself.

Practice Tip

Be sure that the tip of the needle has entered the fluid inside the ampule.

6 Place the dominant hand such that the thumb and forefinger have a firm grasp of the head of the ampule.

7 Use the dominant hand to apply pressure to the neck of the ampule with a quick, snapping motion of the wrist. The ampule should break at the neck.

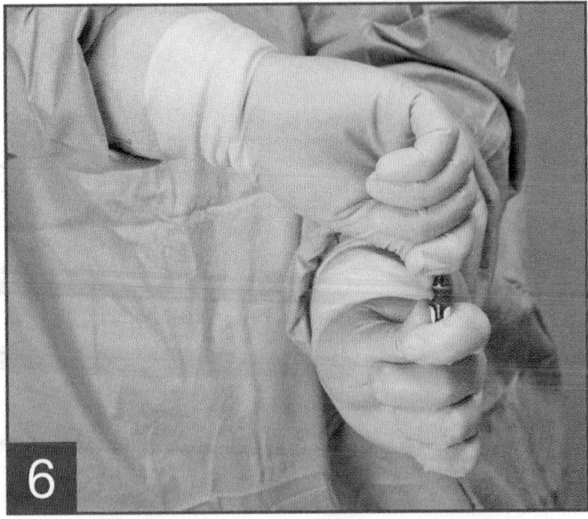

Correct hand placement for breaking a glass ampule

8 Put the head of the ampule into the sharps container, and place the body of the ampule onto the hood surface in an area that receives uninterrupted airflow.

9 Open a new, sterile alcohol swab, and place it on the work surface such that it receives uninterrupted airflow.

10 Hold the barrel of the syringe with the dominant hand, remove the cap of the needle, and place the cap onto the swab, with the opening pointing toward the hood filter.

11 Rotate the barrel of the syringe such that the bevel of the needle is pointing down. Stabilize the ampule with the nondominant hand, and carefully insert the needle into the ampule.

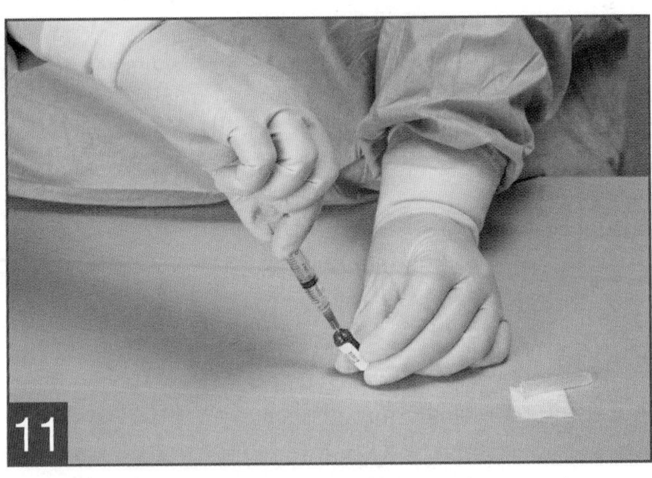

Correct technique for inserting a needle into a glass ampule

© Paradigm Publishing, Inc.

Practice Tip

As you draw up fluid into the needle and the ampule becomes emptier, it may be necessary to tip the ampule slightly to bring the fluid into the shoulder of the ampule, where the tip of the needle can more easily remain in the fluid.

12 Pull the plunger back until the syringe contains approximately 0.5 mL more than what is desired (in the case of the 25 mg dose, approximately 1.5 mL).

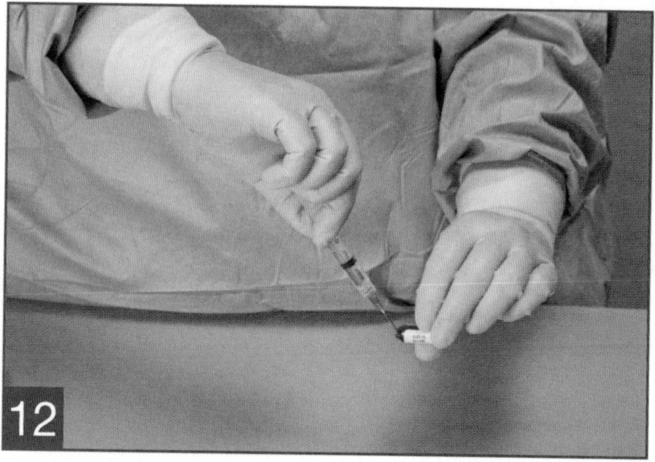

Withdrawal of fluid from the shoulder of a glass ampule

13 Keep hold of the ampule in your nondominant hand. With the fingers of the dominant hand, keep hold of the barrel of the syringe, release the plunger, and then carefully remove the needle from the ampule. Place the ampule on the work surface such that it receives uninterrupted airflow. Turn the syringe so that the needle points upward, and recap the needle.

Safety Alert

Avoid fluid flow into the needle cap by always pulling down on the plunger to remove fluid from the needle *after* tapping the syringe to dislodge air bubbles. Pulling down must be the *last* thing you do before expelling the air from the syringe; do not tap the syringe again.

14 Tap the syringe to force air bubbles up toward the hub. Pull down slightly on the plunger to draw fluid from the needle down into the syringe. (The procedure for expelling bubbles and excess air from a filled syringe is shown in the previous lab in Figure 34.1.)

15 Slowly push up on the plunger to expel all of the air from the syringe. Release the plunger, and hold the barrel of the syringe in the dominant hand.

16 Remove the needle cap, and place it on the alcohol swab.

17 Carefully insert the needle back into the ampule, and use the plunger to push any excess fluid into the ampule. Keeping your eye on the graduations on the syringe barrel, push the plunger down slowly, and stop when you reach the correct volume (in the case of the 25 mg dose, 1 mL).

© Paradigm Publishing, Inc.

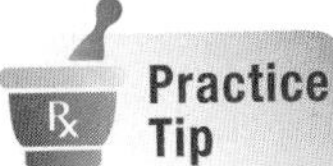

In practice, you may be asked to show the regular needle that has been removed to the pharmacist for verification that the two needle process has been done correctly.

18 While grasping only the barrel of the syringe, remove the needle-and-syringe unit from the ampule. Recap the needle.

19 Pull down on the plunger to clear the needle of fluid. Remove the needle, and place it in the sharps container.

20 Aseptically attach a filter needle to the syringe.

21 Slowly push up on the plunger to expel all of the air from the syringe, and place the capped syringe on the work surface.

22 Repeat the entire procedure (Steps 4–21) for the 10 mg dose. However, note that you should ignore Steps 5–8, because you have already broken open the ampule.

23 Ask for an instructor check of the syringes, the IV bags, and the promethazine ampule.

24 Swab the injection port of a D_5W 50 mL IV bag, and inject the 25 mg dose of promethazine according to accepted protocol (as described in Lab 34, Steps 19–23, pages 324–325).

25 Place the empty needle-and-syringe unit into the sharps container.

26 Squeeze the IVPB to check for leaks, and set it aside.

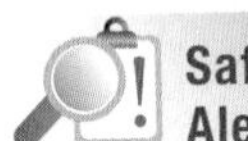

Use caution when cleaning the work surface to avoid injury or product contamination from any small shards of glass that may be present.

27 Repeat the IVPB injection procedure (Steps 24–26 of this lab) using the second IVPB bag for the 10 mg dose.

28 Place the empty needle, syringe, and broken ampule into the sharps container, and clean your work area according to your instructor's directions.

29 **Conclusion:** Go to the Course Navigator, answer all questions in the Lab Review section, and submit your answers to your instructor.

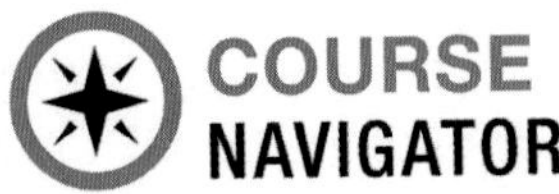

Access interactive chapter review exercises, practice activities, flash cards, and study games.

© Paradigm Publishing, Inc.

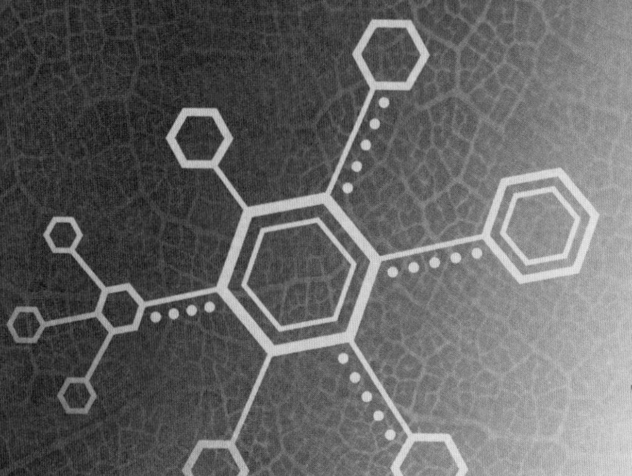

Appendix A

Signa Short Codes

Actions	
Short Code	**Word**
T	Take
N	Instill
I	Insert
IH	Inhale
J	Inject
G	Give
P	Place
PT	Put
U	Unwrap
UI	Unwrap and insert
A	Apply
S	Use
AAA	Apply to the affected area(s)

Quantity	
Short Code	**Word**
H	One-half (0.5)
1H	1.5 (1 and one-half)
1	1
2	2
3	3
4	4
5	5

6	6
7	7
8	8
9	9
10	10
0.5-1	0.5 to 1
1-2	1 to 2
3-4	3 to 4
3-5	3 to 5
4-6	4 to 6

Dosage Forms/Type

Short Code	Word
TAB	tablet(s)
CAP	capsule(s)
GTT	drop(s)
UNI	unit(s)
TBS	tablespoonful(s)
TSP	teaspoonful(s)
TBE	tube(s)
ML	milliliter(s)
CC	cubic-centimeter(s)

Route of Administration

Short Code	Word
PO	by mouth
IM	intramuscularly
SQ	subcutaneously
AU	both ears
AD	right ear
AS	left ear
OU	both eyes
OD	right eye
OS	left eye
V	vaginally
R	rectally
SH	shoulder(s)

© Paradigm Publishing, Inc.

Time-Intervals

Short Code	Word
QD	every day
BID	two times a day
TID	three times a day
QID	four times a day
Q3H	every 3 hours
Q34H	every 3 to 4 hours
Q4H	every 4 hours
Q46H	every 4 to 6 hours
Q6H	every 6 hours
QAM	every morning
QPM	every evening
QHS	at bedtime

Additional Information

Short Code	Word
AC	before meals
PC	after meals
PRN	as needed
ANX	for anxiety
PA	for pain
INF	for infection
X10D	for 10 days
X7D	for 7 days
X14D	for 14 days
FEV	for fever
FLA	for inflammation
ABP	for abdominal pain
HTN	for hypertension

Pre-built Signa

Short Code	Word
ZPAK	Take 2 tablets by mouth on day 1, then take 1 tablet by mouth on days 2 through 5. Take medication for all 5 days.
UUD	Use as directed.
TUD	Take as directed.

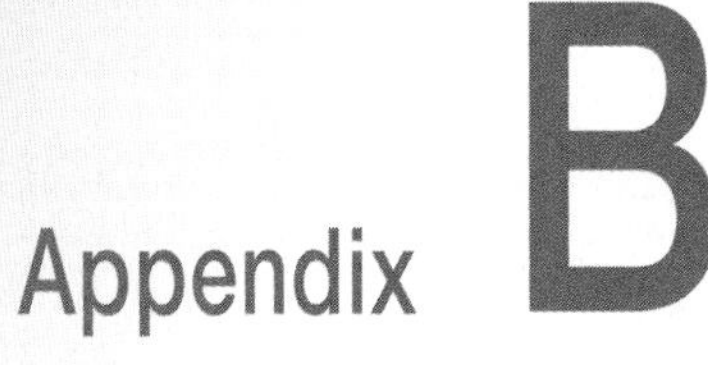

Appendix B

Alternative Recipes

Suggested Alternative Ingredients		
	Original Ingredient	**Alternative Ingredient**
Lab 23 — Reconstituting Powders	Augmentin 125mg/5mL, 100mL bottle	Placebo bottles, 125mg/5mL 100mL bottle, 250mg/5mL or 400mg/5mL KoolAid or Crystal Light drink powder in an amber vial
Lab 24 — Filling Capsules	Metronidazole 500mg tablets	Placebo 500mg tablets Vitamin C 500mg tablets Smarties
	Syrpalta	Simple Syrup (See included recipe) Ora-Sweet Syrup/Ora Plus
Lab 25 — Preparing Suspensions from Tablets	Amoxicillin 250mg capsules	Placebo 250mg capsules Milk Thistle 250mg capsules
Lab 26 — Preparing Suspensions from Capsules	Syrpalta or OraPlus	Simple Syrup (See included recipe) Ora-Sweet Syrup/Ora Plus
Lab 27 — Preparing Creams, Ointments, Gels, and Pastes	Surgical lubricant	KY Jelly Aloe Vera gel Hair gel
Lab 28 — Making Lozenges	Lozenge mold	Mini cupcake liners Miniature silicone ice cube tray
	Benzocaine powder	Corn starch Baking soda
Lab 32 — Preparing Large-Volume Parenteral Solutions	Potassium cholride bulk vial, 250 mL	Potassium chloride, 40 mL vial Dextrose 50%

Suggested Product Sources

Amazon.com	Pocket Nurse	Your local drug or grocery store
MockMeds	Wallcur	
Moore Medical	Healthcare Logistics	

Additional Compounding Recipes

Acne Skin Astringent

Tea tree oil	1 mL
Witch hazel solution	qs 8 oz
Amber vial, 8 oz in volume	1
1 mL dropper or pipette	1

1. Add 1mL tea tree oil to amber vial
2. Using witch hazel solution, fill amber vial to 8 ounces
3. Shake well
4. Label

Beyond use date: 50% of shortest shelf life of ingredients

Alprazolam 1 mg/mL Syrup

		Alternative Ingredients
Rx Alprazolam 2 mg tablets	#60	Miniature Altoid mints
Syrup vehicle	qs 120 mL	Simple syrup
Amber vial, 120 mL in volume	1	
4 oz or 6 oz mortar and pestle	1	

1. Triturate alprazolam tablets using a mortar and pestle
2. Carefully pour triturated tablet powder into the amber vial
3. Using the syrup vehicle as a rinse for the mortar and pestle, gently swish approximately 20 to 30 mL of syrup around the mortar, and pour the contents into the amber vial
4. Rinse the mortar two more times using the syrup vehicle
5. Fill the amber vial to 120 mL with syrup vehicle

Beyond use date: 6 weeks

Benzocaine 5% Ointment

		Alternative Ingredients
Benzocaine	5 grams	Kosher salt
White petrolatum	qs 100 grams	Petroleum jelly
100 gram ointment container	1	
Digital scale	1	

© Paradigm Publishing, Inc.

Mortar and pestle	1
Stainless steel spatula	1
Ointment slab	1

1. Accurately weigh each ingredient
2. Reduce the particle size of the benzocaine to a fine powder
3. Spatulate a small quantity of the petrolatum into the benzocaine and work until very smooth
4. Incorporate the remainder of the petrolatum geometrically and mix well
5. Package and label

Beyond use date: 50% of shortest shelf life of ingredients

Lip Balm

Beeswax	8 oz
Coconut oil	1 pint
Vitamin E 400IU capsules	#45
Preferred flavoring oil	7 to 10 mL
Lip balm containers	#45
Self-stirring hot plate	1
Double boiler or	
500 mL beaker	1
Water for hot bath	1 pint
Prepares:	approximately 45 units

1. In a double boiler, or a beaker in heated water bath, melt beeswax. Do NOT boil
2. Once beeswax is melted, gradually stir coconut oil into melted wax
3. Empty contents of vitamin E capsules into solution
4. Stir until mixture is homogenous
5. Add flavoring oil and stir
6. Carefully pour solution into lip balm containers and allow to cool

Beyond use date: 50% of shortest shelf life of ingredients

Progesterone 5% Cream

		Alternative Ingredients
Progesterone, micronized	5 grams	Corn starch
Glycerin	qs	Mineral oil
Dermabase	95 grams	White petrolaum (i.e. Aquaphor®)
100 gram ointment container	1	
Ointment slab	1	
1 mL dropper	1	
Stainless steel spatula	1	

1. Levigate the micronized progesterone with a small quantity of glycerin to form a smooth paste
2. Geometrically, incorporate the Dermabase and mix until uniform and smooth

© Paradigm Publishing, Inc.

3. Package and label

Beyond use date: 50% of shortest shelf life of ingredients

Simple Syrup

Sucrose	85 grams
Distilled water	100 mL
Amber vial, 120 mL in volume	1
4 oz or 6 oz mortar and pestle	1

1. Geometrically dilute sucrose and water in a mortar and pestle, triturating until dissolved
2. Pour contents into 120 mL amber vial
3. Label

Beyond use date: 30 days from date of preparation

Zinc Oxide Paste

Zinc oxide powder	25 grams
Cornstarch	25 grams
White petrolatum	50 grams
Mineral oil	2 mL
4 oz mortar and pestle	1
Ointment slab	1
Digital scale	1
1 mL oral syringe	1
Stainless steel spatula	1
Ointment jar, 1 oz	4
Prepares:	up to 4, 1 oz jars

1. Weigh ingredients
2. Geometrically dilute zinc oxide using a mortar and pestle
3. Levigate zinc oxide powder and cornstarch powder using mineral oil
4. Spatulate the zinc oxide/cornstarch powder and white petrolatum into a paste
5. Ensure a homogenous mixture by thorough spatulation
6. Weigh and tare the empty ointment container
7. Package the product to 30 grams
8. Label and prepare product

Beyond Use Date: 30 days from date of preparation

 © Paradigm Publishing, Inc.

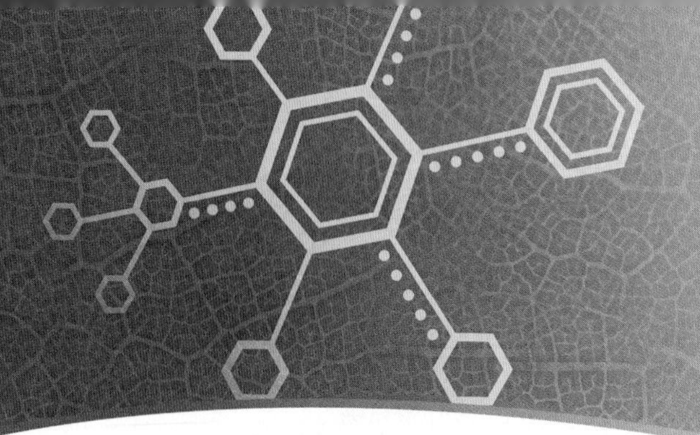

GLOSSARY

A

active ingredient the medication that is added to the base ingredient during compounding

ampules a small, sealed glass vial used to contain a fluid

antineoplastic agent inhibits or prevents the growth or development of malignant cells

aseptic without infection; free of pathogens

aseptic technique clean "without infection" technique that is free of pathogens

B

bacteriostatic diluents with preservatives

base ingredient an inert substance, such as a cream, ointment, gel, or paste, to which an active ingredient is added during compounding

best practice a highly effective process, technique, or activity designed to deliver the best results with little or no margin of error

bioequivalence two preparations of a pharmaceutical product being biologically equivalent and assumed to be the same

C

capturing successfully submitting and obtaining payment on an insurance claim

cash price the price patients must pay when they do not have insurance coverage or their insurance plan is not accepted

chronic condition a health concern that recurs frequently or lasts for an extended time

clean room space where sterile parenteral products are prepared

code a life-threatening situation when a patient is in cardiac or respiratory arrest

compounding preparing individualized medications per prescription order

compounding log official record of the processes and materials used to compound a prescription

contract price significantly lower price than off-contract pricing that wholesalers are able to offer because they deal in bulk and move large quantities of items that are on agreed lists

control number unique number assigned to any monitored prescription for management and tracking purposes

copay the set price often paid by patients having third-party insurance coverage

coring undesired event that occurs when a needle is inserted incorrectly into a rubber stopper atop a solution vial, causing a small bit of the stopper to tear off and contaminate the solution inside the vial

critical sites parts of equipment or supplies that must never be touched and to which airflow from the high-efficiency particulate air (HEPA) filter should never be interrupted

cross-reference directs a reader to another part of the text for related information

customer service the assistance and other resources provided by a company to the people who buy or use its products or services

D

DEA number unique identifier assigned by the US Drug Enforcement Agency to track the prescribing, preparation, and dispensing of controlled substances

designated agent person who is the legal guardian of, or is otherwise designated by the patient to make healthcare decisions on the patient's behalf should the patient be unable to make decisions for himself or herself

dilution injection of a liquid medication into an IV solution such as sterile water or normal saline, which results in a more dilute concentration of the drug

discrepancy disagreement between the actual count of a medication in the ADSDS and the amount displayed on the verification screen

dispensing pin a specialized plastic device that includes a vent, a spike, and a syringe adaptor, and is inserted into the rubber stopper of a vial

drug diversion stealing or otherwise taking or using drugs from the facility illegally

durable medical equipment (DME) reusable items such as wheelchairs, walkers, crutches, and bedpans

E

enteral a route of administration (oral, buccal, or rectal) delivering medication through a patient's gastrointestinal tract

F

filling technician pharmacy technician responsible for prescription counting or pouring, packaging, and labeling during the filling process

floor stock a small supply of medications kept on each floor or unit; also known as *unit stock*

formulary list of approved drugs

G

group monograph discussion of all the drugs in the group

H

Health Insurance Portability and Accountability Act of 1996 (HIPAA) a law passed by Congress that primarily defines the confidentiality of patient medical records as well as prescription records

hood-cleaning log sheet a crucial document for recording who cleaned the hood, the date, and the time

I

in vitro Latin for "in the glass," meaning studies are conducted on a partial or dead organism

in vivo Latin term for "within the living;" in other words, a medication tested on live subjects

incompatibility an undesired chemical reaction between two drugs, or between a drug and its container, negatively affecting drug composition, efficacy, or stability

inventory management refers to a set of activities or procedures that are completed by pharmacy personnel to ensure that medications and supply items are available when needed

inventory technician person who orders pharmacy inventory from the wholesaler

investigational drugs drugs that are being studied in patient trials prior to approval by the Food and Drug Administration

L

lozenge a dosage form that resembles hard candy and is administered orally; also known as a *troche* or *pastille*

M

major contamination a large amount or significant level of contamination of the washed and scrubbed aseptic area

material safety data sheet (MSDS) instructs how to store, handle, and use hazardous drugs and provides the procedures that must be followed when there has been an accidental exposure to or spill of the hazardous material

medication therapy management collaborative oversight of a patient's medications and their delivery to promote a safe, effective plan and encourage targeted outcomes

medication therapy management (MTM) collaborative oversight of a patient's medications and their delivery to promote a safe, effective plan and encourage targeted outcomes

milking technique a process used to ease the negative pressure in a vial or other closed container by adding positive pressure to the system

minor contamination a small amount or low level of contamination of the washed and scrubbed aseptic area

monograph a detailed document containing specific information about a drug product

N

narcotic technician technician who will likely be responsible for entering controlled substances into the pharmacy inventory and storing them under proper security

© Paradigm Publishing, Inc.

negative pressure a quality inherent to vials and some other closed systems, wherein a pressure differential prohibits the withdrawal of fluid from a vial into a syringe

9-point check systematic approach to verifying prescription data during the filing process

non-durable medical equipment disposable medical supply items such as needles, syringes, cholesterol checking supplies, and blood-sugar testing supplies

nonverbal communication composed of a variety of aspects that include eye contact, body language, and appearance

P

par level the total amount of a particular medication that the requesting unit keeps on hand when fully stocked

parenteral any route of administration other than enteral or topical, such as intravenous or intramuscular

particulate a powder or fine-textured material

pastille a dosage form that resembles hard candy and is administered orally; also known as *lozenge* or *troche*

pathogen an infectious agent that can cause disease or illness in a patient

peer-reviewed resource evaluation by experts in the relevant field

perpetual inventory occurs when stock levels are consistently maintained

perpetual log book an official, legal record of all activity relating to medications in the narcotic cabinet

pharmaceutical equivalence occurs when drug products contain the same active ingredient or ingredients, are of the same dosage form and route of administration, and are identical in strength or concentration

pharmacy inventory refers to all the prescription drugs, OTC medications, supply items, durable medical equipment, and non-durable medical equipment that are stocked in the pharmacy

pharmacy wholesaler maintains ample stock of thousands of the most widely used medications and supply items from a variety of manufacturers

point-of-sale (POS) refers to a computerized network of cash registers or computers that accurately record each transaction made

point-of-sale computer systems tracks every item ordered, received, sold, and dispensed by the pharmacy

positive pressure situation that occurs when a small amount of air is introduced into a vial or other closed system, thereby easing the withdrawal of fluid from the vial and into a syringe

professionalism refers to conducting oneself with responsibility, integrity, accountability, and excellence in the workplace

profit margin the difference between the pharmacy's prescription cost and the amount charged to the patient or insurance provider

punch method a technique for filling capsules from a leveled cake of drug powder

R

recipe a listing of the exact quantity of each ingredient and the processes required to compound a particular prescription

reconciling process of checking in the supply order

reconstitute to change into liquid form by adding water or other fluid to a powder

reliable source of information a proven and maintained resource continually updated by an authoritative organization on the subject matter

S

script specific way in which pharmacy personnel should greet customers and answer the phone or drive-through intercom

shadowing form of contamination that results when a worker's hands or their supplies on the hood are incorrectly placed, disrupting sterile airflow from the HEPA filter to the critical site

shipping invoice paperwork used in the reconciliation process

signa a series of abbreviations to communicate prescription and patient directions

signa abbreviations a series of abbreviations used to communicate prescriptions and patient drugs

6-inch rule standard procedure whereby technicians must not work within the outer 6 inches of the hood's work surface

spatulation method of mixing ingredients together into a homogeneous mixture by combining and smoothing them on a slab with a spatula

© Paradigm Publishing, Inc.

stock rotation the process of placing items with the longest expiration dating behind the items that expire earlier

suspension a dispersion of fine solid particles in a liquid

T

tablet trituration diluting a drug powder with an inert diluent powder

therapeutic equivalency (TE) occurs when drug products are pharmaceutically equivalent and are expected to have the same clinical effect with the same safety when administered to patients

third-party adjudication an insurance company determination to pay the pharmacy an amount on behalf of the patient's account

touch contamination form of contamination that results when a critical site, or the hood surface itself, is contaminated through incorrect technique, needlestick, sneezing, or coughing

transcribing transferring information between documents, in electronic or other form

triturate to break up or grind into smaller pieces

troche a dosage form that resembles hard candy and is administered orally; also known as *lozenge* or *pastille*

U

unit dose a medication packaged in a single dose, one-time-use container

unit stock a small supply of certain medications on each floor or unit. Also known as *floor stock*

V

verbal communication type of communication that may take place face-to-face, by phone, or over the pharmacy intercom system

W

want list a log sheet that nearly all pharmacy settings use to keep track of new items that need to be ordered or pharmacy items that are running low

written communication may take the form of a prescription or insurance information presented by a patient

Z

zombie reference still-available reference, originally produced by an unknown source, that has not been updated for a significant period of time

zone of turbulence area behind any item on the hood where sterile airflow is interrupted

© Paradigm Publishing, Inc.

INDEX

D

E

F

G

H

© Paradigm Publishing, Inc.

I

J

L

M

N

O

P

Q

R

© Paradigm Publishing, Inc.

Photo Credits:

1 © istock/sturti; **6** Wendy Almeda; **8** Lisa McCartney; **14** © Shutterstock/Tyler Olson; **17** © Shutterstock/Christy Thompson; **18** © istock/Pamela Moore; **23** © istock/wiliam87; **26** © Shutterstock/Roby Byron; **37** Courtesy of Robert Anderson; **40** © iStock/sjlocke; **70** © istock/YinYang; **178** © istock/sturti; **185** George Brainard; **230** © istock; **247** © istock/luchschen; **281** Image Courtesy of Bibby Scientific Ltd; **283** George Brainard